THE DEATH DOCTORS

THE
DEATH DOCTORS

By

A. MITSCHERLICH AND F. MIELKE

Translated from the German by

JAMES CLEUGH

*(formerly attached to the Office of the
Chief Counsel for War Crimes, Nuremberg)*

ELEK BOOKS
GREAT JAMES STREET, LONDON

CONTENTS

FOREWORD

OF the 260-odd written documents and passages of spoken testimony quoted in this work about 100 were printed in the American transcript of Evidence and Judgment published at Washington in 1947 in two Volumes under the title TRIALS OF WAR CRIMINALS BEFORE THE NUERNBERG MILITARY TRIBUNALS ('The Medical Case').

The passages contained in these two Volumes and quoted in the present work are reproduced by permission of the Library of Congress. They are indicated in the following pages by an asterisk.

The official American transcript of Evidence and Judgment is of course complete and therefore includes the other 160-odd quotations in the work here translated. But these passages, omitted from the two Volumes mentioned above, could not be made readily available for reproduction. They have therefore been retranslated in the following pages, where they differ from the American transcript only in the choice and arrangement of words, not in sense.

J. C.

'Schizophrenia may then occur through which the functionary himself becomes a part of the Id, the affair he is dealing with, and absorbs its characteristic psychological basis which remains independent of his personal attitude as a human being.

"I must get on with the job myself, no one else will do it so well." Such is the common phrase, familiar from totalitarian principles, with which the section of the mind split off by the Id appeases the Ego. The reflection initiates a dissolution of the personality, which totalitarianism then exploits and develops to the point when an essentially good-natured and humane person will, in the service of the Id, perform actions, as a functionary, of the vilest inhumanity. Such deeds are perpetrated because their executant is no longer one but two or more persons.'

ALFRED WEBER
Kulturgeschichte als Kultursoziologie

INTRODUCTION

THE present edition of the documents here collected appears eleven years after the first. The evidence still exceeds in horror anything previously imagined by mankind. No lapse of time will ever mitigate its effect. Today, as during the trials which first revealed these atrocities to the public, such conduct continues to seem utterly unreal. Yet the documents do not record ancient history. They deal with events which actually occurred in our lifetime. They concern ourselves. Innumerable human beings suffered from them. The painful question must be raised of our personal responsibility. Before we can answer that question, which historians will always ask, we must understand what in fact happened. We must identify the infected spots at which human behaviour coarsened into orgies of mania, of the humiliation, the trampling underfoot, of fellow-creatures. We must trace the process by which such seats of infection derived vigour through a sort of vascular and capillary system, radiating from regions apparently distant but invisibly connected with those diseased, so that poisonous matter spread gradually in all directions.

The following pages chronicle crimes of cruelty, malice and blood-lust so reckless, and at the same time organized with such professional bureaucratic efficiency, that the reader can only feel the deepest shame as he realizes that human beings could be capable of such acts. But when the average man hears of modern torture-chambers he declines to allow such alien proceedings to touch him at all closely. He even denies the existence of such barbarous instincts in himself, holding them to have been tamed by civilization or in other words by feelings of sympathy with other people. For civilization tends to discipline inconsiderate and anti-social impulses, to render them less responsive to fear and to transform them into sociability. Yet our moral principles have been founded on permanently volcanic soil. It is therefore not enough to be shocked at the thought that certain deeds can be perpetrated. We must at the

9

same time recognize the fact that they were not committed by beings who were born as monsters. On the contrary, the guilty parties were often rather commonplace people of quite ordinary ability. They had acquired certain technical knowledge and obtained responsible positions in society before they paralysed, as if by a drug, their inherited capacity for humane sentiment and fell back upon a purely instinctive lust for universal destruction. The barbarities carried out in the extermination and concentration camps, dens where civilization had been utterly abandoned, could only have been conceived by minds which had expelled their common humanity and replaced it by the appalling images of a nightmare. A terrible moment in history had decreed that trained subordinate and executive staffs should be available to assist in rendering these dreadful dreams of human sacrifice a reality. Sigmund Freud (*Ges. Werke*, Bd. IX, s. 335) has stated: 'A civilized society which demands efficiency and pays no attention to the instincts on which it must be founded imposes upon great numbers of people a culturally based submissiveness which does not accord with their natural impulses.'

It was hard for us to imagine what combination of circumstances, by paralysing reason and removing normal inhibitions, gave rise to the crimes here to be described, whether perpetrated with or without the excuse of scientific research. But it appeared essential, however distasteful the task might be to moral conviction and self-respect, to trace the relation between 'civilized society' and acts involving the destruction of human life, the suppression of conscience and glaring transgression of the borders of sanity. Our general survey revealed a wide field of distinctions. It stretched from the severest innate forms of degenerate perversion to the 'tolerance' which is a mitigated kind of inhumanity, being characterized on the one hand by both a timidly egotistic instinct of self-preservation and a timidly excessive respect for authority, and on the other by an almost artistic capacity to dismiss personal considerations. These are the regular symptoms of the barbarism referred to by Freud.

The exploration of unsuspected links of this kind is a task imposed upon us, as Germans, by what was done by persons of German nationality, speaking our tongue and trained in our

educational and scientific establishments. We shall have to
solve this problem if we are to succeed in shaping the future
to a more agreeable pattern. The unspeakable misery we inflicted on our neighbours far outweighs that which we brought
on ourselves. The duty to investigate the evil we have done
thus becomes so insistent a moral imperative that our continued
existence as a nation will depend upon its fulfilment. No
'vitality', intellectual ability, talent for organization or material
prosperity will otherwise arrest the course of history. For one
consideration at least remains perfectly clear. It was these very
virtues which voluntarily submitted to degradation in the
service of mania during the Nazi dictatorship.

Feelings of guilt can only be mastered by looking facts in the
face. They must be acknowledged without reservation. A sym-
pathetic attitude to the régime must be seen as such, even if it
amounted only to the 'most harmless' fellow-travelling, the
acceptance of catchwords or the participation in hopes aroused
by official promises. It must be avowed even if it appeared
ethically justified by the principles of faithful service and
obedience to orders. Such habits have in the past admirably
domesticated the national aggressiveness. But they lead imperceptibly to alienation of the self, to a collectively sanctioned
pleasure in the exercise of impersonal, barbarous impulses, to
the rigid formulation of a criminal code of morality and to
mechanical drilling for homicide.

The documents quoted in this volume provide many shocking
examples of the resulting situation, one of which illustrates it
with peculiar force. The evidence will be found in the Chapter
entitled 'Low Pressure and Supercooling Experiments' (p. 23). Dr
Rascher, a staff surgeon of the Luftwaffe, deliberately undertook the extinction of life in a human being subjected to tests
in a low-pressure chamber. He styled this proceeding 'a terminal experiment'. Another doctor participated in the murder,
one committed in the name of scientific research. But he was
then ignorant of Rascher's intention. This assistant stood beside
his principal, watching the victim's heart-beats being recorded
electrocardiographically. In due course he noted that a 'critical
point' had been reached. At his subsequent trial he was asked
by the prosecution why he had not turned to Rascher and
manipulated the control switch so as to heighten the pressure

and save the patient's life. He answered: 'Now that the whole
affair has been examined, it certainly looks like murder. But
at that time I was Rascher's subordinate. He was a staff surgeon
of the Luftwaffe.' The abnegation of personal responsibility,
the intimidation of the man in the presence of his superior, the
murderer, simply because he was the executive member of an
idealized group, can all be understood. But it is more difficult
to comprehend the second abnegation, which completely
elucidated the first and was constituted by the unconscious
temptation to yield to the pleasure of homicide. Such was the
source of the more active principle of obedience, which prevented the man reaching for the control switch. The apparently
rational justification for inaction—'I couldn't suppose that a
Luftwaffe officer could be committing murder'—has to be
compared with the irrational one, the latter being the fact that
homicidal pleasure has still not been eradicated by civilization
in any of us. Many of us, moreover, have little power to resist
its seductions. Only when this comparison is made can there
be any approach to an understanding of the man's otherwise
incomprehensible passivity, which alone made all that followed
inevitable. We must keep that approach to understanding open
if we are not to dismiss the whole appalling business as at
bottom unimportant, simply the result of individual perversity
and nothing more. For if we take that view we shall not only
be affirming that the victim in this case and all the millions of
others sacrificed by National Socialism, including all those who
fell on active service, died entirely in vain. We shall also be
abandoning every reasonable safeguard against a repetition of
such enforced inhumanity.

The whole of this documentary record has been compiled
with the above considerations in mind. The narrative is not
meant to be read primarily as a report of legal proceedings.
It should be taken as a piece of history. The written evidence
was put together with as much objectivity as we could command.
We were careful to stress the significance of the facts disclosed.
But we have also added in every case the arguments adduced
by the defence. For these indicate the context, the conscious
outlook of those who planned, promoted and executed the
outrages as a whole, as well as the attitudes of those who more
or less deliberately ignored what was going on. Some of the

persons involved struggled hard with their consciences. But these conflicts were less acute among high-ranking authorities who could choose between honourable resistance to the demands made upon them, uncompromising refusal to comply and emigration. Such people might have been expected to be capable of judging the issue for themselves. They could have formed a powerful resistance group. But the younger, less eminent doctors found themselves trapped and defenceless in an intolerable situation. Most of them had been brought up to obey implicitly, to idealize and revere, superiors whose behaviour they subsequently considered cowardly, hesitant or criminal. The crushing, practically insoluble dilemma of this younger generation, thoroughly indoctrinated as it had been in youth, was brought home to me in a conversation I had with a British colleague during the trials at Nuremberg. He believed himself to be pointing out a difference in national psychology. 'Let us suppose,' he said, 'that a German colonel sends for a sergeant and gives him the order: "Take Lance-Corporal Schmidt and your platoon to the quarry and shoot him." The German sergeant would reply: "Very good, sir." But an English sergeant would probably have said: "May I see your orders, sir?" ' 'But,' I retorted, 'what would have happened if the arm of that murderer Rascher had been seized by his assistant with a request for the production of the order for the so-called "terminal experiments"? Rascher could have shown him such an order. For the supreme executive authority had sanctioned the tests in question and put the "human material" for them at Rascher's disposal.' In short, the corruption of law, thought and feeling was already absolute.

It is no wonder, therefore, that, after eighteen months' documentary research, overwhelming shame and despair caused us to write, in the preface to the first edition of this volume, that we hardly supposed anyone would reproach us with thinking ourselves any better than those of whom we had to tell. We had no intention of 'proclaiming the guilt of any person to an audience of his fellow human beings. Nor, on the other hand, do we intend to give anyone not named in these documents the cheap satisfaction of feeling that they do not concern him.' The longer we sat in the Court of the Hall of Justice at Nuremberg and the more closely we examined the documentary evidence, the more convinced we grew that we were simply watching a process of taking random samples. The disclosures demonstrated beyond all possible doubt the need for juridical action. When we remembered certain 'judicial' measures taken in the name of Germany, for instance, the special laws passed for application to Poland, we could not refrain from astonishment at the patience and lack of bias displayed by the Court. Here, at any rate, was no case of blind vengeance being executed upon blind hate. On the contrary, painstaking labour had supplied the basis for calm reflection. The proceedings involved not only clarification of the facts upon which judgment was to be delivered, but also the provision of adequate opportunity for the accused to testify to their own feelings and situations. The defendants scarcely ever showed sympathy with their victims even at this late date. They were more concerned with the safety of their own skins than with the misery and death they had inflicted on others. At moments one's disgust with their pedantically solemn eloquence on the subject of their innocence became almost unbearable. Yet the whole affair seemed to us no more than a pointing up and condensation of sinister events on a larger scale. I should be inclined to describe one aspect of this calamity as the concealment of unpalatable truth by rationalization.

The manoeuvres of the accused were extraordinarily varied. One very common expedient was to blame the war for everything. There was a war on, they argued, and one had to take part in it. Those who lived through the years of the dictatorship will remember how hard it was to withstand the impulse to escort the 'ship of state' and not to yield to the temptation to fall into line with the convoy protecting the 'great aims' and the 'absolute necessity of victory in order to eliminate evil elements'. In short, on purely practical grounds one was almost obliged to acquiesce in what was done. The higher a man rose —and every effort was made to rise in order to preserve self-esteem—the nearer he came to crime and the more fiercely he denied the facts. It may well be true that many a letter which resulted in the deaths of thousands, or in only one death, was signed by someone 'not in the know'. He did not or could not foresee the consequences of his action. He affixed his signature not, as was often stated on oath at Nuremberg, because he would otherwise have committed 'dereliction of duty'. For then he would have been aware of the consequences of signing. The real reason was a much simpler one. He had long identified his being with his office, the respect accorded him by others, his rank, his uniform and decorations. In these circumstances it was impossible for him to realize the price he was paying for the macabre feeding of his pride. Even for this development the Nuremberg Trials inspired a formula which could not have been more condensed. It was pronounced by Professor Gerhard Rose, accused in connection with the 'typhus vaccine experiments' carried out in the concentration camps at Buchenwald and at Natzweiler (Struthof). In a single series of such tests at Buchenwald alone 97 persons out of 392 who underwent them were proved to have perished. Rose in his defence cited experiments performed by Richard P. Strong in Manila on criminals under sentence of death who had agreed to take the risk involved. The object was to trace the causes of beri-beri fever. One of the criminals died in the course of the tests. Rose argued, with cunning casuistry, that the natives languishing 'by hundreds of thousands in excruciating pain' owing to beri-beri or the plague were in the same position as typhus-stricken German soldiers. For, while in Manila the distress was caused by endemic disease not consciously introduced by human agency, the German troops suffered as the result of a war planned by Hitler. He had passed special laws, for instance those against Poles and gipsies, under which certain persons had been sentenced to death. The legality of these sentences would at once have been called in question by such a widely travelled man as Rose if he had not been prepared to fly in the face of truth. Strong was seeking to protect people against a species of natural catastrophe that was decimating and tormenting them. Scientists like Rose were working in the jungle of inhumanity created by a dictatorship to maintain its senseless existence. It is perfectly obvious that his ingenious but fallacious comparisons were intended to hoodwink the prosecution and strengthen his defence. But their expression cannot be regarded with indifference. For on the basis of his wide professional experience of emergencies in 'normal' times he proceeded to apply the same considerations to political as to natural disasters, ignoring the difference. He therefore discounted entirely the causes of the war, the brutal ferocity of its aims and the deliberately planned destruction of whole nations. Minds which did not pursue his false reasoning step by step would be left with the comforting reflection that as the best representatives of Germany were in danger it would be preferable to sacrifice in their place persons already condemned to death. It would follow also that the one criminal who died of beri-beri during Strong's experiments had the same significance as the hundreds who succumbed to typhus tests in the concentration camps. Such appears to have been the pretext for the phrase in which Rose seemed to us to reveal the most shocking egotism: 'I hope therefore that my desire for my honour at least to be left to me will be recognized as natural.'

There is no sign in men like Rose of any feeling against a war waged not only for conquest but for the specific purpose of depriving other countries of elementary human rights. Rose and his type showed no true sympathy with those they called 'the pick of the nation', who could only be helped by the quickest possible end to hostilities. No one could have forced the scientists to experiment on the defenceless victims of a terrorist government. In the end those who did so experiment clung to a mere shadow, the ghost of their 'honour', of the human decency they had lost when they struck a bargain with monsters.

I have cited this case first of all because it does not relate to a man who can be dismissed as an adventurer, a psychopath or a born criminal. Professor Rose was a respected scientist who held high academic office. Yet this fact did not prevent his decline from the modest standards of fallible and weak humanity characteristic of most of us into the arrogance, the lust for power, the stupidity and mendacity of a type of scoundrel invariably recognizable by his selfish contempt for others. Rose could have hoped to make some impression if he had said: 'I hope therefore that my desire for some friendly understanding and sympathy will be recognized as natural.' But we live in a world which thinks much more highly of the fetish of 'honour', an idea singularly vague unless we associate it with morbid self-love, than of amiable or humane feelings, which are within the reach of all and peculiarly appropriate to the physician.

Incidentally, the present chronicle itself involves considera-

tions which deserve inclusion in the comprehensive process of
inquiry into the question of guilt which has been going on, or
has been evaded, during the last fifteen years. The authority
exercised in the first place by Hitler and at the other end of
the scale by those who applied torture, some of whom had been
academically educated, was undoubtedly illegal. But the parts
played by the great mass of intermediaries remain disturbingly
obscure. Without their willing, tolerant or apathetic co-
operation the criminal plans and their criminal execution could
never have been carried out. How could these proceedings go
on with such unexampled regularity? Was any serious attempt
made either by individuals or public opinion to investigate the
situation? We found no reason to suppose so nor any convincing proof of reflection on the subject in the evidence given
relating to the cases we examined. Ordinary statistics are
available, of course. There were about 90,000 doctors at work
in Germany under National Socialism. Of these some 350
committed medical crimes. The figure seems pretty high,
especially in view of the magnitude of the illegal acts perpetrated. Though it represents only a small fraction of the whole
medical profession then employed in the country, the realization that one doctor in every three hundred actually incurred
criminal guilt is alarming. Such a ratio would have been
inconceivable at any previous time in Germany. Why, then,
did it exist under National Socialism?

Yet even this question does not probe the heart of the matter
—350 doctors engaged personally in crime. But a 'machine'
existed which enabled them to turn criminals if they liked. It
is true that they did not murder their private patients. They
mostly dealt with 'human material' of a special sort. August
Hirt, for example, Professor of Anatomy at the 'national'
university of Strasbourg, had a collection of the skulls of
'Jewish commissars, showing repulsive but characteristic sub-
human features'. The skulls were supplied to him by the
'machine'. What was its nature? We can only give the right
answer if we realize the extent to which we ourselves formed
part of it. Otherwise we shall have done nothing whatever to
prove our respect for and recognition of the persons who perished in those terrible years. Only through such feelings can we
invalidate for the future the brutish impulses which sacrificed

B

the victims of that period. It is the one gesture of gratitude
to them which we can make, a humble admission on the part
of all of us that we understand and confess the facts. To try to
identify the exceptional cases of morbidity is an obvious and
necessary step. But the attempt will not bring us to the combination of cause and effect, the chain of motive, which originally
rendered such crimes practicable.

The history of the inception of the present work and its
preceding pamphlet, *The Cynical Dictatorship*, is a strange one.
I was at that time Chairman of the German Medical Committee of American Tribunal I at Nuremberg. In that capacity
I was charged by the Study Group of the West German
Chamber of Medicine and by a resolution of the 51st Assembly
of German Medical Practitioners to collect, with the aid of an
assistant, Dr Fred Mielke, the documentary evidence for the
two publications in view. The earlier compilation contained
only an extract from the material at the disposal of the prosecution. The pamphlet was issued during the legal proceedings
themselves, as it was intended primarily to help medical men
to follow the developments in court.

I had been surprised, in the first place, that none of the more
distinguished physicians of Germany seemed able to find the
time to embark upon the painful task of revealing the cruelties
which had been perpetrated under cover what was still being
called research in eugenics or some other branch of medical
science. The late Dr Oehlemann, then President of the Study
Group of the West German Chamber of Medicine, accordingly
nominated me for the job, though I had only just been appointed a university lecturer. It was therefore in the most
unfavourable conditions imaginable that I undertook the work,
in association with Mielke, who was at that time still only a
medical student.

We heard rumours of protests from some of the scientists
mentioned in the documents. We could understand their
astonishment at finding they had been so near to positively
criminal action—described as 'war work'—in the course of
their duties while holding military rank. But not one of those
who served in Hitler's 'machine' used the simple phrase, 'I'm
sorry', in defending himself. It was already evident that
attempts were being made to isolate, so to speak, the guilty and

m plant responsibility solely upon pathological criminals. This proceeding simply encouraged the indifference which I still believe will, if it continues, end the existence of Germany as a nation. The attacks on Mielke and myself eventually reached grotesque proportions. It was often implied that we had invented all we were recording in order to cast aspersions upon the standing of the profession to which we belonged. The hostility of colleagues is not easy to endure, even if the reasons for it seem intelligible enough. The disclosure of all these horrors to the whole world proved an overwhelming shock. For the world was bound to regard them as not simply a series of crimes but as the gravest possible evidence against professional men, in fact a whole nation. New guilty parties had to be found to take the blame for offences which both baffled comprehension and affected one's conscience. Mielke and I were made the scapegoats. We saw little chance of improving the situation through our second publication. But we performed our task, sending 10,000 copies of our documents to the Study Group for distribution to the profession.

The Cynical Dictatorship pamphlet had caused quite a stir. But this further publication was barely mentioned. Readers had no criticisms or comment to offer. In fact, we never met anyone during the next ten years who admitted any knowledge of the book. It might never have been issued. Only one body gave us any reason to suppose it had been received. This was the World Health Organization, which found that our records showed German doctors as a profession to have been unconnected with the crimes committed by the dictatorship. The Organization therefore readmitted them to its ranks. A preface was provided by the Study Group of the West German Chamber of Medicine to the First Edition. It closed with the words:

'The members of the Committee, in particular Privatdozent Dr Alexander Mitscherlich and Fred Mielke of Heidelberg, deserve the thanks of the profession for the objective, scientific and creditable manner in which they carried out their task. It is to be hoped that the result of their labours will contribute to the reinforcement of unblemished humanity and genuine medical rectitude among doctors, to the unswerving maintenance of both the written and unwritten laws of the practice of medicine and to irreproachable social and moral behaviour by all German doctors in both their public and their private capacities, so that the grave stain left upon the profession by certain degenerate members of it may be obliterated.'

After this pronouncement everything seemed to have been forgotten. The amazing recovery of Federal Germany may be regarded psychologically as an example of 'undoing the past', a vast process of eliminating its traces. Mountains of rubble were removed. A new Germany arose, more prosperous than anyone living could remember. No one travelling through the country today could believe that only twenty years ago the gas-chambers were smoking and the mentally afflicted being incinerated in them. Nor would it be credible that barely fifteen years ago the last survivors of millions emerged from the concentration camps and the bodies of young German soldiers, sentenced by their own courts-martial, could be seen hanging from the apple-trees along the main roads. Once more efficiency and talents for organization have thrust horrors into the background. But the efficiency that moved the mountains of debris could not shift the mountain of guilt. In psychological terms its burden was thrown off in the attempt made by the repressive impulse to escape. Such is the position today. But it looks as though what was then repressed is now returning after satisfaction of the flight-impulse and completion of the outward 'undoing of the past'. For as Freud wrote (*Ges. Werke*, Bd. XIV, s. 185): 'That which is repressed is outlawed ... excluded from the comprehensive organization of the Ego.' It cannot be brought within the range of reflection. But if the Ego, or conscious reason, ceases to function, the old murderous and self-abasing instincts do not change. The degradation of the self is simply not consciously acknowledged. The condition has been repressed but not disposed of. It returns. 'Its new course is determined automatically ... it goes the same way as it went before repression.' (Freud, loc. cit.) The impulse which had relieved itself in this way, by a corruption of consciousness, is still present, terrifying as ever. Can there be any end to this process? Will the impulse submit to reason in the new circumstances and consent to be satisfied in ways which the rest of humanity can accept? Or will it again lead men to an utter misunderstanding of the world, dragging reason in its wake, as in the case of the events which our documents record?

No one can be sure that such events will not recur. If they do, and the former symbol of the end of human decency again crops up on German walls, that scrawl will unquestionably prophesy the return of the repressed impulse in its old guise. Yet it will certainly have to compete with other signs which suggest that the conscious mind is confronting the unsolved problems of the past with renewed energy, that the process of coming to terms with guilt has only been interrupted, not terminated. Criminals formerly allowed to remain among us after the death of their instigator are now being unmasked. Professor Werner Heyde, for instance, often mentioned in our records, was not permitted to continue his professional work undisturbed under another name. Germany has been noted in the past as a country without revolutions. But today the nation, after long resistance, will have to embark upon such self-criticism as would mean revolution elsewhere. A powerful movement is afoot to free Germans from the intolerable incubus of the 'Leaders' who involved the country so deeply in their own guilt. There was no revolution after 1945. At that decisive juncture, when revolutionary action might have relieved us of the burden within, we obeyed Allied orders. The trials at Nuremberg and the process of 'denazification' were not initiated by Germans. I doubt very much whether we felt at that time or are even now quite certain that the catastrophe was our own fault. At this very moment of prosperity, of apparent freedom, Sisyphus—to adapt the legend—has actually succeeded in rolling his stone temporarily to the top of the mountain. And yet signs are recurring of the activity of that deadly repressed instinct, accompanied by repressed feelings of guilt. The old phrases are heard again, though only as in a dream. Our future depends, as it did during the preparation of this record, upon whether their return will be dealt with by some genuine effort of conscious intelligence or whether it will remain unaffected, in the nation as a whole, as the trials of individual criminals proceed. Meanwhile little but a transitory variety of attempts to evade the issue can be observed. The future will show whether any truly educative progress has been made, in the sense of recognition and thorough study of the national guilt.

Dr Mielke, my tireless colleague in the years 1947–49, died

at an early age in 1959. His efforts have ensured that the generation which grew up in National Socialist schools and suffered the full impact of a war for which it was not responsible should be able to play its part in the understanding of a situation which must end in deciding Germany's fate. The real decision is in their hands. It is of Dr Mielke and of the courage with which he never ceased to face these horrors, even in his private thoughts, so that Germans might learn to live in a freer and pleasanter atmosphere, that I think as I submit these documents to all his contemporaries.

A. MITSCHERLICH

Heidelberg,
February 1960

A circumstantial record of the evidence submitted at the trials of certain SS doctors, some scientists and three senior Government officials was published by the Office of the Chief Counsel for War Crimes at Nuremberg. A further account of this material was issued in France by Dr François Bayle, Médecin Principal de la Marine and member of the International Scientific Commission, together with exhaustive analyses of the characters of the accused. Other detailed reports of the proceedings are presented in the following chapters.

CHAPTER ONE

LOW PRESSURE AND SUPERCOOLING EXPERIMENTS

THE indicted experiments concerned with the reaction of human beings to (*a*) high altitudes, and (*b*) prolonged supercooling may be considered together. All the persons tested were prisoners in the concentration camp at Dachau. The experiments were all undertaken with a view to improving unsatisfactory results in war operations.

In each series Dr Sigmund Rascher, a former staff surgeon of the Luftwaffe, held a key position. Owing to his rank as SS Untersturmführer he enjoyed direct access to Himmler and was authorized by him to carry out the tests at Dachau.

It appears from the documents submitted that these experiments, begun and executed by Rascher, included the first of a kind which he called 'terminal', i.e. designed to cause the death of the subject.

(i) HIGH ALTITUDE EXPERIMENTS
(*a*) *Captured documents on which the indictment was based*

The following documents are the most striking of the great quantity discovered. They were used by the prosecution in support of charges brought against three doctors, Siegfried Ruff, Wolfgang Romberg and Professor Georg August Weltz, accused of direct participation in an experiment alleged to be criminal.[1]

A letter from Rascher dated the 15 May 1941 was found in Himmler's correspondence. This communication contains Rascher's first request to be allowed to experiment on human beings. As the letter also throws some light on his private personality some introductory sentences are included in the quotation.

1. The services of an examining magistrate are not required by American law. Objective proof of guilt is submitted at the trial itself. (See concluding chapter.)

[DOC. 1602—PS.]*

'Highly esteemed Reich Leader,

My most sincere thanks for your cordial wishes and flowers on the birth of my second son. This time, too, it is a strong boy, though he arrived three weeks too early. I shall take the liberty and send you a small picture of both children some time.

Since I want a third child very soon, I feel very grateful to you that with your help, highly esteemed Reich Leader, the wedding is made possible. Today I was informed by SS Standartenführer Sollman on the telephone that the 165 marks as required for a wedding will be charged to the account "R" and will be transmitted by the "Ancestral Heritage" Community. I thank you heartily! I only need a short certificate concerning Aryan descent for the Luftwaffe, where the permit was already submitted. Tomorrow, prior to my departure, I shall dictate a rough text to Nini D; she will then forward the note to you, highly esteemed Reich Leader.

I also thank you very cordially for the generous regular allowance of fruit; this is at present extremely important for mother and children.

For the time being, I have been assigned to the Luftgau Kommando VII, Munich, for a medical selection course. During this course, where research on high-altitude flying plays a prominent part, determined by the somewhat higher ceiling of the English fighter planes, considerable regret was expressed that no experiments on human beings have so far been possible for us because such experiments are very dangerous and nobody is volunteering. I therefore put the serious question: is there any possibility that two or three professional criminals can be made available for these experiments? The experiments are being performed at the Ground Station for High-Altitude Experiments of the Luftwaffe at Munich. The experiments, in which the experimental subject of course may die, would take place with my collaboration. They are absolutely essential for the research on high-altitude flying and cannot, as has been tried until now, be carried out on monkeys, because monkeys offer entirely different test conditions. I had an absolutely confidential talk with the representative of the Luftwaffe physician who is conducting these experiments. He also is of the opinion that the problems in question can only be solved by experiments on human beings. (Feeble-minded individuals also could be used as experimental material.)'[1]

The following undated reply to this communication was received by Rascher from Dr Rudolf Brandt,[2] Himmler's personal legal adviser.

[DOC. 1582—PS.]*

'Dear Dr Rascher,

Shortly before flying to Oslo, the Reich Leader SS gave me your letter of the 15 May 1941, for partial reply.

I can inform you that prisoners will, of course, be gladly made available for the high-flight researches. I have informed the Chief of the Security Police of this agreement of the Reich Leader SS, and requested that the competent official be instructed to get in touch with you.

I want to use the opportunity to extend my cordial wishes to you on the birth of your son.'

On the 21 March 1942, after the experiment had begun, Himmler expressly stated, through his adviser, that his authorization of them was conditional on Rascher's participation.

[DOC. 1581a—PS.]

Rascher was therefore careful to keep the SS Reichsführer regularly informed of the progress of the experiments. On the 5 April, 1942, he wrote to Himmler, *inter alia*:

[DOC. 1971a—PS.]*

'A few days ago Reich Physician SS Professor Dr Grawitz made a brief inspection of the experimentation plant. Since his time was very limited, no experiments could be demonstrated

1. Professor Weltz deposed in court that Rascher had made a number of incorrect statements in this letter, so as to obtain what he wanted. Volunteers from the Luftwaffe, Weltz stated, had in fact been employed. For many scientists and their colleagues in that arm had performed experiments on themselves without the knowledge or authority of the Director of the Station for High Altitude Experiments.

2. Dr Rudolf Brandt, the lawyer, should be distinguished from Dr Karl Brandt, the physician, formerly Reichskommissar for Health and Sanitation. Both men were indicted at Nuremberg.

to him. SS Obersturmbannführer Sievers took a whole day off
to watch some of the interesting standard experiments and
may have given you a brief report. I believe, highly esteemed
Reich Leader, that you would be extraordinarily interested in
those experiments. Is it not possible that on the occasion of a
trip to Southern Germany you have some of the experiments
demonstrated to you? If the results so far obtained by the
experiments are confirmed by further experimentation, entirely new data will be secured for science; simultaneously,
entirely new aspects will be opened to the Luftwaffe . . .'

This letter was accompanied by a 'First Interim Report on
the Low Pressure Chamber Experiments at Dachau Concentration Camp',[1] given below in full.

[DOC. 1971a—PS.]*

'1. The object is to solve the problem of whether the theoretically established norms pertaining to the length of life of
human beings breathing air with only a small proportion of
oxygen and subjected to low pressure correspond with the
results obtained by practical experiments. It has been asserted
that a parachutist, who jumps from a height of 12 km. would
suffer very severe injuries, probably even die, on account of the
lack of oxygen. Practical experiments on this subject have
always been discontinued after a maximum of fifty-three
seconds, since very severe bends (i.e. air-sickness) occurred.

2. Experiments testing the length of life of a human being
above the normal breathing limits (4, 5, 6 km.) have not been
conducted at all, since it has been a foregone conclusion that
the human experimental subject[2] would suffer death.

Experiments on parachute jumps proved that the lack of
oxygen and the low atmospheric pressure at 12 or 13 km.
altitude did not cause death. Altogether fifteen extreme experiments of this type were carried out in which none of the VPs
died. Very severe bends together with unconsciousness occurred,
but completely normal functions of the senses returned when a
height of 7 km. was reached on descent. Electrocardiograms

1. The prosecution submitted a number of prints [Doc. 610] identified
by the witness Neff from a continuous reel of film found among Rascher's
personal effects at Dachau.
2. Referred to in text as *Versuchsperson*—VP.

registering during the experiments did show certain irregularities, but by the time the experiments were over the curves had returned to normal and they did not indicate any abnormal changes during the following days. The extent to which deterioration of the organism may occur due to continuously repeated experiments can only be established at the end of the series of experiments. The extreme fatal experiments will be carried out on specially selected VPs, otherwise it would not be possible to exercise the rigid control so extraordinarily important for practical purposes.

The VPs were brought to a height of 8 km. under oxygen and then had to make five knee bends with and without oxygen. After a certain lapse of time, moderate to severe bends occurred and the VPs became unconscious. However, after a certain period of accustoming themselves to the height of 8 km. all the VPs recuperated and regained their consciousness and the normal functions of their senses.

Only continuous experiments at altitudes higher than 10·5 km. resulted in death. These experiments showed that breathing stopped after about thirty minutes, while in two cases the electrocardiographically charted action of the heart continued for another twenty minutes.

The third experiment of this type took such an extraordinary course that I called an SS physician of the camp as witness, since I had worked on these experiments myself. It was a continuous experiment without oxygen at a height of 12 km. conducted on a 37-year-old Jew in good general condition. Breathing continued up to thirty minutes. After four minutes the VP began to perspire and to wiggle his head, after five minutes cramps occurred, between six and ten minutes breathing increased in speed and the VP became unconscious; from eleven to thirty minutes breathing slowed down to three breaths per minute, finally stopping altogether.

Severest cyanosis developed in between and foam appeared at the mouth.

At five-minute intervals electrocardiograms from three leads were written. After breathing had stopped, the electrocardiogram was continuously written until the action of the heart had come to a complete standstill. About half an hour after breathing had stopped, dissection was started.

Autopsy Report

When the cavity of the chest was opened the pericardium was filled tightly (heart tamponade). Upon opening of the pericardium 80 c.c. of clear yellowish liquid gushed forth.

The moment the tamponade had stopped, the right auricle began to beat heavily, at first at the rate of sixty actions per minute, then progressively slower. Twenty minutes after the pericardium had been opened, the right auricle was opened by puncturing it. For about fifteen minutes a thin stream of blood spurted forth. Thereafter clogging of the puncture wound in the auricle by coagulation of the blood and renewed acceleration of the action of the right auricle occurred.

One hour after breathing had stopped, the spinal marrow was completely severed and the brain removed. Thereupon the action of the auricle stopped for forty seconds. It then renewed its action, coming to a complete standstill eight minutes later. A heavy subarchnoid oedema was found in the brain. In the veins and arteries of the brain a considerable quantity of air was discovered. Furthermore, the blood vessels in the heart and liver were enormously obstructed by embolism.

The anatomical preparations will be preserved and so I shall be able to evaluate them later.

The last-mentioned case is to my knowledge the first one of this type ever observed on man. The above-described heart actions will gain particular scientific interest, since they were written down with an electrocardiogram to the very end.

The experiments will be continued and extended. Another interim report will follow after new results have been obtained.

(*Signed*) DR RASCHER'

On the 13 April 1942 the following replies were sent to Rascher.

[DOC. 1971*c*—PS.]*
[DOC. 1971*b*—PS.]*
        'Top Secret.
SS Untersturmführer Rascher, M.D.
Munich, Trogerstrasse 56.
Dear Comrade Dr Rascher,
        Your report of the 5 April 1942 has been seen by the Reich

Leader SS today. The tests on which SS Obersturmbannführer Sievers gave a brief report interested him very much.

For the further tests I wish you a continuation of the success you have had so far.

Best regards also to your wife.

Heil Hitler!

Yours,

(*Signed*) B. (R.) BRANDT

SS Sturmbannführer.'

'Dear Dr Rascher,

I want to answer your letter with which you sent me your reports. Especially the latest discoveries made in your experiments particularly have interested me. May I now ask you the following:

1. This experiment is to be repeated on other men condemned to death.

2. I would like Dr Fahrenkamp to be taken into consultation on these experiments.

3. Considering the long-continued action of the heart the experiments should be specifically exploited in such a manner as to determine whether these men could be recalled to life. Should such an experiment succeed, then, of course, the person condemned to death shall be pardoned to concentration camp for life.

Please keep me further informed on the experiments.

Kind regards and

Heil Hitler!

Yours,

(*Signed*) H. HIMMLER'

On the 16 April 1942 Rascher had further reported, *inter alia*:

[DOC. 218.]*

'The experiment described in the report of the 4 April was repeated four times, each time with the same results. When Wagner, the last test person, had stopped breathing, I let him back to life by increasing pressure. Since test person "W——"

was assigned for a terminal[1] experiment, as a repeated experiment held no prospect of new results, and since I had not been in possession of your letter at that time, I subsequently started another experiment through which Test Person Wagner did not live. Also in this case the results obtained by electrocardiographic registration were extraordinary. . . .

Highly esteemed Reich Leader, allow me to close by assuring you that your active interest in these experiments has a tremendous influence on one's working capacity and initiative.'

But the deaths reported were by no means the only fatal results of these experiments. Dr Romberg stated on oath:

[DOC. 476.]

'During the experiments I witnessed the deaths of three persons under test by Dr Rascher. The first death occurred at the end of April. On that occasion I kept the electrocardiogram under observation. After the death of the subject I protested to Rascher and also told Dr Ruff what had happened. Two more deaths took place on separate days in May. I told Dr Ruff about these also. I know that other subjects were killed in this way when I was not present. I estimate the number of these further deaths at between five and ten.'

Himmler had specified that the subjects of the tests were to be persons under sentence of death at Dachau. But Rascher seems to have been in some doubt. On the 20 October 1942 he sent the following express teletype to Rudolf Brandt.

[DOC. 1971d—PS.]*

'Will you please clarify the following case with the Reich Leader SS as soon as possible?

In communication RFSS of the 13 April 1942 under paragraph 3 it is ordered that if prisoners in Dachau condemned to death live through experiments which have endangered their lives, they should be pardoned. As up to now only Poles and Russians were available, some of whom have been condemned to death, it is not quite clear to me yet as to whether the above-mentioned paragraph also applies to them, and whether they may be par-

1. *Translator's note:* 'Terminal' as used here means 'resulting in death'.

doned to concentration camp for life after having lived through several very severe experiments.

Please answer by teletype via Adjutant's Office, RFSS, Munich.

Obedient Greetings,

Heil Hitler!

Yours,

(*Signed*) S. RASCHER'

Brandt at once replied, on the 21st:

[DOC. 1971*e*—PS.]*
'To SS Obersturmführer Schnitzler,
Munich.

Please inform SS Untersturmführer Dr Rascher with regard to his teletype inquiry that the instruction given some time ago by the Reich Leader SS concerning amnesty of test persons does not apply to Poles and Russians.

(*Signed*) BRANDT

SS Obersturmbannführer'

The way in which these scientific proceedings were carried out is strikingly illustrated in another secret report from Rascher to Himmler, dated the 11 May 1942. It is again quoted in full.

[DOC. 220.]*
'Munich, 11 May 1942.

SECRET REPORT

Based on results of experiments which up to now various scientists have conducted on animals only, the experiments in Dachau were to prove whether these results would maintain their validity on human beings.

1. The first experiments were to show whether the human being can gradually adapt himself to higher altitudes. Some ten tests showed that a slower ascent without oxygen taking from six to eight hours kept the functions of the senses of the various VPs fully normal up to a height of 8,000 m. Within eight hours several VPs had reached a height of 9·5 km. without oxygen when bends occurred suddenly.

2. Normally it is impossible to stay without oxygen at altitudes higher than 6 km. Experiments showed however that after ascent to 8,000 m. without oxygen, bends combined with unconsciousness lasted only about twenty-five minutes. After this period the VPs had mostly become accustomed to that altitude; consciousness returned, they could make knees bend, showed a normal electrocardiograph and were able to work (60 to 70 per cent of the cases examined).

3. Descending tests on parachutes (suspended) without oxygen.

These experiments proved that from 14 km. on down severest bends occurred which remained until the ground was reached. The detrimental effects caused by these experiments manifested themselves at the beginning as unconsciousness, and subsequently as spastic and limp paralysis, catotony, stereotypy, and as retrograde amnesia lasting several hours. About one hour after the end of the experiment the VPs for the most part were still disoriented as to time and locality.

The blood picture often showed a shift to the left; albumen and red and white blood corpuscles were regularly found in the urine after the experiment; cylinders were sometimes found. After several hours or days the blood and urine returned to normal. The changes of the electrocardiograph were reversible.

Contrary to descending tests on parachutes without oxygen, descending tests with oxygen were carried out from heights up to 18 km. It was proved that on the average the VPs regained the normal function of their senses at 12 to 13 km. No disturbances of general conditions occurred during any of these experiments. Brief unconsciousness at the beginning of the experiment caused no lasting disturbances. Urine and blood showed only a slight change.

4. As the long time of descent on parachutes, under actual conditions, would cause severe freezing even if no detrimental effects were caused by lack of oxygen, VPs were brought by sudden decreases in pressure with a cutting torch from 8 to 20 km., simulating the damage to the pressure machine of the high-altitude airplane. After a waiting period of ten seconds, corresponding to stepping out of the machine, the VPs were made to fall from this height with oxygen to a height where

breathing is possible. The VPs awoke between 10 and 12 km. and at about 8 km. pulled the parachute lever.

5. In experiments of falling from the same height without oxygen, the VPs regained normal function of their senses only between 2 and 5 km.

6. Experiments testing the effect of pervitin on the organism during parachute jumps proved that severe after-effects, as mentioned under No. 3, were considerably milder. The ability to withstand the conditions at high altitudes was only slightly improved, while the bends, since they were not noticed, occurred suddenly (restraint-loosening effects of pervitin).

7. Dr Kliches, of the Charles University in Prague, reports in the publication of the Reich Research Council: 'By prolonged breathing of oxygen, human beings should theoretically be kept fully fit up to 13 km. In practice, the limit is around 11 km. Experiments which I carried out in this connection proved that with pure oxygen no lowering of the measurable raw energy (ergometer) was noticeable up to 13·3 km. The VPs merely became unwilling since pains of the body cavities grew too severe, due to the lowering of pressure between body and thin air. When pure oxygen was inhaled bends occurred in all twenty-five cases only at heights above 14·2 km.'

As a practical result of the more than 200 experiments conducted at Dachau, the following can be assumed:

Flying in altitudes higher than 12 km. without pressure-cabin or pressure-suit is impossible even while breathing pure oxygen. If the airplane pressure-machine is damaged at altitudes of 13 km. and higher, the crew will not be able to bail out of the damaged plane themselves since at that height the bends appear rather suddenly. It must be requested that the crew should be removed automatically from the plane, for instance, by catapulting the seats by means of compressed air. Descending with opened parachute without oxygen would cause severe injuries due to the lack of oxygen, besides causing severe freezing; consciousness would not be regained until the ground was reached. Therefore the following is to be requested: 1. A parachute with barometrically controlled opening; 2. A portable oxygen apparatus for the jump.

For the following experiments Jewish professional criminals who had committed race pollution were used. The question of

c

the formation of embolism was investigated in ten cases. Some of the VPs died during a continued high-altitude experiment; for instance, after one half-hour at a height of 12 km.

After the skull had been opened under water an ample amount of air embolism was found in the brain vessels and, in part, free air in the brain ventricles.

To find out whether the severe psychic and physical effects, as mentioned under No. 3, are due to the formation of embolism, the following was done: After relative recuperation from such a parachute descending test had taken place, however, before regaining consciousness, some VPs were kept under water until they died. When the skull and the cavities of the breast and of the abdomen had been opened under water, an enormous amount of air embolism was found in the vessels of the brain, the coronary vessels, and the vessels of the liver and the intestines, etc.

That proves that air embolism, so far considered as absolutely fatal, is not fatal at all, but reversible, as shown by the return to normal conditions of all the other VPs.

It was also proved by experiments that air embolism occurs in practically all vessels even while pure oxygen is being inhaled. One VP was made to breathe pure oxygen for two and a half hours before the experiment started. After six minutes at a height of 20 km., he died and at dissection also showed ample air embolism, as was the case in all other experiments.

At sudden decreases in pressure and subsequent immediate falls to heights where breathing is possible, no deep reaching damages due to air embolism could be noted. The formation of air embolism always needs a certain amount of time.

(*Signed*) DR RASCHER'

The low pressure experiments in the camp at Dachau ended in the second half of May 1942.

In addition to the secret reports signed by Rascher alone and addressed to Himmler personally a comprehensive 'Report on High Altitude Experiments', occupying twenty-four typewritten sheets, is signed on behalf of the 'German Experimental Station for Aviation', Registered, by S. Ruff, 'Director of the Institute', Rascher as staff surgeon of the Luftwaffe, and Romberg, the last two signing as 'compilers' of the Report. It was in triplicate, stamped 'Secret for Headquarters' and dated the 28 July 1942. It begins:

[DOC. 402.]*

'I.—Introduction and Statement of the Problem

It is theoretically possible for man to reach as high altitude as he may wish in an aircraft with a pressure-cabin. However, the question must be settled as to what results or effects the destruction of the pressure-cabin will have upon the human being, who in such cases is exposed in a few seconds to the low air pressure and thereby to the lack of oxygen, which is characteristic of high altitude. Of particular practical interest is the question from what altitudes and by what means the safest rescue of the crew can be made. In the work at hand, a report is presented on experiments in which the various possibilities of rescue were studied under special experimental conditions. Since the urgency of the solution of the problem was evident, it was necessary, especially under the given conditions of the experiment, to forgo for the time being the thorough clearing up of purely scientific questions.'

Two Sections follow, entitled *Order of Experiments* and *Results of Experiments* respectively. The extract below, dealing with an experimental descent from a height of 15 km. (*c.* 10 miles) vividly reveals what happened in such tests.

'Descending experiments were made in larger numbers from 15 km. altitude, since it became evident that at this altitude the approximate limits for what was possible in emergencies had already been reached or essentially surpassed. After an ascent made as rapidly as possible, using oxygen apparatus with free flow, the mask was removed immediately upon attaining 15 km. (49,200 ft.) altitude and the descent was begun. Since the results of these descending experiments were very typical and especially impressive it is necessary to present one of these experiments in detail. The record of the experiment is represented as follows:

15 km. (49,200 ft.)   Lets the mask fall, severe altitude sickness, clonic convulsions.

14·5 km. (47,560 ft.) (30 sec.)	Opisthotonos.
14·3 km. (46,900 ft.) (45 sec.)	Arms stretched stiffly forward; sits up like a dog, legs spread stiffly apart.
13·7 km. (44,950 ft.) (1 min. 20 sec.)	Suspended in opisthotonos.
13·2 km. (43,310 ft.) (1 min. 50 sec.)	Agonal convulsive breathing.
12·2 km. (40,030 ft.) (3 min.)	Dyspnea, hangs limp.
7·2 km. (23,620 ft.) (10 min.)	Unco-ordinated movements with the extremities.
6 km. (19,690 ft.) (12 min.)	Clonic convulsions, groaning.
5·5 km. (18,040 ft.) (13 min.)	Yells loudly.
2·9 km. (9,520 ft.) (18 min.)	Still yelling, convulses arms and legs, head sinks forward.
2—0 km. (6,560—0 ft.) (2—024·5 min.)	Yells spasmodically, grimaces, bites his tongue.
0 km.	Does not respond to speech, gives the impression of someone who is completely out of his mind.
5 min. (after reaching ground level)	Reacts for the first time to vocal stimulation.
7 min.	Attempts upon command to arise, says in stereotyped manner: "No, please."
9 min.	Stands up on command; severe ataxia; answers to all questions: "Just a minute." Tries spasmodically to recall his birth date.
10 min.	Typical stereotypes of attitude and movement (catatonia); mumbles number to himself.
11 min.	Holds his head turned convulsively to the right; tries repeatedly to answer the first question concerning his birth date.
12 min.	Questions of the subject: "May I slice something?" (*Note:* In civilian work,

he was a delicatessen clerk.) "May I pant, will it be all right if I inhale?" Breathes deeply, then says, "All right, thank you very much."

15 min.   On being ordered to walk, steps forward and says: "All right, thank you very much."

17 min.   Gives his name; says he was born in 1928 (born 1 November 1908) Experimenter says: "Where?" "Something 1928." "Profession?" "28—1928."

18 min.   "May I inhale?" "Yes." "I am content with that."

25 min.   Still the question continues: "Pant?"

28 min.   Sees nothing; runs against open window sash upon which the sun is shining, so that large lump is formed on his forehead; says "Excuse me please." No expression of pain.

30 min.   Knows his name and place of birth. Upon being asked for the day's date: "1 November 1928." Shivering of the legs; stupor continues; cannot be frightened by the report of a shot. Dark objects are still not discerned; subject bumps against them. Is aware of bright light; knows his profession; spatially disoriented.

37 min.   Reacts to pain stimuli.

40 min.   Begins to observe differences. Falls continually into his previous speech stereotypes.

50 min.   Spatially oriented.

75 min.   Still disoriented in time; retrogressive amnesia over three days.

24 hours   Normal condition again attained; has no recollection of the experiment itself.

The events of the descending experiments from 15 km., as

shown here through this example, repeated themselves in a similar way in all the rest of the experiments.'

The *Results* Section, by way of contrast with the fatal cases specified by Rascher, closes with the words:

'In conclusion, we must make it particularly clear that, in view of the extreme experimental conditions in this whole experimental series, no fatality and no lasting injury due to oxygen lack occurred.'

The *Summary* (Section V) reads as follows:

'V.—SUMMARY

Experiments were instituted upon the possibility of rescue from altitudes up to 21 km. (68,900 ft.).

Without parachute oxygen equipment, rescue in descending experiments is still possible from 13 km. (42,700 ft.), with equipment, from 18 km. (59,100 ft.). The danger arising from cold must be considered.

In falling experiments, rescue from 21 km. (68,900 ft.) altitude with and without oxygen was proved possible. Automatic parachute opening is necessary. Ebullition of the blood does not yet occur at 21 km. (68,900 ft.) altitude.

Oxygen must be breathed before explosive decompression. Abandonment must be by means of the ejection seat. The dive to safe altitude offers good possibilities of rescue if abandonment of the plane is not necessary after loss of the cabin pressure.'

On the 11 September 1942 Rascher and Romberg, according to a report signed by the latter at the time, showed at the Air Ministry a film illustrative of their experiments. Between thirty and forty senior Luftwaffe officers were present. During the interval Rascher called attention

[DOC. 224.]*

'to the strict obligation of secrecy ordered by the Reich Leader SS. After completion of the showing of the motion picture—the State Secretary had not come, as he had been summoned to see the Reich Marshal (Göring)—the persons present still talked a little while about the motion picture, on which occasion less interest was shown in the subject itself than in the place of the experiments and the individuals who had been the subjects.'

A realistic description of the proceedings at the Dachau Experimental Station at that time was given by the witness Walter Neff. Formerly a prisoner and later employed by the camp staff, he had been offered by the latter to Rascher and Romberg as an assistant. He stated [Prot. p. 656] that between 180 and 200 prisoners were subjected to the experiments. These people belonged to every nationality represented in the camp. But they were mostly Russians, Poles, Germans and Jews. He was asked in court how many voluntarily submitted to the tests. He replied that about ten might have volunteered. Only one of the subjects was afterwards released 'as he had taken part in most of the experiments, including one at which the Reichsführer had been present'. This man, named Sobotta, was 'later transferred to the Dirlewanger Group', an organization which the witness believed was 'a SS unit training at Oranienburg for special service . . . the worst thing that could happen to a prisoner was to be sent there'.

Neff was then asked how many prisoners lost their lives in the low pressure experiments. He replied: 'During the altitude flights between seventy and eighty.'

Of these he said that some forty were not under sentence of death.

Neff was also present at the dissections mentioned in the secret reports. He made the following statement:

[PROT. p. 665.]

'In one case it was found that the heart was still beating after the chest and skull had been laid open. I am quite sure of this because I was at once ordered to fetch the electrocardiograph so that the heart action could be recorded on that instrument. This particular experiment was actually the cause of many more deaths, since tests were afterwards repeatedly made with a view to ascertaining how long the heart of a dissected body would go on beating. In these cases part of my work was to hand the rolls taken from the electrocardiograph in the dark room through the window of the dissection room.'

Neff's evidence also suggested that Rascher, in addition to carrying out experiments in collaboration with Romberg, had often acted alone, on his own responsibility.

(*b*) *Low-pressure experiments as illustrated in Court from the cross-examination of witnesses, from documents cited by the defence and from Judgment.*

Judgment on the altitude tests begins:
[Judgment p. 198 f.]*

'The evidence is overwhelming and not contradicted that experiments involving the effect of low air pressure on living human beings were conducted at Dachau from the latter part of February through May 1942. In some of these experiments great numbers of human subjects were killed under the most brutal and senseless conditions. A certain Dr Sigmund Rascher, Luftwaffe officer, was the prime mover in the experiments which resulted in the deaths of the subjects. The prosecution maintains that Ruff, Romberg, and Weltz were criminally implicated in these experiments.'

Investigation of the origin of these experiments showed that in a lecture at a Continuation Course directed by the Munich Headquarters of Aviation Area VII it was explained that 'with the object of determining the effects upon aviators of insufficiency or failure of supplies of oxygen at high altitudes . . . it was necessary to renew tests of the effects of such variations of height upon further groups of air surgeons and pilots'. [DOC. Weltz, 2.]

This statement suggested to Rascher the idea of using professional criminals for the experiments in view. He took advantage of his personal relations with Himmler, as is clear from the documents already quoted, to enlist the latter's interest in this plan and also the powers to execute it of which the Reichsführer disposed.

Rascher also approached Area VII in this connection, though at first without success. In midsummer 1941 Professor E. Hippke, Health Inspector to the Luftwaffe, visited Munich. At a private meeting there he signified his agreement, in principle, to the proposal to use criminals for experimental purposes.

Professor Weltz, in evidence on his own behalf at Nuremberg, described what was being thought of these plans at the time. After Hippke had been told what the Luftwaffe surgeons had by then learned of Rascher's ideas, one of those present at the discussion observed:

[PROT. p. 7138.]

'That in the conditions referred to there could be no objection whatever to such experiments, since after all they would be of advantage to the criminals themselves. And as I considered the wording of the proposed resolution somewhat unfortunate I intervened towards the end of the discussion and tried to define to Hippke my own ideas in this connection.

I was pretty clear myself on the subject because I had recently read de Kruif's book, *The Conquerors of Hunger*.'

Professor Weltz then mentioned Goldberger's experiments in connection with pellagra. They had been carried out in the State of Mississippi, in 1915, on twelve criminals. All the 'condemned volunteers', as de Kruif called them, had withstood the tests without injury to their health and were then set at liberty.[1]

Weltz was asked by his defence counsel why he had quoted de Kruif's work of popularization. He answered:

[PROT. p. 7141.]

'Well, it then seemed to me a perfect precedent, especially useful in its precise statement of the very points with which I was concerned. I accordingly formulated them for Hippke's benefit by telling him that in the first place the tests must have an urgent task in view which could not be solved by experimenting on animals. Secondly, the criminals who came forward for the purpose would have to do so voluntarily. Thirdly, they should be rewarded for their consent. These principles were most scrupulously adhered to in the subsequent operations, far more so than is usually the case in scientific work, where as a rule only summary technical data are requisite, such as the number of subjects, their ages and vital statistics. In de Kruif's book, however, exceptionally

1. Cf. de Kruif, *Bezwinger des Hungers*, pp. 324–8 [Doc. Weltz, 13].

detailed and clear accounts of their personal circumstances were given. I have no reason to doubt the accuracy of his statements. . . . Moreover, the wide public to which such books are addressed is the best indication of what is or is not accept-able by opinion at large. Editions were issued by the million in many languages. Even if the data presented were not correct, of which there is no evidence at all, the book at least proves what is internationally accepted as permissible in the general view.'

At a later conference between Rascher and Weltz the latter rejected the proposal to carry out such experiments on the ground that he did not consider the problem of height varia-tion urgent. He remained of this opinion even after Rascher had been transferred to his Institute in November 1941.

It was not until Weltz heard, in Berlin, of Ruff's experi-mental programme in connection with high altitudes and learned that Ruff had not been able to find enough volunteers for his project at his own Berlin Institute that the professor remembered Rascher, then without employment at the Munich Institute. Weltz and Ruff thereupon decided to take advantage of Hippke's agreement in principle to the plan and of Himmler's authorization of the use of prisoners at Dachau. [PROT. pp. 6622 and 7156.]

The two Institute Directors arranged for future tests to be carried out at both their establishments, Dr Ruff's colleague Romberg to act in Berlin and Rascher at Munich, and the Directors themselves assuming responsibility for the experi-ments. The German Experimental Medical Institute had been set up, under Ruff, in Berlin, at the request of the technical authorities conducting war operations. This Institute was accordingly concerned chiefly with research on practical prob-lems, while that at Munich, under Weltz, for the most part studied questions of theory.

After Ruff, Romberg, Weltz and Rascher had met at Munich to discuss the matter, all four men, accompanied by Himmler's Adjutant, left for Dachau in order to consult the camp com-mandant on the methods to be adopted in executing the plan.

The conditions in which the three defendants who afterwards appeared at Nuremberg were prepared to carry out the tests are evident from the following extract from their cross-examination. Prosecuting counsel asked what arrangements were made to obtain subjects. Weltz replied:

[PROT. p. 7286.]

'We had no difficulty in that connection. For the offer made to us was one of volunteers and we had no reason to doubt this basic condition of the work, which was not even discussed. We had only to take care that the other principles laid down for us were strictly maintained. Accordingly, the question of free will did not come up for serious discussion. It was assumed, without debate, as a necessary preliminary. . . .

Q. I can understand that you had no difficulty in that connection yourselves at the time. But for us here it now constitutes a big problem. You are here for the very reason that you did not consider it as one at the time. But, however that may be, you did go to Dachau. On your arrival you never once raised the question of free will. Be good enough to inform the Tribunal what regulations you found in force for the selection of volunteers. How did you explain to the Camp Commandant what sort of people you required?

A. Schnitzler, the Government's representative, transmitted Himmler's orders to the Commandant in our presence. They were to the effect that (i) Himmler had given his consent to or his instruction for the experiments in question, (ii) we were all to participate in them, (iii) that the subjects must be volunteers and professional criminals. A short discussion followed between Schnitzler, Rascher and the Commandant as to the various Blocks from which the subjects should be taken.'

The court took every conceivable step to ascertain, so far as might still be possible, what sort of persons were chosen to undergo the experiments, how their 'voluntary' agreement was established and by what means they were eventually selected.

[Judgment p. 203 f.]*

'There appear to have been two distinct groups of prisoners used in the experimental series. One was a group of ten to fifteen inmates known in the camp as "exhibition patients" or "permanent experimental subjects". Most, if not all, of these were German nationals who were confined in the camp as criminal prisoners. These men were housed together and were well-fed and reasonably contented. None of them suffered death or injury as a result of the experiments. The other group consisted of 150 to 200 subjects picked at random from the camp and used in the experiments without their permission. Some seventy or eighty of these were killed during the course of the experiments.

The defendants Ruff and Romberg maintain that two separate and distinct experimental series were carried on at Dachau; one conducted by them with the use of the 'exhibition subjects', relating to the problems of rescue at high altitudes, in which no injuries occurred; the other conducted by Rascher on the large group of non-volunteers picked from the camp at random, to test the limits of human endurance at extremely high altitudes, in which experimental subjects in large numbers were killed.

The prosecution submits that no such fine distinction may be drawn between the experiments said to have been conducted by Ruff and Romberg, on the one hand, and Rascher on the other, or as to the prisoners who were used as the subjects of these experiments; that Romberg—and Ruff as his superior—share equal guilt with Rascher for all experiments in which deaths to the human subjects resulted.

In support of this submission the members of the prosecution cite the fact that Rascher was always present when Romberg was engaged in work at the altitude chamber; that on at least three occasions Romberg was at the chamber when deaths occurred to the so-called Rascher subjects, yet elected to continue the experiments. They point likewise to the fact that, in a secret preliminary report made by Rascher to Himmler which tells of deaths, Rascher mentions the name of Romberg as being a collaborator in the research. Finally they point to the fact that, after the experiments were concluded, Romberg was recommended by Rascher and Sievers for the War Merit Cross, because of the work done by him at Dachau.'

The defendants, Ruff, Romberg and Weltz, repeatedly affirmed in their evidence that the tests could only have been applied to volunteers. For otherwise no useful results could have been obtained. It seemed astonishing, all the same, that the entire Luftwaffe, comprising far more than a million members, could produce less than a dozen volunteers. The fact was explained by Weltz, *inter alia*, in answer to his defence counsel, as follows:

[PROT. p. 7332 f.]

Q. Would it not have been possible to continue the series of experiments begun by Ruff and Romberg at Adlershof by resorting to volunteers from the Luftwaffe instead of going to the camp at Dachau? Prosecuting counsel was of opinion, in this connection, that the experiments at Dachau might have been avoided in this way. Please tell me as clearly as you can whether or not you could have obtained the necessary number of subjects, say about fifteen, from the Luftwaffe.

A. There were difficulties in the way of obtaining such a number of volunteers for so long a period. Ruff has already explained the reasons in his evidence. Service personnel could not be released to be put at our disposal. If they were employed at the Institute they had naturally to attend regularly to their daily work, so that in practice, for that reason alone, they were not available. What I was asked was whether enough volunteers would have reported. Luftwaffe volunteers for altitude experiments were always available in great numbers so far as their own inclinations were concerned. If any detachment had been asked which of its members would volunteer for altitude experiments and if it could have been announced that such members would be released from other duties for so long as the experiments lasted, no doubt pretty well the whole detachment would have volunteered. For altitude experiments were familiar to them. They knew that no painful or disagreeable experiences would be involved. They all had personal knowledge of the conditions that would prevail. The reasons, however, why this procedure could not be adopted were altogether different. They were due, of course, to the fact that everyone was overworked during the war. Each department considered it of the greatest possible moment not to lose for a single hour any one of its employees in any category. It was the same in the case of students. . . . This fact accounts for the apparent discrepancy between the statements that we could get as many volunteers as we liked from the Luftwaffe and that in practice none was obtainable.'

Yet it remains astonishing that fifteen Luftwaffe volunteers could not have been released from their duties for the tests. The fact seems to indicate that the trouble was not only due to invincible opposition on the ground of organization but also to the view that the most convenient expedient would be to use concentration camp inmates for the purpose, as had already been suggested.

Not one of the accused ever stated in his defence that he had, for example, tried to convince any responsible Luftwaffe General of the importance of the experiments for the pilots under his command. Nor did any of the defendants express resentment of the fact that, as Ruff put it in answer to his defence counsel, he had been 'subordinate in the camp to the jurisdiction of the commandant and the SS.' Ruff added:

[PROT. p. 6656.]

'That was not a special case. On the contrary, everyone who entered a concentration camp had to acknowledge the fact, by his signature, before he was allowed in.'

If no objection was ever voiced to working in a concentration camp under the remarkable condition just noted, the fact only appears explicable as the result of a tacit acceptance of political exigency. Prosecuting counsel asked Ruff whether he had felt any scruples at being called upon to use the camp prisoners in his experiments. He replied:

[PROT. p. 6748 f.]

'I had no scruples on legal grounds. For I knew that the man who had officially authorized these experiments was Himmler. He was at that time at the Ministry of the Interior. He was Chief of Police and held the highest executive position in the State. Consequently, I had no scruples of any kind in that direction. In the sphere of what one may call medical ethics it was rather different. It was a wholly new experience for us to be offered prisoners to experiment on. Accordingly, both Dr

Romberg and I myself had to get used to the idea. As I have already described under direct examination, we had hitherto experimented almost entirely on ourselves. But we were now called upon to experiment on strangers and prisoners into the bargain. My determination nevertheless to carry out such experiments was due in the first place to my recognition of the importance and urgency of the research involved and secondly to my reading of international literature on the subject, which showed me that my assent to and view of such experiments were at least not contrary to the opinions held in this connection by professional medical organizations in other countries and that no foreign legal, ecclesiastical or political authority had ever taken any kind of exception to such tests. I never heard of any such thing. What I mean is that my knowledge of experiments of this sort carried out abroad gave me the moral certainty that I was not undertaking anything which could have been regarded as immoral anywhere else in the world or in Germany itself.'

At the very start of the tests Rascher had declined, on the strength of a telegram from Himmler, to give Weltz any particulars of them. Weltz then had Rascher transferred from his Institute.

The professor's early withdrawal from the affair is dealt with in Judgment as follows [p. 202]:*

'There is evidence from which it may reasonably be found that at the outset of the programme personal friction developed between Weltz and his subordinate Rascher. The testimony of Weltz is that on several occasions he asked Rascher for reports on the progress of the experiments and each time Rascher told Weltz that nothing had been started with reference to the research. Finally Weltz ordered Rascher to make a report; whereupon Rascher showed his superior a telegram from Himmler which stated, in substance, that the experiments to be conducted by Rascher were to be treated as top secret matter and that reports were to be given to none other than Himmler. Because of this situation Weltz had Rascher transferred out of his command to the DVL branch at Dachau. Defendant Romberg stated that these experiments had been stopped soon after their inception by the adjutant of the Reich War Ministry, because of friction between Weltz and Rascher, and that the

experiments were resumed only after Rascher had been transferred out of Weltz's Institute.

While the evidence is convincingly plain that Weltz participated in the initial arrangements for the experiments and
brought all parties together, it is not so clear that illegal experiments were planned or carried out while Rascher was under
Weltz's command, or that he knew that experiments which
Rascher might conduct in the future would be illegal and
criminal.'

The experiments were stimulated by the development of jet
fighters capable of a ceiling of 18,000 metres (c. 11 miles). At
the Berlin Institute Ruff had already proved, in experiments
carried out on himself and other members of the establishment,
what effects on the human organism might be expected at
altitudes of 7 to 8 miles and also if pressure suddenly dropped
owing to leakage in the pressure cabin. Consequently, when he
and Romberg arrived at Dachau, they had already determined
their programme. They intended to extend the tests so as to
take in the higher altitudes now attainable. The suspicions
aroused by the transfer of the Station to Dachau and the use
of a different type of subject for the experiments are expressed
by the following exchanges at the trial.

[PROT. p. 6772 ff.]

'*Prosecuting Counsel:* Why could you not have undertaken this
investigation of effects at altitudes between 12,000 and 20,000
metres in Berlin instead of Dachau?

Ruff: We could have undertaken it in Berlin. I have already
stated why I agreed to the suggestion to conduct the second
series of tests at Dachau.

Q. So it was not because your colleagues or yourself, as
appears to be the case, hesitated to experiment with such altitudes as you intended to reach with the prisoners?

A. No, that was not the reason. For, as I have already explained under direct examination, we had previously undertaken, on ourselves as before at our Institute, one part of these
tests at greater heights, that part, namely, which precedes the
jump, the pressure-drop, as it is called. In my direct examination
I only gave a very brief account of a few series of experiments

conducted over a period of ten years at my Institute. If I had then been allowed more time, I don't think the question would have been raised of any hesitation on our part to attempt such altitudes.

Q. Well, Doctor ... your report No. 402 shows that your colleagues, Rascher and Romberg, made a distinctly tentative attempt to go up to over 12,000 metres. They did reach 12,500 or 13,500. But then, according to the report, they discontinued the test, owing to the severe pains they experienced. Isn't that so? ... The last third of the page states: "At the same time very severe pains in the head began, as if one's skull were being blasted open. The pains continually increased, so that eventually it became necessary to give up the experiment." So it appears, doesn't it, that Rascher and Romberg had to stop when they reached 12,500 and 13,500 metres?

A. That is correct in one sense but not in another. I don't think I made myself quite clear in this connection yesterday and I should therefore like to repeat what I then said. In such experiments there is a fundamental distinction between the case of a person who remains for 100 seconds, let us say, above 12,000 metres and that of one who stays at such a height, as in the present instance, for forty minutes. The tests which Rascher and Romberg carried out on themselves are in no way related to the true parachute jump experiments subsequently undertaken with other subjects. I explained yesterday why my colleagues undertook these pioneer experiments on themselves. It was because they had found, while they were present several times a day in the same room as the actual subject of experiment, that pain and discomfort were experienced at the second or third ascent but not at the first. The discomfort experienced by those in charge of the experiment therefore increased with the number of ascents made in one day. They wished, accordingly, to determine whether the pains were simply due to the numbers of ascents made or whether they might be caused by remaining at great altitudes for a longer period. It was for this reason that they undertook the tests on themselves, which proved that discomfort in fact occurred or might occur. The tests were described in the report in order to account for certain phenomena which took place in the persons subject to experiment. That is why Romberg and Rascher conducted these tests.

D

There would have been no point in conducting them with other subjects, for in the first place the latter experienced no discomfort since they were only at the altitude in question for a very short time and secondly——

Q. One moment. I hope you realize that I am a very simple person and therefore find it difficult to understand some of these things. If you could express yourself more briefly I might be able to understand better. I take it that the object of the experiment by Rascher and Romberg was to determine how long they could stand the height in question. Was that what they wanted to find out or was it something else?

A. No, it was not that we wanted to determine how long one could remain at such a height. We only wished to know whether, if one remained for a longer period at such a height, pains would be experienced similar to those which occurred when such ascents were made several times a day for short periods.

Q. It was the period, then, which was in question?

A. We wished to find out whether the pains experienced by those in charge of the tests while undergoing them in person were influenced in any way by the number of ascents made or whether the period spent at the altitudes concerned during the separate ascents increased the severity of the discomfort experienced.

Q. So you were really anxious to discover means of undertaking special research on the question how long human beings could remain at such heights?

A. No, there is no doubt whatever about the time ratios involved in the problem of survival at great heights. If a man who jumps from an aircraft at any height whatever does not open his parachute, he falls some 1,000 metres in ten seconds. On the other hand, if he opens his parachute at once, he falls 1,000 metres in one minute. These time ratios are solidly based on flying experience. There are no grounds for altering them in any way.

Q. Well, when those fatalities occurred during Rascher's experiments, what do you consider, according to your information, their origin could have been? You probably have no idea, as you were not present when they occurred at Dachau. But does your acquaintance with the relevant papers throw any light on the causes of these deaths?

A. In the case of the first death of which I heard probably neither I nor anyone else can tell you for certain how it was caused. I am convinced today, from the present state of my knowledge, that is, dating from about 1946, I personally take the view, that it was a case of death occurring in consequence of prolonged retention of the subject at altitudes between 12,000 and 14,000 metres, when one or more small gas-bubbles formed in the blood-vessels . . . I have been led to this opinion by the study of accidents to American aircraft personnel during retention at great heights.'

The experiments then carried out by Rascher alone prove that he continued them beyond the point at which he and Romberg had abandoned tests on their own persons at Dachau. It is no secret that, owing to the prosecution's failure to put medically precise questions at this and other stages of the trial, the ultimate intentions of those in charge of the experiments could not be brought out with the necessary decisive clarity.

According to Romberg both he and Ruff 'considered that altitude experiments would not normally cause death and as a matter of fact no deaths so caused had hitherto occurred.'

After the first fatality had taken place in Romberg's presence owing to Rascher's ruthlessness the former returned to Berlin to inform his chief of what had happened. 'But as Rascher had conducted the experiment at Himmler's orders on a man already sentenced to death, we did not see how we could in principle give any official reason for obstructing his work.' Romberg's behaviour as an eyewitness of the death of a person undergoing an experiment was fully discussed in court. The decisive exchanges were as follows:

[PROT. p. 7018 ff.]

'*Prosecuting Counsel:* Well, what were you personally doing while these fatal experiments were being carried out? Did you simply stand by and look out of the window or did you handle any of the apparatus for Rascher?

Romberg: No. I have already told you that in the first case when death occurred I was watching the electrocardiogram, actually the point of light by which the heart action——

Q. So you were studying the electrocardiogram, working

with Rascher at Ruff's orders. Did you assist Rascher in the experiment by studying the electrocardiogram?

A. No. Nor was I working with Rascher on this occasion. I was present by chance, looking at the electrocardiogram. And as soon as I saw that a critical moment had been reached at which I myself would have discontinued the experiment, I informed Rascher accordingly.

Q. Well, what action was necessary to discontinue the experiment at that critical point? On the assumption that you were controlling the lever that Rascher had in front of him, or those of the low-pressure chamber, at that critical and fatal moment which you had noticed on the electrocardiogram while you were studying it, what would you have been able to do if you had been experimenting, so as to discontinue the test and save the subject's life? What would have been the quickest course of action? Would you have opened a valve or what? I'm asking you a simple question, Doctor, and I believe you can answer it briefly. Could you have turned a handle, pressed a button, pulled out a plug or opened a valve or how could you have saved that man's life?

A. Do you mean, if it had been my own experiment?

Q. I'm asking you what could have been done to discontinue the experiment at that critical point. How would you or anyone else have discontinued it? What could you have done with the apparatus so as to discontinue the experiment and prevent the death of the subject? Was there any special wheel handy that you might have turned?

A. I understand. Rascher had his hand on a tap by which he could regulate altitude. By turning it he could either raise or lower pressure in the chamber.

Q. Well, as to the low-pressure chamber, you were of course well acquainted with the entire mechanism, were you not? It was perfectly familiar to you, wasn't it?

A. Yes.

Q. You had used it yourself for experiments?

A. Of course.

Q. You had been connected with the Institute for Aviation Medicine?

A. Yes. I had myself worked with Ruff.

Q. You could tell by the electrocardiogram that the subject in that special low-pressure chamber had at that moment reached an altitude that was very likely to cause death? You could tell that from your own experience in the field of aviation medicine, could you not?

A. I could not, of course, be sure when death would be likely, as I was not acquainted with any case of death from altitude. I have already stated that I myself, if the experiment had been my own, would have discontinued it in this case.

Q. That's the first I've heard of any such statement. It doesn't appear in your affidavit and it was never made during any of your earlier examinations. It was only just now, in your direct examination, that you stated for the first time that you had warned Rascher. You said: "Here, Sigmund, be careful. Let's be careful. You're going too high." Was that what you said? If you did say it, did you know for certain that death was imminent?

A. No. I didn't know that for certain. I only knew that it was a critical moment. And I naturally didn't call him "Sigmund". I addressed him as "Herr Rascher". Moreover, so far as I remember, I did say in my preliminary hearing that I had called Rascher's attention to the state of affairs. This is not the first time I have said so.

Q. Well, could Rascher, while he was working the apparatus, see the electrocardiogram himself?

A. Yes. He could see it too.

Q. Will you please indicate by a gesture how far away the apparatus was from the electrocardiogram? Was Rascher standing in such a way that he could see and study it?

A. Well, the window at which Rascher was watching the experiment was somewhere about here. To the left, about as far away as the window, was the tap on which he had his hand in order to regulate altitude. The electrocardiogram stood to the right of it.

Q. Why couldn't you simply reach over, turn the tap and thus save the subject's life?

A. I told Rascher he ought to turn it down.

Q. I'm putting a question to you. Why couldn't you do that? You were standing close to the electrocardiogram. You weren't ten miles away. Why couldn't you simply reach over, turn that tap and save the subject's life? You could have done that, couldn't you?

A. After I had told him what to do and he didn't do it, I couldn't have done any good even by force. I should have had to knock him down or shoot him down or something of that sort.

Q. I agree with you, Dr Romberg, that scientists are seldom good at wrestling. But Rascher wasn't a Nordic six-footer. He was smaller than you are. You were physically the stronger and you could have very easily reached over, turned the tap and saved the subject's life. You could have discussed the matter with him later. As you say, words are extremely important, and more effective than bodily effort. After taking the action I have suggested you could have talked the question over with him intelligently, by word of mouth. Then, if you couldn't make any impression on him orally, you might have gone back to Berlin and let him do as he pleased. Now, you were in a position to turn the tap, were you not?

A. No. Since I had told him what should be done and he didn't do it, he obviously did not intend to go lower, and if at that point I had made some sort of physical assault on him——

Q. But there was no need for you to assault him physically. You only had to reach over and turn the tap. You didn't need to touch him, except to put your hand over his and turn the tap. Perfectly simple. He had his hand on the tap, hadn't he?

A. Yes, he had his hand on the tap. But as he did nothing after I had spoken to him, he wouldn't have done anything if I had tried to turn the tap. He would have merely gone on with the experiment.

Q. You were bigger than Rascher, weren't you?

A. Possibly. Well, yes, I was probably a bit bigger.

Q. You ridicule the suggestion that after the death of the subject you should have reported Rascher to the police for committing murder. Why did you not do so? It was surely the logical thing to do after a murder had been committed. It is not such a ridiculous action to hand over a murderer, is it?

A. The question of murder certainly seems now to have arisen. Now that all the facts are known it is possible to judge. But at that time, so far as I was concerned, Rascher was a Captain in the Air Force Medical Service.

Q. Allow me to ask you a question. When you saw that dead man, how did the matter strike you then? Here, in this Court, it may not look like murder. But when you saw the dead man lying there, what did you think then?

A. That it was an experiment which had ended fatally. Such experiments do occur in this world at times, without being described as murders.

Q. You were also present at the dissection, were you not? Did you dissect the corpse?

A. Do you mean, was the man dissected?

Q. Yes.

A. Certainly, I have already said so.

Q. And did you, after having, as you say, protested while the man was in the chamber and altitude was being increased and after having again protested after he was dead, did you nevertheless watch the dissection? Do you consider it was decent, after your dispute with Rascher, to sit there with him and watch the dissection?

A. No, I wasn't at all happy about it. But in my view Rascher had simply prolonged the experiment until the man died. I was obviously in no position to say whether he had consciously intended to murder him or anything like that. In any case an experiment had ended fatally and that was the reason why I watched the dissection.

Q. Now, when this fatality occurred, was Rascher still in the Air Force?

A. Yes.

Q. You were also in the Air Force, were you not, as a civilian employee?

A. No. I was a civilian employee at the Aviation Research Institute. That was not part of the Air Force.

Q. But you were under Air Force patronage?

A. No. The Institute was, legally speaking, a Registered Company. It did not belong to the Air Force. For that reason we did not wear uniform.

Q. But you did work for the Air Force?

A. To some extent we did, just as we did for civil aviation.

Q. So you reported this fatality, in common with all others, to Ruff. But this was the first and you reported it to him at once, did you not?

A. Yes.

Q. What did he then do? Did he call the police?

A. No. I have already myself stated that he did not. The police as such were of course not competent to deal with Rascher, since he was a member of the Air Force. In this case he was answerable only to Air Force jurisdiction. Ruff accordingly reported the matter to Rascher's immediate superior, Hippke, Chief of the Air Force Medical Service.

Q. Well, I should like to know why, after this first fatality, Dr Romberg did not turn up his coat-collar, leave the building, jump into the trailer that brought the chamber and drive it to Berlin. Why didn't you immediately remove the chamber? You had seen the deaths it caused. Why did you stay there?

A. Well, we had a long talk about it. Ruff himself has already stated that we considered what we ought to do. Ruff had reported the matter. That was quite in order of course and did not require any further consideration. On the other hand, we knew perfectly well that we should make no impression whatever on Himmler by going to him and saying that Rascher had conducted an experiment which ended fatally. For Himmler would probably then have simply said: "He was acting under our orders. It's nothing to do with you."

For this reason we resolved that I should return to Dachau and conclude our experiments, so that we could say: "The experiments are finished and the chamber will not be needed any more." Then, as a result of the conclusion of the experiments, Rascher and Himmler would both agree to the removal of the chamber, it could be taken away and further work with it rendered impossible. This was what in fact actually happened.

Q. The sophistry in the whole of this story is traceable to the fact that you had plenty of opportunity, for example, not to have repaired the barometer. You were on the spot and had been considering how that thing, that chamber, could be quickly got away from Dachau. And there was actually a broken component of it which could only be repaired in Berlin and one would have to go to Berlin to fetch a replacement. Yet Neff[1] has stated that he was very disappointed when you returned with the repaired component after he had damaged it. But your story is even more fantastic. You have said that you

1. A concentration camp prisoner who had been appointed by Rascher as his technical assistant and stated in court, as a witness, that he had rendered the low-pressure chamber unserviceable by an act of sabotage.

hurried back almost at once, in five days or less, not two weeks as Neff states. You dashed back immediately, so as to put the chamber to rights. And then, after you had set it going again, two people died. That was a somewhat strenuous way of bringing Rascher's work to an end, wasn't it?

A. I believe that a study of Rascher's intentions as described in the documents I read today, all that he meant still to do, will show that it was a very effective method.

Q. It certainly was. And then, Doctor, after you had at last left Dachau and the chamber had been taken back to Berlin— it may have been in May, July or August—you continued to maintain relations with Rascher and sent him reports. You reported on the film and lamented the fact that Milch had not been present at its showing in September. So you were still on friendly terms with Rascher in September and continued to collaborate with him, with the man who had proved himself a murderer under your very eyes?

A. It was not quite clear at that time that he was a murderer, as I have already stated today. It is still not clear, either in a moral or a legal sense . . .'

Further discussion of such an incident in the present connection can only be justified in the interests of a deeper understanding of it. The effort is necessary because existing tendencies in historical and scientific development render the recurrence of similar episodes quite likely. Accordingly, such attempts at analysis are only made to bring out, by reference to the behaviour of the eyewitness of this fatality, the pattern of a tense situation, not without a truly tragic element.

Romberg was asked by his defence counsel:

[PROT. p. 7043.]

'Since you were opposed to Rascher's experiments, can it be correctly assumed that you now regard these three fatalities as sheer murder?'

'No. I cannot regard them as sheer murder. For he had been officially ordered by his highest superior in that connection to conduct these experiments. But I did not myself wish to have anything to do with them and that was why I made my report to Ruff.'

Does a murder cease to be reprehensible when it is committed at the order of higher authority? It is clear that no such question would be asked except under war conditions. War as a function might actually be defined as murder at the instance of higher authority. The greater, more direct responsibility was Rascher's alone, since he initiated the 'lethal experiment' in question. Himmler's permission to act in that way was merely an authorization obtained by Rascher.

There might have been several very different reactions to this embarrassing situation. Romberg's actual behaviour and his reasons for it are clearly apparent from the records quoted above. Questions based on hypothesis and theoretical principle were addressed to Professor Ivy, the prosecution's expert in these matters.

[PROT. pp. 9206 and 9213.]

'Q. If one of your colleagues deliberately killed someone in your laboratory and another colleague reported the fact to you, what would you do?

A. I would cause a perfectly impartial investigation to be made of the report, to see if it were true. I would notify the police that I had done so. . . .

Q. Is it not the usual practice in any laboratory for the senior scientists to take responsibility, especially where life may be endangered?

A. Certainly.

Q. The senior in rank has the greatest responsibility, has he not?

A. In my opinion, yes.

Q. Let us assume for the moment that I was working as your assistant in a certain laboratory, for instance Wright Field in the United States, dealing with altitude tests, and sent a man up, by way of experiment, to a height of 18,000 or 20,000 metres and left him there until he died. And let us also suppose that during the course of the experiment you were in a position to watch the electrocardiogram recording the experimental conditions. Would you then have taken the responsibility of telling me to discontinue the test?

A. Undoubtedly.

Q. It would be your duty to order me to desist?

A. That's how I should see it.

Q. But if we assume that you were not my superior, I mean that I would not be working as your assistant, but that you were simply an observer with more scientific experience. In the same situation would you still feel it your duty, as a scientifically more experienced investigator, to order me to stop, in case life might be endangered?

A. I think it would be my moral duty . . .'

The need for special care in proceeding to practical action after theoretically accepting a moral obligation is evident from the following answers given by Professor Ivy to the question what demands those responsible for waging war are justified in making on scientists and also from the professor's definition of the difference between therapy and experiment.

[PROT. p. 9429.]

'*Defence Counsel:* I take it then, Professor Ivy, that you recognize the needs of war as justifying experiment?

A. Yes.

Q. Well, Professor, that is admitted in the United States and I believe you will be prepared to grant Germany similar grounds for undertaking experiment?

A. Certainly.'

After a discussion of the Oath of Hippocrates the record goes on:

'*Q.* You have confirmed today your opinion that experiments on criminals condemned to death, provided they volunteer, should be regarded as ethically permissible even when dangerously excessive doses of drugs are given them which may have serious consequences. This question has been raised in the case of Professor Rose, in which poison was administered to a volunteer. But does not such an experiment run counter to the following sentence in the Oath of Hippocrates: "I would never administer deadly poison to anyone, even if the patient asked for it"?

A. I should say that this sentence refers to the therapeutic, not to the experimental, function of a doctor. The part of his function to which the Oath refers is his duty to respect human life and that of his patient.

Q. You consider then, Professor, that a distinction should be drawn between the doctor as therapist, concerned with healing, and the doctor as scientific investigator? And you therefore concede that in each category different precepts and sections of the Oath of Hippocrates apply?

A. Yes, quite positively.'

Professor Ivy accordingly recognized as valid for medical action certain guiding principles in addition to those of aid to the patient. In the case of war, for example, the doctor should place at the service of the militant arm his knowledge of the functional relations of the human organism. But this idea strikes at the root of medical freedom in the sense of a doctor's duty, overriding political loyalties, to come to the assistance of suffering humanity.

It is clear that the distinction between medical research and medical practice, if it is taken right down to this basic obligation, itself invalidates medical action, since the right hand would then really not know what the left hand was doing. For the knowledge obtained by medical research helps a political party to injure persons belonging to other parties, while practical medicine then tries to heal their injuries. Thus Professor Ivy paralysed, in the domain of theory itself, any really universal validity for the 'moral duty' he had previously mentioned.

It is therefore of fundamental importance—and, obviously, not only in Germany—to recognize that as a result of technical developments and the rise in modern times of such gigantic social units as certain nations of today doctors have reached a position in which literal fidelity to the formula of Hippocrates in its original significance is no longer practicable, or at any rate only if all the possible consequences under modern conditions can really be ascertained. Unless some unifying formula can be devised to apply to all medical men without exception, it must be acknowledged that the distinction between research and practice, each with a different moral code, not only abolishes the present conception of the medical profession as a whole but also implies two diverse conceptions of the humanitarian ideal. For it is after all quite out of the question for an experimental scientist to be allowed, in an extreme case, deliberately to cause death, a proceeding absolutely forbidden to the practising doctor and in fact, under the still prevalent moral code of Christianity, to anyone.

Yet it cannot be denied that such a temptation is one that may arise anywhere at the present stage of history. The dictatorship merely rendered the temptation more acute and gave it more opportunities.

Such, then, were the 'interior' circumstances in which Romberg played his part, or rather played no part at all, as he watched the luminous play of the electrocardiograph. A further theoretical question is whether a colleague could reasonably take offence 'morally' at the intentional and actual destruction of human life during an experiment conducted by so experienced a scientist as Rascher. It is however an eminently practical question when we observe how a man behaves when he is faced with the choice between serious danger to himself and peril equally serious to another, in this case the subject of the experiment. In the present instance the destruction of life appeared to be sanctioned by the highest authority. Accordingly, if due account is taken of such a situation, in which scruples were not in question and criticism both impotent and dangerous, one's judgment of and dealings with it will be so much the more adequate. This consideration brings us closer to the root of the trouble. It may be deplorable for an individual to come to his own decision in such a case. But it remains easy to understand his feelings, all the more so since Romberg was found not guilty. A perfectly resolute attitude in such a matter may be a virtue. But it is no part of the duty of a citizen. Yet something can be done to rectify this situation, for it is at all times subject to public opinion.

Ruff and Romberg stated during the hearing that after the discovery of Rascher's unscrupulous use of the low-pressure chamber in Romberg's absence they took steps to have the chamber returned to Berlin with all possible speed. The following extract from the proceedings at their trial again shows the consequences of transferring a department of scientific research to a concentration camp.

[PROT. p. 6899 f.]

'*Defence Counsel:* What led to the experiments being permanently discontinued?

Romberg: The basic reason was of course the agreement

between Hippke, Ruff and myself to put forward an urgent plea,
so to speak, for the removal of the chamber and thus an end
to the experiments. But the practical difficulty was that neither
Himmler nor Rascher could be told that the ground for the
proposal was the fatalities caused by Rascher. In these circumstances, as I have already stated, the excuse that the chamber
was needed in connection with accidents to pilots did not seem
weighty enough to justify the interruption of experiments
concerned with the rescue of personnel at great heights, which
the Luftwaffe considered so important. In fact, when I returned
from Berlin and dropped my first hints on the subject to
Rascher, to the effect that the chamber was needed elsewhere,
and told him that we should soon have to put a stop to the
experiments, he not only would not hear of any such thing but
said he would immediately obtain from Himmler or Milch the
necessary permission to go on using the chamber. He did
actually secure such permission. But by the time Milch's orders
to continue arrived the chamber had already been removed.
Accordingly, the primary condition for removing the chamber
and getting it back into our possession was an accelerated but
duly complete conclusion of the high-altitude experiments, as
well as the shooting of the film of them which had been ordered
by Himmler, I believe, when he visited Dachau. It was only
by arranging for both these demands by Himmler to be met
that I was able to induce Rascher actually to agree to the temporary removal of the chamber. I persuaded him that there
would really be little point in contriving to retain the chamber
for possibly another two or three weeks, telling him that its
dispatch to the front would certainly not be postponed any
longer. I suggested that it would be far more satisfactory to
have the chamber or a replacement of it sent back to Dachau
later on for use over an extended period, as on the one hand
the high altitude experiments could then be further developed
and on the other hand Rascher himself could get on with the
work Himmler had instructed him to do. I told him that I
myself would also again take part in the altitude experiments.
It was only by adopting such tactics that I could prevent
Rascher from opposing the removal of the chamber and obtaining orders, through Himmler, from Milch or Göring in
time to counteract us.

In conclusion I should like once more to state positively in this connection that no one, not even Hippke or Milch, would ever have been able to get that chamber out of the camp at Dachau against Rascher's and Himmler's wishes.'

According to the Works Records of the Berlin Institute the chamber had been reinstalled there by the 23 May 1942. The accused subsequently saw to it that no further apparatus of this kind should be sent to Dachau.

At the beginning of July Rascher and Romberg together drew up a final report, which Ruff also signed, on the high-altitude experiments. As already noted, no reference was made in this report to fatal results. The reason given by the accused in court was that such fatalities only occurred in Rascher's experiments. These last, the defendants asserted, unlike their own, were concerned with the question of human resistance to prolonged location in high altitudes, a problem which had not been mentioned even among those raised with scientists by the military authorities. The prosecution tried to establish a correspondence between the report signed by Ruff, Romberg and Rascher and the reports to Himmler signed by Rascher alone. But Professor Ivy himself could find no necessary connection between Rascher's experiments and the research data in the report signed by all three men. Judgment was therefore given as follows:

[Judgment p. 204 ff.]*

'The issue on the question of the guilt or innocence of these defendants is close; we would be less than fair were we not to concede this fact. It cannot be denied that there is much in the record to create at least a grave suspicion that the defendants Ruff and Romberg were implicated in criminal experiments at Dachau. However, virtually all of the evidence which points in this direction is circumstantial in its nature. On the other hand, it cannot be gainsaid that there is a certain consistency, a certain logic, in the story told by the defendants. And some of the story is corroborated in significant particulars by evidence offered by the prosecution.

The value of circumstantial evidence depends upon the conclusive nature and tendency of the circumstances relied on to establish any controverted fact. The circumstances must not only be consistent with guilt, but they must be inconsistent with innocence. Such evidence is insufficient when, assuming all to be true which the evidence tends to prove, some other reasonable hypothesis of innocence may still be true; for it is the actual exclusion of every other reasonable hypothesis but that of guilt which invests mere circumstances with the force of proof. Therefore, before a court will be warranted in finding a defendant guilty on circumstantial evidence alone, the evidence must show such a well-connected and unbroken chain of circumstances as to exclude all other reasonable hypotheses but that of the guilt of the defendant. What circumstances can amount to proof can never be a matter of general definition. In the final analysis the legal test is whether the evidence is sufficient to satisfy beyond a reasonable doubt the understanding and conscience of those who, under their solemn oaths as officers, must assume the responsibility for finding the facts.

On this particular specification, it is the conviction of the Tribunal that the defendants Ruff, Romberg, and Weltz must be found not guilty.'

(ii) PROLONGED SUPERCOOLING EXPERIMENTS

Rascher took steps, dictated at bottom by personal ambition, to exploit his freedom to experiment on human beings by undertaking a fresh series of such tests. His plans were in accordance with the desire of the Luftwaffe for further experimental data to meet the requirements of war operations.

The unfavourable impression created by the Luftwaffe's continued support of the same man in the same place was not removed by the proceedings in court. For it remained an open question whether the competent authorities acted in this way through mere ignorance of what had hitherto occurred or whether they suppressed any moral scruples they may have felt in the interests of practical needs.

In common with the previous experiments at Dachau those undertaken after the 15 August 1942, which subjected human beings to supercooling, were designed to elucidate problems which had arisen as a result of aviators being precipitated into the sea. Effective protective clothing was one objective. Others

LOW PRESSURE AND SUPERCOOLING EXPERIMENTS 65

were various means of restoring warmth. As early as the 24 February 1942 the Health Inspector of the Luftwaffe had charged Professor Holzlöhner of Kiel to examine 'the effect of supercooling on warm-blooded mammals'. [Doc. 286.] The Air Ministry adviser on aviation medicine wrote on 8 October 1942:

[DOC. 286.]*

'At the proposal of Stabsarzt Dr Rascher appropriate examinations were made of human beings, and in agreement with the Reich Leader SS suitable SS facilities were used for the examinations.

In order to carry out these examinations a research group "Hardships at Sea" was set up, consisting of Professor Dr Holzloehner as leader and Stabsarzt Dr Rascher and Dr Finke.

The leader of this research group has reported that the examinations have been concluded.'

In July 1942 Rascher and Romberg reported to Himmler on their high altitude experiments at Dachau. A long discussion followed between Himmler and Rascher on the current importance of supercooling experiments. In this connection Romberg gave the following answers to his defence counsel:

[PROT. p. 6907 ff.]

'*Defence Counsel:* Did Himmler say anything more about supercooling experiments at this meeting?

Romberg: Yes. He began by saying that the experiments were of the greatest importance to the Army, Air Force and Fleet. He proceeded to talk at considerable length about such tests and how they should be conducted. For example, he instructed Rascher to find out how rescues of shipwrecked crews in the Baltic were carried out and the methods in use by the coastal population to revive the half-frozen men saved. He added that country people often knew excellent remedies which had long proved their worth, such as teas brewed from medicinal herbs and perhaps rum, ordinary tea and coffee were also administered. At any rate in his view such popular remedies should be by no means overlooked. He said that he could also well

E

imagine that a fisherman's wife might even take her half-frozen husband to bed with her after he had been rescued and warm him up that way. For, as everyone knew, animal warmth differed in its effects from that produced artificially. He told Rascher that he must certainly experiment in that direction as well as in those, already mentioned, of popular remedies and drugs.

Q. And what was your personal reaction to these remarks by Himmler?

A. I had no great hopes of any sensible and practical application of such somewhat mystically based expedients and therefore raised objections both to them and to the experiments in view. I said that the main thing was to warm the subject quickly. Prolonged research would only result in casualties. A painful silence ensued, which showed me that disagreement and similar expressions of opinion were not welcome.

Q. Did anyone argue against your objections?

A. No, not verbally. But the silence that then fell was far more eloquent than any words. Later on Rascher reproached me in the strongest terms for my behaviour. He asked me whether I had gone completely mad in contradicting "Reichsheini", as he called Himmler, like that.

Q. Did Himmler add anything more at these discussions?

A. Yes. As soon as that painful pause was over he began talking about the demands of total war. He said that it certainly would not be asking too much to require concentration camp prisoners, who could not be sent on active service on account of the crimes they had committed, to participate in such experiments. He declared that in that way they would be able to rehabilitate themselves, those sentenced to death could be reprieved and given an opportunity to go to the front. People who could not see this point, he said, had not yet grasped the fact that Germany was engaged in a life or death struggle. He went on to expatiate again on the losses of the troops in the East, especially of the SS, and told us that his heart bled every time he heard that more thousands of his gallant boys had fallen.

Q. What impression did you receive from these remarks?

A. They were statements with which one could not be wholly out of sympathy in the grave emergency of those days. All the same, I was absolutely determined never to work again with Rascher.

Q. What impression did you receive from the discussion with Himmler as a whole?

A. I must confess that at the time it made quite an impression on me. His serious talk about the losses of the troops and the strength of our adversaries afforded so strong a contrast with the optimistic propaganda of the Press, which obscured all causes for anxiety, that I might even have been ready, from a sense of duty, to participate in the proposed supercooling experiments if I had not felt so deep a repugnance to Rascher's experimental work and his obvious lack of scruple in dealing with men's lives. This feeling remained despite the facts that Himmler had authorized the tests, that the subjects were in any case under sentence of death and that they had freely volunteered to submit to the experiments. Accordingly, when Himmler requested me to participate in them, I tried to get out of it and in fact succeeded in doing so.'

Rascher also informed the Luftwaffe Health Inspector, Professor Hippke, of the orders he had received from Himmler. At Milch's trial Hippke declared in this connection:[1]

[PROT. p. 817.][2]

'This question was already under consideration. But a practical solution of it had now become urgent. I was myself well aware of its pressing nature and I therefore had to come to a decision at once.'

During the conversation it was decided that Professor Holzlöhner should take charge of the whole experiment. Rascher intimated that the subjects would be criminals who volunteered from prison.

In reply to prosecuting counsel Hippke stated that it had been proposed to invite a pathologist to participate 'as one of the subjects might die'. But this proposal was discarded as Holzlöhner did not consider it necessary. [PROT. p. 878.]

During the course of these experiments Rascher reported

---

[1] The prosecution stated that Hippke would have been in the dock if he could have been located before the trial started.

[2] From the record of General Field-Marshal Milch's trial at Nuremberg.

progress personally, as before, to Himmler. On the 10 September 1942 he sent the Reichsführer an 'Interim Report on the Intense Chilling Experiments at Dachau Concentration Camp'.

[DOC. 1618—PS.]*

Experimental procedure.

The experimental subjects (VP) were placed in the water, dressed in complete flying uniform, winter or summer combination, and with an aviator's helmet. A life-jacket made of rubber or kapok was to prevent submerging. The experiments were carried out at water temperatures varying from 2·5° to 12° C. In one experimental series, the occiput (brain stem) protruded above the water, while in another series of experiments the occuput and back of the head were submerged in water.

Electrical measurements gave low temperature readings of 26·4° in the stomach and 26·5° C. in the rectum. Fatalities occurred only when the brainstem and the back of the head were also chilled. Autopsies of such fatal cases always revealed large amounts of free blood, up to one-half litre in the cranial cavity. The heart invariably showed extreme dilation of the right chamber. As soon as the temperature in these experiments reached 28° C., the experimental subjects died invariably, despite all attempts at resuscitation. The above discussed autopsy finding conclusively proved the importance of a warming protective device for head and occiput when designing the planned protective clothing of the foam type.

Other important findings, common in all experiments, should be mentioned, marked increase of the viscosity of the blood, marked increase of hemogoblin, an approximate five-fold increase of the leukocytes, invariable rise of blood sugar to twice its normal value. Auricular fibrillation made its appearance regularly at 30° C.

During attempts to save severely chilled persons it was shown that rapid rewarming was in all cases preferable to slow rewarming, because after removal from the cold water, the body temperature continued to sink rapidly.

I think that for this reason we can dispense with the attempt to save intensely chilled subjects by means of animal heat. Rewarming by animal warmth—animal bodies or women's bodies—would be too slow. As auxiliary measures for the prevention of intense chilling, improvements in the clothing of aviators come alone into consideration. The foam suit with suitable neck protector which is being prepared by the German Institute for Textile Research, Munich-Gladbach, deserves first priority in this connection. The experiments have shown that pharmaceutical measures are probably unnecessary if the flier is still alive at the time of rescue.

(Signed) Dr S. Rascher
Munich—Dachau, 10 September 1942.'

On the 22 September 1942 Himmler replied as follows:

[DOC. 1611—PS.]*

'I have received the intermediate report on the chilling experiments in Camp Dachau.

Despite everything, I would so arrange the experiments that all the possible measures of prompt warming, both medicinal and animal, are taken in prescribed series.'

The data of Holzlöhner's experiment were to be submitted to a conference called by the Health Inspector of the Luftwaffe to take place in Nuremberg on the 26 and 27 October 1942 on the subject of 'Medical Problems of Service at Sea and in Winter'. For this reason, on the 10 October 1942, the group consisting of Holzlöhner, Rascher and Finke prepared in Berlin a 32-page report, stamped 'Secret, for Headquarters' and entitled 'Chilling Experiments on Human Beings'.

Rascher dispatched it to Himmler on the 16 October 1942 together with the following personal note:

[DOC. 1613—PS.]*

'Highly esteemed Reich Leader!

Permit me to submit the attached final report on the supercooling experiments performed at Dachau. This report does not contain the course and results of a series of experiments with drugs as well as experiments with animal body heat which are now being conducted. Likewise this report does not contain the microscopic pathological examinations of the brain tissues of the deceased. I was surprised at the extraordinary microscopic findings in this field. I will carry out experiments before the start of the conference at which the effect of cooling will be discussed and I hope to be able to present further results by that time. My two co-workers left Dachau about eight days ago.

In the hope that you, highly esteemed Reich Leader, will be able to spare a quarter of an hour to listen to an oral report, I remain, with the most obedient regards and

Heil Hitler!

Yours respectfully,

(*Signed*) S. RASCHER'

The closing summary of the report reads:

[DOC. 428.]*

'X. SUMMARY

1. The curve of rectal temperature of human beings chilled in water of 2° C. (35·6° F.) to 12° C. (53·6° F.) shows a gradual drop to about 35° C. (95° F.), after which the drop becomes rapid. Death may occur at rectal temperatures below 30° C. (86° F.).

2. Death results from heart failure. The direct damage to the heart becomes evident from the total irregularity observed in all cases, setting in at approximately 30° C. (86° F.). This cardiac damage is due to overloading of the heart, caused by the marked and regular increase in the viscosity of the blood, as well as by the marked throttling of large peripheral vascular areas; besides, a direct injury to the heart by cold is also probable.

3. If the neck is also chilled, the lowering of the temperature is more rapid. This is due to interference with the temperature-regulating and vascular centres; cerebral oedema also makes its appearance.

4. The blood sugar rises as the temperature falls, and the blood sugar does not drop again as long as the body tempera-

ture continues to fall. This fact suggests an intermediary disturbance of metabolism.

5. Respiration of the chilled subject is rendered difficult due to the rigor of the respiratory musculature.

6. After removal from the cold water, the body temperature may continue to fall for fifteen minutes or longer. This may be an explanation of deaths which occur after successful rescue from the sea.

7. Intensive rewarming never injures the severely chilled person.

8. Strophanthin treatment was not observed to have been successful. The question of the use of strophanthin remains open, however. Remedies which influence the peripheral circulation are definitely not advisable.

9. The most effective therapeutic measure is rapid and intensive heat treatment, best applied by immersion in a hot bath.[1]

10. By means of special protective clothing, the survival time after immersion in cold water could be extended to double the survival time of subjects who were immersed without protective clothing.

11. Certain proposals for improvement of life jackets are being made.'

It is repeatedly evident from the descriptions given that these experiments too were arranged with a view to observation of 'terminal conditions'. In Section III, for instance ('The Clinical Picture of Chilling'), it is stated:

'If the subject was anaesthetized before being placed in the water, certain signs of returning consciousness were observed ... defensive movements ceased after about five minutes. Increasing rigor ensued, especially in the muscular system of the arms, which stiffened in a bent position close to the body. As refrigeration proceeded, the rigor increased, interrupted occasionally by spasmodic muscular contraction and relaxation. But when body temperature fell still lower, the rigor suddenly

1. The same experimental result was attained by Professor Weltz and his colleagues in tests on animals at their Munich Institute, as reported by them to the Nuremberg conference held by the Luftwaffe on chilling in October 1942.

stopped. These cases ended fatally, attempts at revival having failed. . . . Generally speaking (in six cases) death ensued at temperatures between 24·2° C. and 25·7° C.'

Section VII ('Pharmacological Influence and the Problem of Alcohol') contains a description of death after an intracardiac injection of ·25 mg. of strophanthin.

Rascher urged Himmler to release the data of this experiment. Holzlöhner also referred to the case at the Nuremberg conference, and Rascher added some remarks of his own. According to witnesses Rascher's explanations somewhat obscured the true facts of the case. But the official report of the conference includes the following passage from a speech by Holzlöhner:

[DOC. 401.]

'. . . Men who had been rescued after prolonged immersion in cold water were the only possible subjects of a series of investigations. We owe the relevant data to the researches of Captains Rascher and Finke of the Air Force Medical Service. These data are based on immersion in water of temperatures between 2 and 12° C.' (38·6 and 53·6 F.)'

While this document was being read Mr McHaney, representing the prosecution, observed:

[PROT. p. 361.][1]

'It might perhaps have been implied that the experiments had been conducted with subjects who really had been rescued after shipwreck. But the witness Lutz has told us it was made perfectly clear that the tests in question were made on persons who had been deliberately exposed to ice-cold water. The fact is quite evident in the following extract from the report, for the simple reason that it would have been physically impossible for any scientist to draw up so detailed a clinical report on the basis of isolated cases of rescue at sea.'

The document goes on:

'The rapidity with which numbness set in was remarkable. It was found that between five and ten minutes after immersion an increasing stiffness of the skeletal muscular system began,

[1] In this connection the statements of Dr Becker-Freyseng (see next chapter) are also important.

rendering arm movement, in particular, more and more difficult. This condition affected breathing. Inhalation deepened
and exhalation slowed down. In addition, much mucus was
secreted. . . . On a fall of rectal temperature to 31° C. (87·8 F.)
consciousness grew dim and a further drop below 30° C. (86 F.)
induced a profound general anaesthesia due to chilling. . . .
But any fall of rectal temperature below 28° C. (82·4 F.) might
lead to sudden heart failure due to loss of rhythm. . . .

After Holzlöhner had finished speaking Rascher intervened.
(See Weltz's description of the conference, about to be quoted.)

Judgment summed up this matter as follows:

[Judgment p. 57 f.]*

'During the meeting and after Holzlöhner had made his
report, Rascher also made statements before the meeting concerning these experiments, from which it was obvious that
statements contained in the reports were based upon observations made by experimenting on human beings. From the two
reports it was clear that concentration camp inmates had been
experimented upon and that some deaths had resulted.'

The question therefore arises whether those at the conference
could suppose Holzlöhner and Rascher to have deliberately
and ruthlessly frozen the subjects of their tests to death or
whether the audience could believe that the data related to
shipwrecked soldiers. Consequently, opinions may differ as to
why none of the ninety-five persons present, some of them well-
known men of science, protested in any such way as might have
been expected from people of that eminence.[1]

All the accused and witnesses repeatedly affirmed that no
such protest was raised. The defence tried to make use of this
very point, maintaining that no protest could have been made
because the experiments in question could not have been regarded as criminal at that time. Such, for example, was Becker-
Freyseng's attitude.

[PROT. p. 8022 f.]

'*Defence Counsel:* One final question, witness. You have stated

---

1. Such a public protest, clearly remembered by all witnesses, is quoted
hereafter in connection with the typhus experiments.

that this was a meeting concerned with medical questions arising from the incidence of distress at sea and in winter. In other words it was simply a discussion of chilling phenomena by experts. You told us just now that you were not an expert in this field, having had no practical experience of distress at sea and not having conducted any experiments in connection with it. But I can no doubt assume that the leading experts of the Air Force and also of other military organizations were present at the meeting. You cannot, of course, tell us what these experts concluded from the speeches made. But I should very much like you to enlighten me on one point. Did anyone present at that meeting, either during the discussion that followed Holzlöhner's speech or at any later stage, publicly protest to the assembly against the statements he made?

Becker-Freyseng: No. And I must say that at that time any such protest would have been utterly unintelligible to me. I might also add that, according to the document before the Court, the meeting was attended by fifty-five members of the Air Force, twelve representatives of the Army, four of the Fleet, four of the Waffen SS and police, and nineteen civilians, comprising university professors and others.

Q. You say, therefore, if I may briefly recapitulate your evidence, that you would have thought any protest pointless, since you had heard no statement of any kind that had even hinted at criminal conduct. Nor, obviously, had any of the leading German experts on chilling who were undoubtedly present noticed any such statements, for none of them protested. Is that correct?

A. That is correct.'

This line of defence was undoubtedly weak. At any rate it did not apply to all the specialists in this field of research who were listening to Holzlöhner's speech. One scientist wrote in an affidavit on behalf of Weltz:

[DOC. Weltz 14.]

'At the Nuremberg meeting on chilling at the end of 1942 Weltz reported on chilling experiments with animals, after Holzlöhner and Rascher had previously reported on experiments with prisoners. I remember that immediately after these speeches I discussed the questions therein treated with Weltz. Though I cannot now recollect exactly what we said, I do know that we came to the general conclusion that Weltz had obtained more valuable results with his animals than Rascher had with his prisoners.'

Weltz himself described the conference in a dialogue with his defence counsel.

[PROT. p. 7197 ff.]

'I naturally listened very closely to Holzlöhner's speech and gathered by inference that he had implied at least one fatality. But I could not make out whether this case had resulted from rescue at sea or whether it occurred at Dachau. Holzlöhner had run together in so inextricable a fashion his data drawn from the sea-rescue service on the one hand and from Dachau on the other that even experts on questions of chilling could not understand either how many deaths had occurred or whether the one death which certainly had occurred transpired in the course of sea rescue or of experiments at Dachau.

Q. Did you have any conversation with Holzlöhner after he had finished his speech?

A. Yes, I talked to him. It turned out from a consideration of each of our speeches that although we had both experienced the same practical results we differed in our theories of the way in which death could be caused by chilling. I told Holzlöhner that I should of course be much interested in the reasons for his own opinion and said that I would for my part place my notes on the experiments with animals at his disposal. I asked him to send me, in his turn, his own experimental records. I knew, of course, that he was not in a position to give me a more detailed account of the matter without permission. For Rascher had explained, after Holzlöhner's speech, that these experiments were secret, that they were officially confidential matters of State. I therefore requested Holzlöhner to forward me his records through Service channels, in support of his theoretical opinion. I also sent him my own records for study. He agreed to my proposal. But I never heard anything more about it. I never received any such reports from him.

Q. It would also be interesting to know what Rascher's attitude was after Holzlöhner's speech.

A. That has already been described by Lutz in his evidence. After Holzlöhner had finished speaking Rascher began by making a few technical observations of little consequence. He then expressed himself in a most unfortunate way, which has already been several times referred to in this Court, to the effect that the experiments had been rendered possible by the action of Himmler himself, that they must be kept secret and that the subjects were volunteers, criminals previously sentenced in the regular courts of law. These were the statements which have so often been discussed in the present Court.

Q. Did you also discuss these two speeches with other persons who attended the meeting?

A. Yes. We naturally talked about what had been said. . . . We were all of the opinion that Rascher had expressed himself in an extraordinarily unfortunate manner. He had cast his statements in so frivolous a form that we all felt him to have been guilty of great tactlessness.

I must insist that Holzlöhner's own attitude was entirely different. He had spoken with great earnestness. We naturally discussed his speech too. Büchner and Knothe were of opinion that he had not added anything particularly novel to what we had already discovered from experiments with animals. For this reason they were unwilling to allow his experiments any importance.

Q. Well, didn't any of those at the meeting criticize Rascher at all? After all, some of them had been extremely indignant about his speech and general attitude. It would surely have been natural for them to have taken some such action.

A. It would be an exaggeration to say that they were extremely indignant. I heard no expressions of opinion from the majority. I can only speak of those who were near me at the time and with whom I talked on that particular subject. These were Knothe, Büchner and Werz. They all condemned what had been said. To what extent they really understood the point at issue I don't know. At conferences of this kind one is stuffed so full with speeches and erudition and one thing and another that one isn't inclined to give very close attention to everything that is said unless one is specially interested in the subject. I can very well imagine that some people missed this particular point altogether and didn't think it mattered much.'

If the experiments of Holzlöhner and Rascher had really met with scathing criticism at that time, the former would probably never have repeated his speech in December 1942 at a conference in Berlin of Army medical advisers.[1] Professor Hippke, the Health Inspector, was present at that meeting. He declared on oath:

[Interrogation 1306A.]

'Neither at this meeting nor at any later time did any of those present, any of the speakers or any of the medical advisers protest in my hearing against any speech by Professor Holzlöhner or any fact that he mentioned. I am perfectly sure of this, as I relied on my medical advisers and if any of them had protested I should have at once acted.'[2]

1. The statement of the editors in an earlier documentary record that none of the ninety-five persons who attended the Nuremberg conference had protested was twice publicly challenged. In the first case a provisional order of the court prohibited further circulation of the objection. For proceedings at the trial had clearly proved our statement to be true. Consequently our opponents expressly agreed in Court to let the matter drop. Secondly, an article in the *Göttinger Universitäts Zeitung* (No. 18/18, 1947) contended that it was a question of conscience for us to decide whether we would stick to our statement or not, since it 'deprived' our collection 'of any documentary character'.

But no such question of conscience can arise for a chronicler whose reconstruction of the facts is guaranteed by recorded history. His conscience only begins to operate when he has to estimate the importance of what happened. Critical contemporaries will not be able to evade such stirrings of conscience nor will, in our opinion, the participants in the conference find it any easier to do so. At any rate it is a logical deduction from the allegation by some of the audience that a protest of some kind had in fact been made by them to infer that Holzlöhner's speech and Rascher's subsequent remarks had convinced listeners that the experiments described were in direct contravention of medical ethics. In this connection we may refer to the statement by Professor Rose quoted in the next chapter. Rose had himself questioned Holzlöhner at the conference.

2. The 'protest' here referred to would be one made on formal Service grounds. Professor Hippke, after his release, added the information, in a letter to us, that he 'afterwards remembered that one of the doctors present had in fact disagreed with what was said in the lecture'. But Hippke had not understood this disagreement in the sense of a 'formal protest'. At the conference Holzlöhner, in reply to questions, had 'expressly denied' that fatal results occurred at Dachau.

Further details of the duration and character of the experiments were given by the witness Neff, formerly Rascher's technical assistant. They are illustrated by the following extract from his examination by Mr McHaney, prosecuting counsel.

[PROT. p. 672.]*

Q. Now, you have stated that you can divide the freezing experiments into two groups, one where Holzlöhner and Finke were working with Rascher and then the period after Holzlöhner and Finke had left?

A. Yes.

Q. Now, will you tell the Tribunal approximately how many persons were used over the whole period? That is, including both groups that you have mentioned.

A. Two hundred and eighty to three hundred experimental subjects were used for these freezing experiments. There were really 360 to 400 experiments that were conducted, since many experimental subjects were used for more than one such experiment—sometimes even for three.

Q. Now, out of the total of 280 or 300 prisoners used, approximately how many died?

A. Approximately eighty to ninety subjects died as a result of these freezing experiments.

Q. Now, how many experimental subjects do you remember that they used in the Holzlöhner–Finke–Rascher experiments?

A. During that period of time approximately fifty to sixty subjects were used for experimental purposes.

Q. Did any of these experimental subjects die?

A. Yes. During that period of time there were about fifteen, maybe even eighteen cases of death.

Q. When was that experimental series concluded?

A. It was concluded in the month of October. I think it was at the end of October. At that time Holzlöhner and Finke discontinued these experiments, giving the reason that they had accomplished their purpose and that it was useless to carry out further experiments of that kind.

Q. And then Rascher continued experiments on his own?

A. Yes. Rascher continued these experiments, saying that he

had to give them a scientific basis and was preparing a lecture for Marburg University on the subject. . . .'

Holzlöhner's own condemnation of the chilling tests is clear from a letter written by Rascher to Himmler on the 9 October 1942.

[DOC. 1610—PS.]

'As Professor Holzlöhner declines to make any scientific use of the experiments, so as not to depreciate his scientific renown (fancy using human subjects, fie for shame!) I will undertake their evaluation at the University College of Professor Pfannenstiel, SS Obersturmbannführer.'

Statistics by Dr Rascher of Seven Fatal Refrigeration Experiments

EXITUS

Experiment No.	Water Temperature (C.)	Body Temperature on removal from water (C.)	Body Temperature on time of death (C.)	Period of Submersion (Minutes)	Time of Death after Submersion (Minutes)
5	5·2	27·7	27·7	66	66
13	6	29·2	29·2	80	87
14	4	27·8	27·5	95	100
16	4	28·7	26	60	74
23	4·5	27·8	25·7	57	65
25	4·5	27·8	26·6	51	65
—	4·2	26·7	25·9	53	53

The experiments conducted by Rascher alone from the 9 October 1942 until May 1943 included some in which the restoration of warmth to chilled persons by 'animal heat' was observed. These series of tests were undertaken in response to a personal request by Himmler, who wrote to Rascher on the 24 October:

[DOC. 1609—PS.]*

'I am very curious as to the experiments with body warmth. I personally take it that these experiments will probably bring the best and lasting results. Naturally, I could be mistaken.'

In the same letter Himmler again lent his authority to Rascher's experiments on human beings.

'I regard as guilty of treason and high treason people who, still today, reject these experiments on humans and would instead let sturdy German soldiers die as a result of these cooling methods. I shall not hesitate to report these men to the offices concerned. I empower you to make my opinion on this known to the offices concerned.'

For the production of 'animal heat' four women were brought to Dachau from the concentration camp at Ravensbrück. [DOC. 295.]

When the women arrived at Dachau Rascher made a disturbing discovery. On the 5 November he announced it in a 'Report, as requested, on Concentration Camp Prostitutes'.

[DOC. 323.]*

'For the resuscitation experiments by animal warmth after freezing as ordered by the Reich Leader SS I had four women assigned to me from the women's concentration camp Ravensbrück.

One of the assigned women shows unobjectionably Nordic racial characteristics: blonde hair, blue eyes, corresponding head and body structure, 21¾ years of age. I asked the girl why she had volunteered for the brothel. I received the answer: "To get out of the concentration camp, for we were promised that all those who would volunteer for the brothel for half a year would then be released from the concentration camp." To my objection that it was a great shame to volunteer as a prostitute, I was told: "Rather half a year in the brothel than half a year in the concentration camp." Then followed an account of a number of most peculiar conditions at camp Ravensbrück. Most of the reported conditions were confirmed by the three other prostitutes and by the female warden who had accompanied them from Ravensbrück.

It hurts my racial feelings to expose to racially inferior concentration camp elements a girl as a prostitute who has the appearance of a pure Nordic and who could perhaps by assignment of proper work be put on the right road.

Therefore, I refused to use this girl for my experimental purposes and reported accordingly to the camp commander and the adjutant of the Reich Leader SS.

(Signature) Dr S. Rascher'

The results of this method of restoring warmth were summarized by Rascher on the 12 February 1943 in a secret report to Himmler.

[DOC. 1616—PS.]*

'Experiments for rewarming of intensely chilled human beings by animal warmth

(*a*) Purpose of the Experiments

To ascertain whether the rewarming of intensely chilled human beings by animal warmth, i.e. the warmth of animal or human beings, is as good or better than rewarming by physical or medical means.

(*b*) Method of the Experiments

The experimental subjects were cooled in the usual way—clad or unclad—in cold water of temperatures varying between 4° C. and 9° C. The rectal temperature of every experimental subject was recorded thermoelectrically. The reduction of temperature occurred within the usual span of time varying in accordance with the general condition of the body of the experimental subject and the temperature of the water. The experimental subjects were removed from the water when their rectal temperature reached 30° C. At this time the experimental subjects had all lost consciousness. In eight cases the experimental subjects were then placed between two naked women

F

in a spacious bed. The women were supposed to nestle as closely as possible to the chilled person. Then all three persons were covered with blankets. A speeding up of rewarming by light candles or by medicines was not attempted.

(c) Results

1. When the temperature of the experimental subjects was recorded it was striking that an after-drop of temperature up to 3° C. occurred, which is a greater after-drop than seen with any other method of rewarming. It was observed, however, that consciousness returned at an earlier point, that is, at a lower body temperature than with other methods of rewarming. Once the subjects regained consciousness they did not lose it again, but very quickly grasped the situation and snuggled up to the naked female bodies. The rise of body temperature then occurred at about the same speed as in experimental subjects who had been rewarmed by packing in blankets.

Exceptions were four experimental subjects who, at body temperatures between 30° C. and 32° C. performed the act of sexual intercourse. In these experimental subjects the temperature rose very rapidly after sexual intercourse, which could be compared with the speedy rise in temperature in a hot bath.

2. Another set of experiments concerned the rewarming of intensely chilled persons by one woman. In all these cases rewarming was significantly quicker than could be accomplished by two women. The cause of this seems to me that in warming by one woman only, personal inhibitions are removed, and the woman nestles up to the chilled individual much more intimately. Also in these cases, the return of complete consciousness was strikingly rapid. Only one experimental subject did not return to consciousness and the warming effect was only slight. This person died with symptoms suggesting cerebral haemorrhage, as was confirmed by subsequent autopsy.

(d) Summary

Rewarming experiments of intensely chilled experimental subjects demonstrated that rewarming with animal warmth was very slow. Only such experimental subjects whose physical condition permitted sexual intercourse rewarmed themselves remarkably quickly and showed an equally strikingly rapid return to complete physical well-being. Since excessively long exposure of the body to low temperatures implies danger of internal damage, that method must be chosen for rewarming which guarantees the quickest relief from dangerously low temperatures. This method, according to our experiences, is a massive and rapid supply of warmth by means of a hot bath.

Rewarming of intensely chilled human beings by human or animal warmth can therefore be recommended only in cases in which other possibilities for rewarming are not available, or in cases of specially tender individuals who possibly may not be able to stand a massive and rapid supply of warmth.

As, for example, I am thinking of intensely chilled small children, who are best rewarmed by the body of their mothers, with the aid of hot water bottles.

Dachau, 12 February 1943.

(*Signature*) DR S. RASCHER
SS Hauptsturmführer.'

Rascher remarked in an accompanying note that it would be simplest if

'. . . I went to Auschwitz with Neff and put on a big serial experiment so as to reach a quick solution of the problem of people frozen on land. Auschwitz is in every respect better suited than Dachau for such an experiment, as the climate is colder and the camp itself is so extensive that less attention will be attracted to the work. For the subjects howl so when they freeze!'

This plan, obviously, was never carried out.

But Rascher was able to report further progress to Himmler's personal adjutant on the 4 April 1943.

[DOC. 292.]*

'The question of the saving of people frozen in the open air has in the meantime been cleared up, since, thank goodness, there was once again a period of heavy frost weather in Dachau. Certain people were in the open air for fourteen hours at −6° C., reached an internal temperature of 25° C. with peripheral freezings, and were ALL able to be saved by a hot bath. As I said: it is easy to contradict! But before someone does so, he should come and see for himself. Moreover, a report about freezing in the open air will be sent to the Reich Leader in the next few days.'

The report on 'open air freezing' referred to in this letter was never found. But the witness Neff gave a clear account of these 'dry freezing' experiments.

[PROT. p. 681.]

'A first experiment was carried out in which the prisoner was placed naked on a stretcher in front of the block one evening. He was then covered with a sheet. But every hour a bucket of cold water was poured over him. He lay there in the open under these conditions until shortly before dawn. These subjects had their temperatures taken by thermometer.

Later on Dr Rascher said it would be wrong to cover the person concerned with a sheet and pour water over him, as in those circumstances air could not reach the subject. In future, subjects must not be covered.

The next experiment consisted of a series of tests on ten prisoners, who were also laid out naked one after the other. One of them was checked by galvanometer and the rest by thermometer. But I can't quite remember how many, if any, deaths occurred in connection with these experiments. Speaking with due reserve, I should say that there were about three fatalities at that time.

On one of the following days Rascher called me up and said that Dr Grawitz had visited him and told him that at least 100 tests of this kind must be carried out. . . .'

Neff also reported that subjects were 'kept out of doors' from 6 p.m. till 9 a.m. Their lowest temperature was 25° C., (77° F).

The witness was asked by prosecuting counsel whether the subjects had suffered much. He answered:

[PROT. p. 683.]

'Yes. For at first Rascher would not allow the tests to be carried out after the subject had been rendered unconscious. But the persons concerned screamed so loudly that he found it impossible to continue the series unless they were drugged.'

The supercooling experiments were now mainly conducted by prolonged exposure of the subjects in the open air. But at the same time Rascher continued the tests in icy water. The 'worst ever made' was described by Neff as follows:

[PROT. p. 675 f.]*

'It was the worst experiment which was ever carried out. Two Russian officers were carried out from the bunker. We were forbidden to speak to them. They arrived at approximately four o'clock in the afternoon. Rascher had them undressed and they had to go into the basin naked. Hour after hour passed and while usually after a short time, sixty minutes, freezing had set in, these two Russians were still conscious after two hours. All our appeals to Rascher asking him to give them an injection were of no avail. Approximately during the third hour one Russian said to the other, "Comrade, tell that officer to shoot us." The other replied, "Don't expect any mercy from this Fascist dog." Then they shook hands and said "Goodbye, Comrade." If you can imagine that we inmates had to witness such a death, and could do nothing about it, then you can judge how terrible it is to be condemned to work in such an experimental station.

After these words were translated for Rascher in a somewhat different form by a young Pole, Rascher went back into his office. The young Pole tried at once to give them an anaesthetic with chloroform, but Rascher returned immediately and threatened to shoot us with his pistol if we dared approach these victims again. The experiment lasted at least five hours until death occurred. Both corpses were sent to Munich for autopsy in the Schwabing Hospital.'

Romberg was asked by his defence counsel what he thought of this description.[1]

[PROT. p. 6896.]

'I am not an expert in chilling. But I consider this description of the experiment at the very least greatly exaggerated.

1. This quotation is given in order that our extracts in this case may not appear one-sided. But Romberg's statement does not alter the material facts in any way.

It is in fact impossible for the events to have taken the course described. For this reason I have myself examined the records before the Court dealing with chilling experiments. According to these descriptions of other chilling experiments the numbness or rigor produced by cold occurs in a very short time, within about ten or twenty minutes, whereupon it renders movement or speech by the subject impracticable. Moreover, after an hour at latest unconsciousness sets in, though Neff has stated in his evidence that the two Russian officers talked to each other after as long as three hours, were fully conscious and then actually shook hands. I can't imagine such a time elapsing. This view is also supported by American researches on chilling, which likewise record that in sea-rescue cases numbness begins after an extremely short interval, about ten minutes, whereupon the person concerned is rendered incapable of, for instance, boarding a dinghy. It is invariably pointed out that account must be taken of such numbness.'

Until Rascher was finally transferred from the Luftwaffe to the SS the controversy about his character grew more and more acute. The SS reproached Hippke with not having supported Rascher to the extent that the importance of his experiments demanded. Hippke replied to this point, among others, on the 6 March 1943 in a letter addressed to the chief of Himmler's personal staff, Obergruppenführer Wolf.

[DOC. 262.]

'. . . As a matter of fact you are wrong in supposing that in my capacity as director of all medical research I took any exception whatever to chilling experiments on human beings and thus obstructed the development of such tests. On the contrary, I at once agreed to them. For our own previous experiments on large animals had been suspended and required completion. It would also surely be most improbable for me, as the responsible authority for the development of every possible resource for the saving of our pilots' lives, not to have taken every possible step to promote research in this direction. As soon as Rascher told me what he wanted to do at that time I immediately fell in with his views. . . .'

Both Professor Holzlöhner, who had been in charge of the Dachau supercooling experiments, and Rascher himself, at the time of the trial, were dead. Finke had disappeared. Consequently only two of the accused could be called to account for their part in facilitating the tests. They were Rudolf Brandt and Wolfram Sievers, neither of them a doctor. Further details of their activities will be given in later chapters.

Sievers described as follows an experiment he had witnessed

[PROT. p. 5752 f.]*

'together with Dr Hirt, whom I had to accompany by order of Himmler, as he had been included in Rascher's experiments with Himmler's approval. Himmler probably had realized in the meantime that Rascher alone would not be sufficient in order to clarify these scientifically very extensive and difficult questions. Hirt could only come to Munich for one day because of his state of health and for that reason asked that everything be prepared beforehand, so that he could gain insight into all the work results which had been obtained so far. I told Rascher to prepare everything according to Hirt's desire. A professional criminal was presented for the purpose of this experiment.

Q. Was that a professional criminal who had already been condemned to death, and how did you know whether it was such a criminal?

A. Before the experiment started Hirt wanted to look at the files because there was a possibility that this experiment would end fatally. The sentence was furnished by the Criminal Police Department of the Camp Administration. We saw that this was a sentence which had been passed by a regular court, and it became evident therefrom that this man had served more than ten years' penitentiary, and had been recently sentenced to death because of murder and theft. Hirt furthermore asked the man whether he knew that this experiment might end fatally, whereupon the man answered that he was well aware of it. He said that he would have to die anyway for he was a confirmed criminal, and he just could not stop his criminal activity; therefore he deserved death.

Q. Did you convince yourself of that by asking the experimental subject whether he was actually a volunteer?

A. After Hirt's questioning I personally asked the man whether he agreed to that experiment. He thereupon said that he was in full agreement, providing it didn't hurt him. This assurance could be given to him because the experiment was carried out under complete anaesthesia.'

At this point we may briefly examine the circumstances which must have existed to allow so psychologically abnormal a personage as Rascher to pursue his private aims under the cover of scientific research, with the support of the highest authority, and thus to satisfy his perverse instincts in activities which he described to his taskmaster as scientific. Rascher would never have been able to carry out his purpose in such positively ideal conditions if he had not found in the most eminent of his chiefs a man of fundamentally the same tendencies as himself. Professor Gebhardt, one of the accused, noted the relationship between Himmler and Rascher in the following terms:

[PROT. p. 4167 ff.]

'. . . On the other hand Himmler, a most remarkable man, who collected all sorts of persons, good and bad, about him, seized upon every idea that was brought to his notice. Although I had a great deal to do with Himmler, both medically and socially, I never met Rascher. Himmler knew perfectly well that I would have objected to a man of that sort and naturally there had always been rows whenever our spheres overlapped. But Himmler's plan was simply to have at his disposal an academically trained physician, a strange man like Rascher and a biochemist. He had got everything possible together for the purpose. Consequently, all Service channels were circumvented, so that the experiments, for example those in the Air Force, which had been officially sponsored and terminated, were pursued, so far as I can see, on lines which had never been intended. . . .

Himmler's pet project was the development of a purely SS

science. That was the root cause of all the trouble. People coming fresh from the universities or experienced senior officers of the Medical Service were naturally opposed to the radical innovations of the Third Reich and might be expected to raise the question of interference with the spirit and substance of an instrument already in existence.

A group of Third Reich personalities which included Himmler and Hess was frankly of the opinion that no further new and vigorous life could emerge from the tired soil of middle-class civilization and that future progress was only to be looked for among young, hitherto obscured talents. Himmler openly avowed his adherence to this view.

He became, I am now told, President of *"Ahnenerbe"*,[1] the Ancestral Heritage Community. He was the centre of two groups, to neither of which I ever belonged. I had been friendly with him, you might say, for family reasons, ever since my young days. But I never belonged to the so-called "Friends of Himmler" circle which he founded. It was a dangerous mixture of eccentric individuals and industrialists. From that quarter he obtained both the funds and the encouragement to undertake the thousand and one schemes in all directions which he put into operation. I have an idea that the extraordinary newly founded scientific Institute where all these scientific friends of his met was in fact the "Ancestral Heritage" Community. Himmler, in a word, as I have often pointed out, was attached to a crazy, completely false notion of antiquity. Although the whole tendency of modern research is to specialize in separate fields and branches of knowledge, he was devoted to the conception of "universality", represented by his "Circle", his "Militant Medical Institute" and his "Ancestral Heritage" Community. I really can't remember all the names he gave it ... its various branches included ... physicists, doctors of medicine, "nature healers" and all sorts of others. He did a certain amount of good with these people but also a very great deal of harm. The danger lay in the fact that it was always he who made the decisions. The positive tragedy and disaster for us all was that, owing to his personal participation

1. For further details of 'Ancestral Heritage', the SS research and study community, see the chapter on 'Mustard Gas and Phosgen Experiments' (p. 213).

as President in the activities of that extraordinary social group, his executive capacity in it as, for instance, directly controlling the concentration camps, and his supreme command of it, everyone could be brought into mutual conflict, as in fact happened, as soon as any private notion was put forward.

All the same, I had no idea of all this at the time.

I should here emphasize that our present unhappy position is highly advantageous in one respect. I have never felt so intellectually independent as now, when I can of course see what an extraordinary collection of teams and inter-related machinery, which couldn't work, we represented. But it was yet another characteristic of the Third Reich to try to harness the instinct of a typical outsider to university organization, time-honoured army institutions and many other German traditions and to make a complete mess of the attempted unification.

In our own case the two activities were always parallel.

Rascher succeeded at a certain point, through his private relations with Himmler, in gaining access to this strange circle of pseudo-antiquarian studies and in persuading Himmler that relentless adherence to the plan at all costs, disregarding all obstruction by the university and military authorities, etc., might indeed entail sacrifices but would certainly result in Himmler obtaining the free hand which he had always aimed at. Accordingly, Rascher was suddenly taken up by the pedants in question. He was seconded for duty with us because in wartime he had to remain a soldier of some sort. But I should, of course, point out that I never succeeded in acquiring control over that particular surgeon. Before I could do so he was ordered to the Ahnenerbe Institute and went on with his work there.'

As early as 1939 Rascher had been able, through the contacts of his wife with Himmler, to undertake researches, concerned with blood crystallization, at the Dachau concentration camp. Some of these investigations, as well as others, were based upon plagiarism. They were all designed to launch him on an academic career. He took the formula of Polygal, a haemorrhage astringent, from a Jewish chemist imprisoned at Dachau, Dr Robert Feix, with a view to exploiting it commercially himself. The murders committed in connection with the

manufacture and testing of this remedy were referred to in a
sworn statement by Rascher's uncle.

[DOC. 1424.]

'During my nephew's absence I found, by chance, a paper
in his desk reporting on the shooting of four persons with the
object of trying out the haemorrhage astringent known as
"Polygal 10". So far as I recall the victims included a Russian
commissar and a congenital idiot. But I don't remember who
the other two were. The Russian was shot through the right
shoulder by a SS man standing on a chair to his right. The
bullet came out near the spleen. The report stated that the
Russian gave a convulsive start, dropped into a chair and died
in about twenty minutes. The dissection record mentions lacera-
tion of the lungs and aorta, adding that the lacerations had
been plugged by hard blood-clots and that it was only for that
reason that relatively prolonged survival after the shot could
be accounted for. After reading this first statement I was so
shocked that I read no more. I took a sample of the astringent
out of the desk at the time, and enclose it.

On the way back to Munich after this last visit of mine to
Dachau I spoke to my nephew about my discovery. He was
very angry when he learned that I knew of the affair. But after
I had appealed to his conscience as a scientist and thinker he
broke down and exclaimed, "I'm not allowed to think! I'm
not allowed to think!" When we reached Munich I went on
talking to him all night. He then admitted that he had taken
the wrong road, but said that he could see no chance of
abandoning it.'

This statement also reveals that Rascher and his wife were
arrested in 1944 for child abduction. Rascher '. . . was shot at
Dachau before the Americans arrived. His wife was hanged at
Ravensbrück or in Berlin at Himmler's suggestion.'

CHAPTER TWO

TESTS OF THE POSSIBILITY OF DRINKING SEA-WATER

EVER since 1941 the Luftwaffe had reported that, with the intensification of air operations over the Mediterranean and Atlantic, cases of distress at sea were multiplying. In warmer areas the chief danger was thirst. In view of the lack of possible counter-measures Dr Konrad Schäfer was requested in 1942 to examine the problem from the scientific angle. He developed a new process by which, if a rubber boat were available, salt could be extracted from sea-water and its magnesium sulphate also eliminated. In December 1943 he demonstrated the process and the Technical Department of the Luftwaffe ordered mass production of the requisite materials by I.G. Farben.

At the same time Berka, a Luftwaffe engineer, produced at Vienna a specific which was also supposed to make sea-water drinkable. The Schäfer process involved actual removal of the salt. Berka's system merely improved the taste of the water and allegedly facilitated, through the Vitamin C content of the agent, the secretion of salt by the kidneys. A Luftwaffe doctor had experimented with this medium in a Viennese hospital. Dr Schäfer stated in reply to his defence counsel in court:

[PROT. p. 8504 f.]

'*A*. On my arrival in Vienna Herr von Sirany, wearing the uniform of a colonel in the Medical Service, accompanied me to the ward in which the patients, the subjects who had undergone the experiments, were accommodated.
Q. Were they soldiers?
A. Yes, they were soldiers. Herr von Sirany observed laconically: "Good stuff that Berka-water, eh? You're none of you thirsty, what? Isn't that splendid!" The soldiers all answered: "Yes, sure, Colonel. It went down jolly well." But I was in mufti. I asked Herr von Sirany to permit me to examine the men one by one. I told them they might explain to me what

it had really been like, adding that I was a scientist and had nothing to do with the military authorities otherwise. The following medical history was then disclosed. Most of the men declared that the more they drank the more thirsty they became. Both Hlava and Winter, for example, said so. "Thirst was only quenched quite momentarily," they explained. Many of the subjects had had diarrhoea. That was the general picture, as one might have expected of Berka's remedy.'

Dr Becker-Freyseng, at that time consultant for aviation medicine under the Health Inspection Department of the Luftwaffe, explained:

[PROT. p. 8110 f.]

'The chief danger in drinking sea-water in circumstances of distress at sea arises from the fact that the recipient is already in a parched condition. He is drinking sea-water after he has been thirsty for two or three days. . . . According to all experts in this field the organism when parched to this extent actually runs a most serious risk from sea-water and may be harmed by it. The danger of Berkatite was evident to us from the following experience. Berkatite is a drug resembling sugar. It has the quality of suppressing the disagreeable, bitter, salt taste of sea-water so as to render it, in fact, drinkable. Accordingly, anyone wrecked at sea will at once be able to provide himself, as soon as he feels thirsty, with a certain quantity of potable liquid by means of Berkatite. But as this substance does not eliminate the actual content of salt in the water, he will soon feel thirsty again and apply himself once more to the Berkatite in order to make the sea-water palatable. He will thus in time absorb a large quantity of salt which his body will have to get rid of and as the amount of water which he takes in with the sea-water and its salt does not suffice to quench his thirst it will continue to increase as he goes on drinking more and more sea-water treated with Berkatite. If he then drinks at one time more than 300 cubic centimetres of it (about half a pint) diarrhoea must certainly result. He will then not only be losing water by urination but also by excretion, with the consequence that his thirst and also of course its accompanying danger to life will continue to increase.'

The Health Department accordingly rejected the Berka specific in no uncertain terms.

But meanwhile the Technical Department of the Luftwaffe, which alone could authorize the introduction into the Service of medical supplies as an item of equipment, had made other plans. It reported to Himmler on the 15 May 1944:

[DOC. 184.]*

'With reference to the inter-office conference between Oberstingenieur Christensen and Haupsturmführer Engineer Dohle regarding the above-mentioned matter, it is announced that two processes have been worked out by the office to render sea-water potable:

1. The I.G. method, using mainly silver nitrate. For this process quite a large plant needs to be set up, which would require about 200 tons of iron and cost about 250,000 RM. The amount of the product needed by the Luftwaffe and Navy requires 2·5 to 3 tons of pure silver a month. Besides, the water which is rendered potable by this preparation has to be sucked through a filter in order to avoid absorption of precipitated chemicals. These facts make the application of this process practically impossible.

2. The second process which was worked out is the so-called Berka method. According to this method, the salts present in the sea-water are not precipitated, but are so treated that they are not disagreeable to the taste. They pass through the body without oversaturating it with salts and without causing an undue thirst. No special plants are necessary for producing preparations needed for this process; nor do the preparations themselves consist of scarce materials.

It can be presumed that this method will be introduced in the Luftwaffe and the Navy in a short time. Now that German technical science has actually succeeded in rendering sea-water potable for people in distress at sea, in accordance with the above, the knowledge as to how foreign countries intend to solve this problem is no longer of prime importance. Naturally the office is very much interested in ascertaining how, above all, the United States has solved this problem, and it is requested that this information be sought, without, however, compromising any person or any office too much.'

Dr Becker-Freyseng, in reply to his defence counsel, commented on this report as follows:

[PROT. p. 8096 f.]

1. 'Two hundred tons of iron may seem quite a large quantity to a goldsmith or a housewife. But to the Air Force, which after all had to reckon continuously with many total losses of its machines, 200 tons could really not have appeared a prohibitive quantity, even in 1944. Again, the 250,000 marks required for the installation of works to manufacture Schäfer's remedy would naturally be regarded as a large sum by a private investor. But when one reflects that the training of a pilot until he is ready for active service in fighters or bombers used to cost the State between 50,000 and 100,000 marks, inclusive of the costs of all training accidents, ground organization, fuel and so on, and when one realizes that by the use of Schäfer's remedy two or three pilots who come to grief at sea could be saved, it is obvious that an expenditure of 250,000 marks by the Air Force on the production of the remedy would be worth while. The size of the sum in question does not therefore constitute a practical objection to the introduction of Schäfer's specific. As to the 2·5 to 3 tons of pure silver which were alleged to be needed every month, this estimate, as I hope to prove beyond doubt later on, was most grossly exaggerated. This quantity was that required for the so-called primary installation. During the ensuing months certain additions only would be necessary to it, to replace quantities lost in the previous month by accidents at sea or total wreckage of aircraft. The Technical Office appeared to assume in its calculations that either every pilot would come to grief at sea every month or else that every aircraft would become a total loss every month. To deal, finally, with the last argument advanced by the Technical Office, to the effect that a filter would be necessary in using Schäfer's preparations, it is surely obvious even to those who are not chemists that this perfectly simple matter could easily be arranged and would in no sense be a valid argument against the introduction of the specific in question.'

2. 'Your question suggests that this is a purely medical statement which the Technical Office was not in a position to make, since it was primarily a purely engineering establishment. I have already pointed out that at the beginning of May 1944 a very definite and elaborately supported rejection of the Berka process was passed to the Technical Office. The latter nevertheless referred this document on the 15 May to Himmler. . . . The fact that no special plant would be required to manufacture the preparation was actually an advantage, for Berkatite could be made up in any sugar refinery. As to the assertion that preparations would not involve any materials in short supply, I had better tell you that the essential ingredient was grape-sugar. It was characteristic of the narrow specialist outlook of the Technical Office that it alleged the requirement of 200 tons of iron to be an insurmountable obstacle, while making no reference to the bottleneck in the supply of grape-sugar. I don't think I shall be betraying any secret if I say that in 1944 grape-sugar, which as everyone knows is manufactured from maize, was unquestionably, as a whole, in short supply with us. It could only be obtained for the use of invalids and even for them in extraordinarily limited quantities. I may add now, when there is so much talk in the newspapers about calories, that during our dispute with the Technical Office about the introduction or rejection of Berkatite the Office claimed priority for the Air Force commissariat to the extent of the first ton of grape-sugar made available. Fortunately we discovered this fact in time to prevent the claim being met. One ton of grape-sugar contains four million calories. When one reflects that at the present time 2,000 calories per day per head are regarded as essential, it is evident that the ton of grape-sugar demanded by the Technical Office in this instance could feed a family of four, naturally only on the basis of calorie intake, for fully 500 days. Yet the Technical Office did not refer to this bottleneck in the supply of grape-sugar. . . .

The Technical Office alone was competent to decide whether an item of equipment should be produced or not. I should perhaps add that such a specific, designed to render sea-water potable, did not come under the heading of victuals in the German Air Force lists of materials and apparatus. Consequently the Commissariat would not have been competent to

G

claim it. Nor would the decision to adopt it be one for the
Director of the Medical Service. For it was an item of equipment and thus a matter entirely for the Technical Office to
dispose of.'

In order to reach a practical solution of the dispute between
the Technical and Health Departments conferences were held
on the 19 and 20 May 1944. The representatives of the Health
Department made the dangers of Berka's remedy perfectly
clear. The Technical Department, on their side, insisted that
the Schäfer process was impracticable for the reasons given
in their letter of the 15 May. As no agreement could be
reached, it was suggested that Sirany's experiments should be
repeated and the question raised of using for the purpose the
prisoners at that time employed in Berlin on clearing debris
and missiles which had failed to explode. Becker-Freyseng
commented:

[PROT. p. 8130 f.]

'It was of course clear to all those present that experiments
could not be carried out on prisoners in any place of confine-
ment whatever. I was probably asked at the time how, in these
circumstances, I supposed that the tests could be performed.
No doubt I answered by representing what I knew to be the
fact, viz. that the concentration camp at Dachau had laboratory
accommodation where, if prisoners could be made available,
I thought that the experiments might be conveniently conducted. The existence of this laboratory accommodation had
been made known to me at the Nuremberg conferences on
distress at sea and chilling. . . .'

After the Technical Department had called attention to the
approval of Berka's specific by Professor Eppinger of Vienna,
it was decided to postpone final decision to a further conference
on the 25 May, to be attended by experts. The refusal to use
the Schäfer process appeared to leave only two alternatives
open, either to expose the aviators to thirst at sea or else to
supply them with the Berka drug. Professor Eppinger added a
further clinical consideration when he said that having studied
the records of the experiments carried out by Chief Surgeon
Sirany in Vienna he thought it possible that kidney secretion

might be stimulated by Berka's method. Becker-Freyseng commented as follows:

[PROT. p. 8140.]

'Professor Eppinger considered, against my own judgment, that further experiments would be required in order to ascertain whether Berkatite should be adopted or rejected. There is probably no need for me to go into all the scientific arguments which Professor Eppinger advanced at that time. I need only briefly mention that he had watched Professor Sirany's experiments in Vienna. He stated at the meeting in Berlin on the 25 May that he had noticed during Sirany's tests that one or more of his subjects had passed urine with a higher salt concentration than would have been assumed as normal in the state of scientific knowledge at that time. He proceeded to adduce a whole series of scientifically grounded reasons for supposing that the body would be able to digest, without injury, by the aid of Berkatite, quantities of salt as great as would be absorbed by drinking sea-water. Eppinger maintained his theory with the greatest tenacity and succeeded in obtaining general support for it from Professor Heubner, the other scientific authority present. . . .'

At the conference on the 25 May the medical side drafted a detailed programme of experiments. Professor Beiglböck, Eppinger's head physician, was to be in charge. On this occasion nothing was said about the use of prisoners as subjects.

It was no longer easy at this period to obtain the necessary forty subjects from military establishments. The Health Inspection Department of the Luftwaffe made inquiries of both the Military Academy and the Luftwaffe hospital at Brunswick. But replies were negative. Becker-Freyseng accordingly suggested to Professor Schröder, his chief at that time, 'to try to obtain prisoners as subjects, an idea then entirely new to Professor Schröder.'

Becker-Freyseng continued:

[PROT. p. 8147.]

'In connection with this question I told him what I myself

already knew at that time, viz. that international medical
literature provided many instances of experiments having been
carried out on prisoners. I added that in the time of his prede-
cessor, Professor Hippke, such tests had also been conducted by
Holzlöhner. Finally I pointed out that the proposed sea-water
experiments were perfectly safe, that nothing could happen to
the subjects and that I was sure that enough volunteer prisoners
could be found to undergo the tests if only because they would
then be guaranteed a specially nourishing diet both before and
after experiment. Professor Schröder then asked me if I could
tell him in greater detail how Holzlöhner had been led to perform his experiments. I was unable to answer this question,
but could only say I knew that Rascher had mentioned Holzlöhner's tests at the Nuremberg meeting, declaring that the
prisoners in question had been put at Holzlöhner's disposal by
the Chief of Police. Schröder then said he would discuss the
matter with the Head of the Police Health Service.'

In the course of this interview with Dr Grawitz, Chief
Physician of the SS and Civil Police, Schröder, in giving
evidence in his own defence, said that he proposed the recruitment of subjects from the group of those adjudged 'unfit to
bear arms'. After Grawitz had agreed in principle that something should be done, the Health Inspection Department
approached Himmler for his approval in the following letter:

[DOC. 185.]*

'Highly respected Reich Minister!
Earlier already you made it possible for the Luftwaffe to
settle urgent medical matters through experiments on human
beings. *Today I again stand before a decision which, after numerous
experiments on animals as well as human experiments on voluntary
experimental subjects, demands a final solution.* The Luftwaffe has
simultaneously developed two methods for making sea-water
potable. The one method, developed by a medical officer,
removes the salt from the sea-water and transforms it into real
drinking water; the second method, suggested by an engineer,
leaves the salt content unchanged, and only removes the unpleasant taste from the sea-water. The latter method, in contrast to the first, requires no critical raw material. From the

medical point of view this method must be viewed critically, as the administration of concentrated salt solutions can produce severe symptoms of poisoning.

As the experiments on human beings could thus far only be carried out for a period of four days, and as practical demands require a remedy for those who are in distress at sea up to twelve days, appropriate experiments are necessary.

Required are forty healthy test subjects, who must be available for four whole weeks. As it is known from previous experiments that necessary laboratories exist in the concentration camp Dachau, this camp would be very suitable.

Direction of the experiments is to be taken over by Stabsarzt Dr Beiglböck, university lecturer and in peace-time Chief Physician of the Medical University Clinic in Vienna (Professor Dr Eppinger). After receipt of your basic approval, I shall list by name the other physicians who are to participate in the experiments.

Due to the enormous importance which a solution of this problem has for shipwrecked men of the Luftwaffe and Navy, I would be greatly obliged to you, my dear Reich Minister, if you would decide to comply with my request.

Heil Hitler!

(*Signature*) Schröder'

The English translation of one sentence, the second, in this document was repeatedly the subject of dispute during the trial.

The prosecution insisted that the sentence meant that prisoners were now to be substituted for voluntary subjects, while the accused maintained that it merely stressed the need for a final solution of the problem, going beyond the results hitherto obtained, through experiments on voluntary subjects.

In the Judgment on Schröder's case this point was referred to as follows:

[Judgment p. 89 f.]*

'In fairness to the defendant it should be stated that he contests the translation of the second sentence in the first paragraph of the letter written by him to Himmler, which the prosecution interprets as meaning that experiments could no

longer be conducted on voluntary subjects, and that the words
"demands a final solution" meant that involuntary subjects in
concentration camps should be employed. Regardless of
whether or not the letter quoted by us is a correct translation
of the German original, the evidence shows that within a
month after the letter was sent to Himmler through Grawitz,
sea-water experiments were commenced at Dachau by the
defendant Bieglböck.'

The accused defended their decision to undertake the experiments in a concentration camp on the ground that the tests
could not be properly carried out in Berlin owing to the daily
air raids. They also repeated that they had not been able to
find any suitable subjects there. The prosecution fastened on
this very point in its examination of Becker-Freyseng.

[PROT. p. 8309 f.]

Q. You could surely have made a broadcast appeal and so
obtained a few volunteers out of the millions of Berlin citizens
to undergo a perfectly safe experiment for the benefit of the
German Air Force. You could have said, for example, "It is
your patriotic duty to volunteer for this experiment", or something of that sort. Would you not then have obtained at least
forty volunteers in the whole of Berlin?

A. I have already stated under direct examination that I
was sure we could have obtained forty subjects for these
experiments in Berlin. But they would not have been such
subjects as we could have used. The prosecution could easily
have obtained enough witnesses to testify that in Berlin in the
summer of 1944 there could not possibly have been forty
healthy young men between 20 and 30 years old with so much
time to spare that they could undergo experiments lasting a
whole month. Such a situation would have been utterly out of
the question in Berlin in 1944.[1]

1. It was also very difficult to obtain suitable subjects for medical experiment in the United States at that time, according to the following evidence
of the prosecution's expert, Professor Ivy of Chicago.
Prosecution Counsel: 'Were those who refused field service obliged to
volunteer for medical experiments?
Professor Ivy: Certainly not.
Q. But they were obliged, were they not, to undertake work in national
establishments if required?

Dr Grawitz, who had received Schröder's letter to Himmler for editing before dispatch, wrote to the Reichsführer on the 28 July 1944:

[DOC. 179.]

'Reichsführer.

The Chief of the Medical Service of the Air Force requests permission in the enclosed paper to carry out experiments on prisoners in order to test two apparently promising and simple processes for the rendering of sea-water potable. In accordance with your order of the 15 May 1944 I have ascertained the views of SS Gruppenführer Professor Gebhardt, SS Gruppenführer Glücks and SS Gruppenführer Nebe. They are stated as follows:

1. SS Gruppenführer Professor Gebhardt.
"I consider it very proper to support the Air Force in every respect and to appoint a specialist in internal diseases from the Waffen SS to supervise the experiments."

2. SS Gruppenführer Glücks.*
"You are informed that I have no objections whatsoever to the experiments requested by the Chief of the Medical Service of the Luftwaffe to be conducted at the Rascher experimental station in the Dachau concentration camp. IF POSSIBLE, JEWS OR PRISONERS HELD IN QUARANTINE ARE TO BE USED."

A. Yes, they were bound to undertake some kind of national service.

Q. Well, you then discovered that you needed subjects for experiment. How did it happen that those who refused field service were put at your disposal?

A. So far as I remember, the National Research Council, finding that students of medicine and dentistry were being drafted into the Army and could therefore no longer serve as subjects for experiment in the universities and at the Medical School laboratories, consulted the Director of the Civilian Public Service. The latter then decided that conscientious objectors would be given permission to volunteer for such work at the Medical Schools and Research Institutes.'

Reference has already been made in the last chapter to Professor Ivy's recognition of the 'needs of war as the fundamental reason for experiment'.

3. SS Gruppenführer Nebe.*

"I agree to the proposal to use for this purpose the asocial gipsy half-breeds. There are people among them, who, although healthy, are out of the question as regards labour commitment. Regarding these gipsies, I shall shortly make a special proposal to the Reich Leader, but I think it right to select from among these people the necessary number of test subjects. Should the Reich Leader agree to this, I SHALL LIST BY NAME THE PERSONS TO BE USED."

With regard to the proposal by SS Gruppenführer Nebe to use gipsies for these experiments I venture to raise the objection that owing to their racial composition being in some cases alien the results of experiment on such gipsies might not be applicable with perfect confidence to our own people. It would therefore be desirable for only such prisoners as are racially comparable with the European population to be made available.

I respectfully request permission for the experiments to proceed.'

Himmler annotated this document in his own hand: 'Gipsies and for checking three others.'

In conformity with this decision of the Reichsführer the defendant Sievers, in his capacity as business manager of the 'Ancestral Heritage' Community, a SS institution to which the Department for Practical Research on Military Science was attached, arranged for equipment of the research station at Dachau. He wrote in his report to Dr Grawitz:

[DOC. 182.]*

'I hope that this arrangement may permit a successful conduct of the experiments. When the results are reported at the proper time, please arrange to point out the participation and assistance of the Reich Leader SS.'

Although these experiments for the rendering of sea-water potable were eventually carried out at Dachau, they were entrusted to another group. The SS doctors neither attended nor supervised them. Professor Beiglböck was in charge. He had at first refused to work in a concentration camp. But after he, like others, had failed to find suitable accommodation and subjects for experiment in the hospital department which he had hitherto directed, he finally agreed to the Dachau solution and was ordered by Becker-Freyseng to proceed to the camp.

Beiglböck gave a clear description in court of the nature and object of the experiments.

[PROT. p. 8142 f.]

'The order stipulated that these experiments were to be performed with four separate groups of subjects. One group was to be made hungry and thirsty, another was to be given ordinary sea-water to drink and another sea-water with Berkatite added, one section taking 500 cubic centimetres of the mixture per day and the other 1,000. As in these three cases loss of water had to be taken into consideration and all the subjects were on a diet to which they were not used, it was necessary to determine how much water would be lost. Accordingly, a fourth group was collected, the members of which were given an ordinary amount to drink but otherwise put on the same diet as the other groups. So far as I know, this last group was at first given ordinary drinking-water. But later Schäfer-water was administered to its members, in order to provide a further check on the assumption that no untoward consequences would follow even on the use of this water in normal conditions.'

Details added by Becker-Freyseng to Bieglböck's statement were to the effect that all the subjects were fed on full pilots' rations amounting to 3,000 calories daily for ten days before the test and that during the experiment participants in the group numbered two to four were given Luftwaffe marine distress diet.

Beiglböck's statement continues:

[PROT. p. 8825 ff.]

'I was also given precise instructions as to the conditions under which these experiments were to proceed. They provided us with a rather full programme and we had plenty to do at this time. A very great deal of blood-analysis had to be carried out, not concerned with quantity, but with the determination of individual components. The most exact analyses of urine were also required, so that we could ascertain with a high degree of probability the course of alteration in the water content of the body. This was the extent of my orders. I knew nothing of the discussions on the 19th and 20th, so often referred to at the present hearing. I was only aware of the conference on the 25th, so far, that is, as it concerned myself. I mean its unfortunate choice of myself to direct the experiments and the above-mentioned prescriptions, which it then adopted, for the work to be done.

The plan and object of the experiments were as follows. I was first made acquainted with the results so far attained by Messrs. Schäfer and Sirany. I was also given the opportunity to study their records. I was then informed, in so many words, that Sirany's experiments were unsatisfactory in the sense that they constituted no sort of a proof of the practical utility of Berka's specific. Above all, Sirany had only tested it over four days, whereas the Air Force required a drug which would be effective for a long period of distress at sea. They could not consider the introduction of a short-term agent. A period of twelve days was mentioned as requisite at the time, as there had been some recent cases in which men had been rescued after twelve days of distress at sea. Accordingly, we were told, in order to avoid misunderstanding, that the specific needed should last twelve days in its effect without injurious consequences to the subject. The conditions of the experiment were to resemble as closely as possible those experienced in marine distress, though only so far as the supply of water and victuals was concerned. For of course there could be no question of reproducing the other disagreeable features of such a situation, including for example climatic conditions of cold, heat and adverse weather, the encrusting of the skin with heavy deposits of salt carried by flying spray, the uncomfortable postures and sleeplessness enforced by occupation of a dinghy and so on. I proceeded to discuss in detail, with Dr Becker-Freyseng, all these important points relating to my experiment. We also talked over its theoretical bases. Dr Becker-Freyseng drew my special attention to Dr Schäfer's explanations of his process, impressing on me that Schäfer had calculated the quantities of sea-water which would last twelve days, though not of course without certain variations of intake. The question arose whether small quantities of sea-water could be taken over a longer period, how long, for instance, 500 cubic centimetres might last a man. For at that time our pilots were issued with a small ration of drinking-water, enough for two days. But if a man were able to assuage extreme thirst by imbibing small quantities of sea-water for another eight or ten days he could of course survive at sea for twelve days without serious risk to health, assuming, naturally, that he had not been issued with Schäfer's specific. Dr Becker-Freyseng told me, accordingly, that while efforts should be made in one way or another to aim at this upper limit of twelve days, such endeavours should not of course be pressed too far. I was only, in the case of each group, to get as near to this goal as my medical responsibility for the state of health of the subject would permit. We next considered exactly when the dangerous degree of loss of water would be reached in ordinary circumstances and when there would ordinarily be a risk to the life of the subject. In the interval between the points of danger and of actual menace to life it would happen that, owing to previous evacuation of water, only freely available water from the tissue would at first be released, whereas between the tenth and twelfth days up to 22 per cent of the water in the cells might also be given off, with consequent affection of the intra-cellular water. I stressed at the beginning of our conversation that I would in no circumstances carry out experiments which might involve injury to health or actual survival. I said I would refuse to do any such thing. Dr Becker-Freyseng at once replied that he shared my views in this respect and that of course possible fatalities must be ruled out in every case. The limit must be set, he said, wherever injury to health might be apprehended. At the same time the experiments would have to be carried far enough to enable unmistakable signs of thirst to be recognized which would render comparison between the two groups feasible. I was to go as far as my sense of medical responsibility allowed, so far, that is to say, as I could go without injury to the subject's health. We also agreed at that time that we must clearly recognize the fact that experiments concerned with thirst are very disagreeable to the subject, making very high demands on his strength of will, since he would be required to feel thirst for several days. We determined that for this reason the consent of the subject must be obtained beforehand and that if anyone volunteered he should be told what to expect. In order to spare the feelings of the subjects as much as possible, we arranged that they should spend the time in bed. This prescription had two further grounds.

In the first place the pilot forced to take refuge in his dinghy can only lie down and secondly any kind of movement or walking about increases evaporation of water through the lungs. Consequently, a quiet recumbent position with as little movement as possible conserves the water in the body to some extent. Accordingly, as already stated, exterior conditions in these cases were of such a character as to preclude so far as possible sensations of discomfort in the subject, with the exception of hunger and thirst. The object of the tests was quite definitely to elucidate the following questions:

1. Whether it would be better to go without liquid altogether or drink sea-water.

2. Whether the Berka specific, contrary to expectation, might improve the digestibility of sea-water.

3. Whether the Schäfer specific would last twelve days without any ill effects. The group undergoing this experiment would be retained for twelve days if the specific clearly proved not to be dangerous.

4. The opportunity would be taken to study the metabolism of those enduring thirst or drinking sea-water with a view to obtaining data if possible of any internal changes since such data might prove to be of use in the treatment of persons rescued at sea.

Q. Who, then, was to decide when the experiments should be discontinued?

A. That decision was of course reserved to my own professional judgment. I can assure you, in this connection, that I discontinued the experiments in every case before the critical line was crossed. I naturally also took subjective phenomena into consideration. But in view of the general character of the tests I could only do so to a certain extent, since thirst was actually an indispensable condition for their performance.'

The Court was much concerned with the extent to which the prisoners exercised free will in consenting to the experiments.

At Nebe's suggestion the SS had paraded about a thousand

gipsies at the camp in Buchenwald and asked for volunteers to join a 'superior labour force' at Dachau. Many stepped forward. Forty-four were selected. The gipsies believed at that time that a bomb disposal force was being recruited. But the main reason why they volunteered was the general recognition by prisoners that Dachau was preferable to Buchenwald as a camp. At Dachau the gipsies were passed on by the camp doctor, Dr Ploetner, to Professor Beiglböck, with the intimation that they were volunteers.[1] Beiglböck informed the gipsies of the nature of the tests they were to undergo. After medical and X-ray examination of them he dismissed those he considered unsuitable subjects. He also questioned those he retained as to their willingness to participate in the experiments.

Some of the witnesses who gave evidence in Court had only indirect, second-hand knowledge of the tests carried out. Others were vague about the voluntary participation of the subjects. Apart from these there remained three witnesses for the prosecution and three who favoured discharge of the accused. All six witnesses had been present at the experimental station. But only two had themselves undergone the tests, allegedly against their will. One of these gave convincing evidence. But the testimony of the other, a confirmed criminal, appeared unreliable. He attempted to attack the defendant Beiglböck in court and was sentenced to three months' imprisonment for unseemly conduct on that occasion.

Accordingly, two situations had clearly to be distinguished. In the first place the gipsies at Buchenwald had voluntarily agreed to join a labour force. Secondly, after they had been told by Beiglböck the real reason why they had been brought to Dachau, they were asked to signify their consent to participation in the experiments. As to whether they did so or not the evidence was contradictory.[2]

1. Ploetner, in his capacity as camp doctor, had assisted Professor Schilling in the latter's experiments with malaria at Dachau. But he had later told Himmler that he would have nothing to do with any experiments on human beings. This refusal did not affect his continued activity at the camp.

2. Beiglböck's defence counsel, in dealing with the erasures mentioned below, made by his client in the records of the experiments which had been submitted as in Beiglböck's favour, declared that the defence knew the names, also erased in the records, of the subjects of the tests. But counsel added that he was not prepared to disclose these names 'because he did not

It is clear, however, that the gipsies had to give their
decision at Dachau in the atmosphere of a concentration camp
and that to have accepted any offer of release from the tests
which Beiglböck may have made to them would have seemed
undesirable to them on account of the treatment they could
then have expected from the SS. The readiness of most of the
gipsies to participate was found to be by no means unqualified
as the tests proceeded. The fact proves on the one hand that
their initial agreement was only obtained under the pressure of
their situation as prisoners and on the other that they were all
unsuitable subjects. Both documents and oral testimony show
beyond doubt that it was a mistake of the Health Inspection
Department to order the experiments to be carried out in a
concentration camp. In particular, the Department must have
known, as can be deduced, if not proved, from various points
made in the evidence submitted, even that of the defendants
themselves, that highly suspicious, if not downright criminal,
experiments connected with altitude and refrigeration had
already occurred in secret at Dachau as the result of collaboration with the SS. Nor could the appointment of a well-known
hospital physician to conduct the tests themselves in the absence
of the SS guarantee the proceedings as unexceptionable from
the standpoint of medical ethics or even scientifically. Only the
urgency of reaching a decision on the question of employing
the Berka specific can account in any way for the renewal of
close relations between the Luftwaffe and the SS. Even if in
this case the latter exercised no further influence on the course
of the actual experiments, the method of choosing subjects and
the state of mind of those chosen, which had so much effect in
determining their attitude, depended wholly on the measures
taken by the SS as a closed institution. Consequently, the
influence of National Socialist racialism on the choice of the
participants and the pressure of a concentration camp environ-

feel justified in aiding the prosecution's researches ... the subjects of the
experiments were simple, primitive people, often belonging to families
stigmatized as anti-social by the authorities.' Counsel went on to say that
if he called these people as witnesses he would be obliged to obtain a police
report upon each of them. But he would give their names to the Tribunal
if so desired. [Prot. P.9489.] According to Judgment he added to his final
plea the sworn statements of further witnesses (see below).

ment were decisive factors in the organization of the tests. Even the fair treatment of the subjects by Beiglböck, which was acknowledged by almost all the witnesses, could not compensate for this fundamental blunder.

Beiglböck denied that any seriously prejudicial results occurred during the experiments. Yet while under arrest he had made certain erasures in their records as collected by his defence counsel with a view to his exoneration. These erasures were afterwards, on their discovery, reinstated by the defendant himself. For example, on the back of the record dealing with subject 23 the following shorthand note on a phase diagram appeared:

[PROT. p. 9081 ff.]*

'The thirst assumes forms difficult to endure. The patient lies there quite motionless with half-closed eyes. He takes little notice of his surroundings. He asks for water only when he awakes from his semi-conscious condition. Outward aspect much deteriorated but general condition nothing to worry about.'

But the note had originally read:

'He takes no notice of his environment . . . in his stupefied condition . . . general condition gives cause for anxiety.'

Beiglböck excused himself with the observation that:

[PROT. p. 9102.]

'People unacquainted with the symptoms of intense thirst would derive a much more serious impression from this description than corresponds with the facts.'

Professor Andrew Conway Ivy, the prosecution's expert, after examining these records and their subsequent alteration, declared that on conclusion of the tests some of the subjects showed symptoms of illness, e.g. were feverish, very weak and apathetic, could no longer stand.

The expert for the defence, Professor Volhard of Frankfurt, had been the first to examine the records, which he obtained from counsel before they were altered. He gave his opinion in some detail in Court, emphasizing the obvious fact that 'prolonged thirst is a thoroughly disagreeable experience.' But he said that in the experiments there had been no question of any injury to the subjects' health and certainly no fatal results.

In reply to defence counsel he stated, *inter alia*:

[PROT. p. 8543.]

'Such an experiment can only be performed on volunteers, since the collaboration of the subject is essential. But this circumstance does not mean that they will not attempt to mislead the director of the experiment, just as many patients, even educated persons, when undergoing cures of this kind, try to deceive their doctor. In the case in question several subjects could not help breaking down and secretly contriving to obtain drinking-water. . . . Well, of course a certain amount of personal endurance is necessary and I can very well imagine that uneducated, somewhat unstable and weak-willed persons lost interest in further collaboration.'

Under cross-examination by prosecuting counsel he retorted:

[PROT. p. 8580.]

'*Q*. Professor, are you giving evidence as an expert or in order to justify these experiments at Dachau?

A. I am only giving evidence to the effect that from my personal observation there can be no question of any crime against humanity in connection with these experiments.'

His attitude was based on the assumption that all the subjects were volunteers. In studying the records he had in mind experiments with thirst which had been undertaken in his own hospital.[1]

At Dachau the periods averaged between five and seven days. The longest, according to Beiglböck, took nine and a half days. Professor Ivy made it ten days. But he admitted that this was a case in which the subjects had interrupted the course of the experiment by drinking water.

1. These consisted of eleven tests on three groups, directed by Dr E. Schütte, university lecturer in physiological chemistry. In every case the subjects were volunteers, doctors and medical students, who continued their professional work while under test. The experiments lasted five and a half days. One series was carried out in very hot weather. Dr Schütte reported that no after-effects or delayed injury to health took place.

The Viennese medical student Fritz Pillwein, employed as a male nurse at the station, described the tests as follows.

[DOC. 912.]

'The experiments themselves were carried out in the following way. During the first three days the subjects were put on marine distress diet, consisting of a slab of choco-kola, some dextropur and a few rusks, between ten and twelve small pieces. Furthermore, from the first to the last day of the experiment the participants were given doses of salt water four or five times a day amounting to half a litre in all. The forty-four subjects were divided into five or six groups. Two of these were given pure sea-water. Two more received pure sea-water with a preparation of salt added. The fifth group took distilled sea-water without any admixture. From the start, samples of blood were drawn daily from the subjects. Some patients were so severely afflicted by bodily weakness and especially by thirst that after a few days they could no longer get out of bed. I can remember one who fell into screaming fits. Such patients, at times when they were left without supervision, quite often drank from the sewage pails used by the nursing staff, or took water from the air-raid fire-buckets in the corridor. Some also, when the floor was washed, sucked up the water thrown over it. I had to weigh the subjects daily and found that their daily loss of weight amounted to about a kilogram (2·2 lb.). When Dr Beiglböck discovered one day that some of the patients had been taking liquids not prescribed for them, the male nurse on duty, also a prisoner, was dismissed from the sick bay.

During the process of recruiting subjects for these experiments promises were made that they would receive better food for a while. But in fact only the first group was put on an improved diet. All the rest, for two days after the experiments ended, were given only drinking-water and skim milk, after which, from about the third day onwards, they were put back on the ordinary camp diet. The first group received for some four or five days a little sausage, bread, butter, cheese and jam, as well as two cigarettes. I can remember that some disagreement arose between the camp administration and the Air Force authorities concerned, as the latter did not make enough victuals available for the diet. The sufferers from this dispute were naturally the subjects who had undergone the experiments.'

He added later, *inter alia*:

[DOC. Beiglböck 32.]

'I know for certain of two prisoners who reported voluntarily for the tests. They were Dachau men, German gipsies who had been relieved of duty in the so-called punishment squad on account of having participated in the experiment. I think the others were also "volunteers", because when Beiglböck found out that some of the gipsies had been drinking water he flew into a rage and reproached them with having first reported for the tests and then disobeyed the rules while under experiment. . . .

I am of opinion that there were no true volunteers in the camp, even if they had been induced by promises to report for the tests, so as to obtain some alleviation of their unhappy position. I am bound to assume this from my personal acquaintance over a period of years with the sufferings undergone in the camp. It is, however, quite likely that Beiglböck, who was ignorant of the conditions at the camp, believed that he was dealing with true volunteers.

He treated the patients well, in striking contrast with the way in which the SS men in the camp dealt with us prisoners. Beiglböck really only lost his temper when the gipsies lied to him about their water-drinking and he detected the fact when he examined their blood-samples. He used his influence on behalf of Taubmann and his friend, the other German gipsy, and also arranged for the transfer of the French doctors from the labour blocks to service in the sick bay.'

The results permitted a practical solution of the main problem. Beiglböck himself commented:

[PROT. p. 8890 f.]

'It was proved that in cases of normal thirst a greater quantity of sea-water was of no advantage and might sometimes be actually disadvantageous. It also appeared that kidney concentration capacity was far higher than had hitherto been assumed. It might rise in practice, in any one case, to about 2·4 per cent and often to 3 per cent and more. This capacity was not substantially affected by the administration of vitamins. It was also found that sea-water taken at dispersed intervals did not bring on diarrhoea. The subjective phenomena occurring after drinking salt water, that is to say, feelings of thirst, closely resembled those of thirst in normal conditions. But objectively the administration of small quantities of liquid, even if salt, has the best effect. It was established that even minute quantities of fresh water drunk at intervals were extraordinarily beneficial. The Schäfer specific produced perfectly acceptable drinking-water, while the Berka proved unserviceable. . . .

I am aware that these experiments did not demonstrate so much as might have been expected if the subjects had co-operated correctly, mainly because the data they afforded were distorted by their drinking of fresh water, kidney concentration capacity in particular being thus liable to much variation. Strictly scientific evaluation of the tests was therefore only possible to a very limited extent. But results were sufficient to enable us to come to a practical decision. And the principle thereby discovered agreed with what was later recognized by British and American scientists, viz. that small quantities of sea-water are to be preferred to no water at all.'

In a discussion with Professor Ivy he admitted that he would not have been able to give an account of the tests in a scientific periodical.

Schröder was sentenced to imprisonment for life, the Tribunal declaring that he had also been responsible for other experiments on human beings. Becker-Freyseng was given twenty years and Beiglböck fifteen.

The final plea on behalf of the accused included certain affidavits additional to the evidence already before the court. They had not been available during the taking of testimony. The statements were signed by two subjects who had swallowed 500 cubic centimetres of sea-water, one who had swallowed 1,000 cubic centimetres, and one other subject. All four declared that they were volunteers. One affidavit swore to the voluntary consent of all the other participants. An exceptional statement was made by a French medical student, a prisoner in the Dachau camp who had acted as a male nurse at the experimental station. He referred to Beiglböck's attitude as 'consistently irreproachable' and added, *inter alia*:

'The nature of the proposed experiments was explained to all the gipsies on their arrival at the centre. They were put on a copious and rich diet for some days. Then they were examined to see whether they were physically capable of undergoing the experiments. Throughout the tests they were kept under close observation by Professor Beiglböck. I can state positively that none of them died during the experiments, that they were given plenty of food for a considerable time after termination of the tests and that they were all in good, sound physical condition when they left the centre. ... I can also state with equal confidence that on the advice of a professional oculist— also a prisoner—who checked the posterior part of the retina in each subject Professor Beiglböck brought the experiments to an end prematurely, thus sparing the subjects further discomfort and also, what was more important, preventing possible future ill effects or injury.'

The Tribunal, as explained in its General Principles, only pronounced a defendant guilty when there was not the slightest doubt that experiments had been carried out on unwilling subjects. The fact that they had been undertaken in a concentration camp did not influence the verdict, as is proved by the acquittals granted in the case of the low pressure tests. Accordingly, the declarations of voluntary consent submitted after Judgment had been pronounced should probably be checked in relation to the whole question of the sea-water experiments. The affidavits seem to render it doubtful whether the definition of these tests as of a 'characteristically criminal nature' can be upheld. If so Judgment would appear to require revision in this case.[1]

1. Several eminent scientists and doctors submitted their views of the Dachau sea-water experiments to the German Domestic Medical Congress. In May 1948 the Congress appointed a committee under the chairmanship of Professor Oehme of Heidelberg, assisted by Professor Heilmeyer of Freiburg and Professor Schoen of Göttingen, 'to investigate the question whether, from the standpoints of medical science and ethics, the sea-water experiments should be regarded as "of a characteristically criminal nature" and consequently as war crimes and crimes against humanity, with the result

CHAPTER THREE

TYPHUS VACCINE EXPERIMENTS

TYPHUS experiments on human beings are proved to have taken place in Germany during the war at two places, the concentration camps at Buchenwald and at Natzweiler (Struthof).

A. Data concerning the typhus experiments at Buchenwald were obtained for the most part from the diary kept at the experimental station of the SS Hauptsturmführer Dr Ding-Schuler, who worked at the camp, as well as from the evidence of several European scientists, prisoners in the camp, and of Dr Eugen Kogon, who was examined by the prosecution at the trial on the 6 and 7 January. He was responsible for recovery of the diary, having acted as Dr Ding-Schuler's station clerk. The 'Department for Typhus and Virus Research', run by Dr Ding-Schuler at the camp, was part of the Institute of Hygiene of the *Waffen* (Military Branch) of the SS in Berlin, headed by SS Oberführer Professor Mrugowsky, one of the accused.

A typhus station was first set up at Buchenwald in order to produce, as ordered by the SS Dr Grawitz, Senior State Physician, a 'special SS vaccine' for the protection of the SS troops in the East against typhus. The Institute was established in a concentration camp so that foreign scientists imprisoned there could be employed in the work. They included Professor Ludwig Fleck of Lemberg, Professor Balachowsky of the Pasteur Institute in Paris, Professor van Lingen of Amsterdam and others.

---

that the Judgment pronounced should be maintained.' The committee took full account of all the material produced at the trial and based their conclusion upon careful consideration of the ten governing principles of the Tribunal. Their general inference was that 'mistakes were made in the method of choice and recruitment of subjects' and in the selection of a concentration camp as an experimental station, but that such mistakes did not constitute crimes. The report added: 'Not one of the subjects suffered any injury, in spite of the fact that their freedom of choice in the matter left something to be desired.' The report was dispatched to General L. D. Clay, the American Military Governor of Occupied Germany.

At first, however, the Institute did not concentrate on developing the 'special SS vaccine' but on checking those already available. This process was carried on at Block 46 of the camp.

Two discussions at the Ministry of the Interior on the 29 December 1941 preceded the organization of the station.[1] One of the conferences had been called to lay down regulations for production of the vaccine. But opinions differed as to the value of the various vaccines concerned and no agreement could be reached. Professor Gildemeister stated that during the discussion 'a proposed plan for experiment in collaboration with Dr Mrugowsky was rejected.' [DOC. Mrugowsky 63.]

Methods of work and location were not mentioned. The second conference, held on the same day and attended by Dr Conti, Secretary of State for Hygiene in the Ministry of the Interior, Dr Linden, Professor Gildemeister and Professor Reiter among others, continued to debate the problem of typhus. According to a sworn statement by Professor Reiter experiments in infection were advocated by Conti, who in doing so exchanged

[DOC. 265.]

'significant looks with Dr Linden of the Ministry of the Interior, who was present, and I had the impression at that time that neither of these two gentlemen intended to respect the views of the opposition, but would favour experiment by infection.'

At Conti's suggestion the whole business was handed over to the SS for organization, whereupon Dr Grawitz, in agreement with Himmler, ordered the experiments to be carried out.

The following example, taken from the series of tests, incidentally shows Dr Ding-Schuler to have been associated with the experiments.

'6 January 1942:*
1 February 1942:*

    1. Dr Ding-Schuler made notes [Doc. 265] about one of these discussions on the introductory page of the Experiments Diary. But they have been left out of account, as he himself was not present at the meeting and his enumeration of those who attended it does not agree with that in other relevant documents.

TYPHUS VACCINE, RESEARCH SERIES 1

Vaccination for immunization against typhus using the following vaccines:

1. Thirty-one persons with Weigl vaccine from the intestines of lice from the Institute for Typhus and Virus Research of the Army High Command, Krakow.

2. Thirty-five persons with vaccine from vitelline membrane cultures made by the Cox, Gildemeister, and Haagen process.

3. Thirty-five persons with vaccine "Behring Normal" (one egg in an emulsion of 450 c.c. vaccine. Mixture of 70 per cent Rickettsia Mooseri and 30 per cent Rickettsia-Prowazeki).

4. Thirty-four persons with "Behring Normal" "Behring Strong" (one egg emulsified in 250 c.c. solvent).

5. Ten persons for control.

3 March 1942:

All persons vaccinated for immunization between 6 January 1942 and 1 February 1942, and the ten control persons were infected with a virus culture of Rickettsia-Prowazeki in the presence of Professor Gildemeister. SS Haupsturmführer Dr Ding infected himself in the process (laboratory accident).

17 March 1942:

Visit of Professor Gildemeister and Professor Rose (Head of the Department for Tropical Medicine in the Robert Koch Institute) to the experimental station. All persons experimented on fell sick with typhus.

19 April 1942:

Final report on the 1st typhus vaccine research series:
Five deaths (three control persons, one "Behring Normal", and one "Behring Strong").[1]
Professor Rose, giving evidence on his own behalf, described the visit he paid to Buchenwald at the time, together with the circumstances that preceded and followed it, in these terms:

[1]. It is interesting to find that these facts, including Dr Erwin Ding's infection, are given in the version intended for the public. (See *Zeitschrift für Hygiene und Infections-krankheiten*, Vol. 124, 1943, p. 670 ff.)

[PROT. p. 6231 ff.]

'During a visit to the Robert Koch Institute, probably at the beginning of March 1942, I looked up Professor Gilde-meister ... he told me that on the initiative of Dr Conti the prophylactic efficacy of the various typhus vaccines was to be tested in comparative experiments on human beings at the Buchenwald concentration camp near Weimar. He said that this was to be done on account of the irreconcilable differences of opinion on the merits of the different manufacturing processes concerned. He added that the experiments were to be performed on criminals sentenced to death. I was much surprised at this information and expressed my disapproval with considerable warmth. I said I thought such plans would prejudice deliveries of the vaccines to be tested, and that I considered experiments on animals adequate even in relation to typhus. I exclaimed angrily that if this example were followed we might as well hand over all questions of immunization to public executioners and start a school for these gentry in the Institute as soon as possible. Gildemeister was obviously annoyed at the pointed way in which I had rejected the idea, especially as our personal relations were not friendly. He informed me that he had been invited to inspect the place at which the experiments were to be carried out in Buchenwald and that before I took such a tone I had better go there myself and see what was to be done and how the tests would be conducted. . . .

A few days later I accompanied Gildemeister, by train, to Weimar and thence by car to Buchenwald. We were met by a doctor who took us to the sick bay, this building being separated by barbed wire from the rest of the camp. We were shown a number of different departments. I cannot now remember the name of the doctor who guided us nor those of the other persons who were introduced to me at Buchenwald. But I am sure that he was not Dr Ding. For we were told that he was himself ill with typhus, having infected himself during the experiments. The doctor who accompanied us explained that various groups had been first treated with different typhus vaccines and subsequently infected with the virus. But one group had been infected without previous vaccination. The patients in this group looked very ill indeed. Their whole ward was typical of those reserved for serious cases of typhus elsewhere. In the other wards the overall impression was one of lighter cases. We then went to the laboratory, where we were shown the patients' fever charts. The curves already indicated very clearly, as had the wards, the difference in the course of the disease with and without vaccination. Since it is extraordinarily difficult to compare 140 curves by eye alone, the people at work in this ward prepared, overnight, average curves based on the individual curves of patients in the various groups. We examined these average curves the following morning. They showed even more clearly the difference already noted. We were lodged in a hut outside the camp. Next day we inspected the patients again. On this occasion the doctor in charge of the hospital showed us two prisoners belonging to the unvaccinated group who had not fallen ill. The doctors taking part in the experiment had at first been greatly surprised by this fact. For all the 120 or so persons who had been vaccinated were sick. But a further investigation of the medical history of the two prisoners concerned revealed that they had suffered from typhus while imprisoned in Berlin awaiting sentence. On their first interrogation at Buchenwald they had described this illness as influenza. The doctor added that this discovery had originally caused much vexation, because the reason for selecting German criminals only to undergo the experiments had been the probability that criminals from the East had already once suffered from the disease. It had been supposed that in the case of Germans this possibility could be ignored. But it turned out that the two men who had not been ill were of great value in the subsequent assessment of the results of the experiment. For their cases proved that natural immunity to artificial infection was effective, while none of the vaccines had afforded any protection. The vaccines had merely imparted a decisive mitigation to the course of the disease and prevented a fatal outcome.

    ... After my return to Berlin ... I called on the Secretary of State (Dr Conti), gave him a brief account of what I had seen and added that I had not called to discuss the details of the experiment with him but rather the fundamental problems of a general character involved. Professor Gildemeister had told me that the experiments had been performed at Conti's suggestion. I represented to the latter that experiments on human beings were no novelty in themselves but that in this case the adoption of the vaccines was to be made dependent on their effect on the human organism. This experiment therefore differed from all others of its kind in risking men's lives. The question of vaccine testing had been before hygienists for forty years and the accepted method of procedure was to check tolerance by the organism and the protective effect of such inoculations by experiment on animals. If such experiments turned out satisfactorily, the next step was to test tolerance by human beings and thus determine the doses required. In this process serum was used in order to establish from dermal changes the nature of the transformation induced. The line was drawn there, although it was perfectly well known that no reliable criterion could be acquired by such means. For the rest, the automatic grouping of the patients would show the epidemiological position, which could be assessed by comparison of vaccinated with unvaccinated groups. Artificial infection has of course been practised occasionally for centuries. But it never involved danger to human life. So complete a divergence from hitherto accepted procedure caused me to feel it necessary that such authorities on typhus as Professor Gildemeister, Otto Eyer, Haagen, Bickhardt, Bieling and Wohlrab should at least have been asked beforehand whether they considered so serious a step absolutely essential. . . . Conti replied that he, too, had not decided upon this measure without very careful reflection. But he added that the gravity of the menace of typhus necessitated extraordinary and unprecedented action.

He said that in occupied Poland a serious epidemic of typhus had already broken out, while Germany itself had been affected by the disease to a considerable extent owing to the influx of Russian prisoners of war. Local epidemics were already in evidence in all the German camps and prisons. As for conditions in the Army, he was sure I knew them better than he did. But even he had heard extraordinarily disturbing rumours. The experience of the last war proved that hundreds of thousands of men's lives were at stake. It was he, therefore, as Secretary of State, not the scientists, who must bear the responsibility for the steps that must be taken. In view of this calamity he had been obliged to set aside the scruples which he, in common with myself, had felt. He could not afford to wait for epidemiological statistics which might not make the matter clear for years or even, depending on what happened, for decades.

Such delay was unacceptable when the opportunity existed to discover the right way to save hundreds of thousands of lives by risking so few. He declared that he was as good a doctor as I was and put an equally high value on human life. But in wartime, when millions of our best men, of wholly innocent character, had to sacrifice their lives, those who injured the community had also to be required to make their contribution to the common good. As for the objection I had raised, that the opinions of specialists should have been obtained direct, he had considered it sufficient to consult his own staff in the matter. He would, however, be very ready in future to bear my suggestion in mind should the appropriate circumstances arise. . . .

I am bound to admit at this point that, as the subsequent experiment proved beyond doubt, my assumption in what I said to Conti at that time was erroneous. For the tests at Buchenwald certainly made a most important and new contribution to the knowledge we had already acquired by experiment.'

He also touched upon the question whence the many criminals under sentence of death were obtained.

[PROT. p. 6242.]

'*Defence Counsel:* I should like to put another question in connection with your visit to Buchenwald itself. Did you not wonder at that time whence so great a number of criminals sentenced to death had been obtained? Were there not nearly 150 of them?

Professor Rose: In view of subsequent events the question appears perfectly natural. But the answer was given to me at that time from a source which I considered absolutely trustworthy. I had no reason to doubt it then. With regard to the figure quoted, one has to remember that we were living in those days under martial law. Many special regulations were then in force and so many offences were punishable with death that I was not in the least surprised at the numbers of men under capital sentence. I can give some examples of such cases. They included crimes committed under cover of darkness, profiteering in foodstuffs on a fairly large scale, serious cases of illicit slaughtering of cattle, looting in the course of air-raids, refusal of military service, espionage and much else. Nor was the slightest hint ever dropped in Buchenwald that the subjects of the experiments were long-established prisoners in the camp.'

Rose also gave good reason to suppose that Professor Gildemeister, too, was not conversant with all the phases of the experiments carried out at Buchenwald, since these soon became exclusively the affair of the SS Institute of Hygiene. [PROT. p. 6247 ff.]

We append a summary, based on Dr Ding-Schuler's station diary, of all the vaccine tests performed. (See Table 1.)

After vaccination, subjects were artificially infected with fresh blood from diseased persons or with the cultivated virus produced by the Rickettsia-Prowazek process.

The figures in this diary were stubbornly contested by the defence, intelligibly enough, since at first it was the only piece of documentary evidence which incriminated five of the accused. Handwriting experts thought it doubtful whether entries had been made literally every day. The document as produced may have been a fair copy, in which, however, all the entries were countersigned by Dr Ding-Schuler himself. But the experiments as noted in the diary were corroborated by many other documents and statements. Consequently there could be no doubt about its evidential value.

The third business meeting of Army medical consultants was held in the Hygiene Section in May 1943. Dr Ding-Schuler addressed it on the subject of 'Recent Tests of Various Vaccines against Classical Typhus'. A summary of the lecture is contained in the report on the meeting preserved in the Academy of Military Medicine, Berlin, p. 108. At the close of the lecture, which gave a veiled account of the experiments, Professor Rose protested to the assembly against the use of human beings for such tests. He was aware, of course, of the true state of affairs. Rose was interrupted by the chairman, Professor Schreiber.

TABLE I

Typhus Vaccine Experiments

Subjects artificially infected		Subjects taken ill	Deaths	
Vaccinated by the under-mentioned processes	Not vaccinated (checking personnel)		Vaccinated subjects	Checking personnel
Weigl 31				
Cox–Gildemeister–Haagen 35	10	143		3
Behring normal 35			1	
Behring strong 34			1	
Durand and Giroud 20	19	59		4
Combiescu and Zotta 20				
Giroud 20	6			
Weigl 25	10	5		
Zürich 20	—	—	—	—
Riga 20	—	—	—	—
Asid 20	10	70	18	8
Asid Adsorbat 20			18	
Weigl 20			9	
Kopenhagen (Ipsen) 17	9	26	3	3
Weimar 5	5	20	1	3
Giroud 5				
Asid 5			1	
Weimar 20	20	60		19
Weigl 20			5	
Total 392	89	383	57	40

[PROT. p. 6252.]

'Schreiber said he would have to take exception to the kind of criticism I was expressing and added that if those present wanted to talk about fundamental moral questions they could do so during the interval.'

Professor Walter Schnell wrote in a sworn statement:

[DOC. Rose 6.]

'We all felt the warmest sympathy for Rose's indignation when, during the questions that were asked and answered immediately afterwards, it was quietly whispered among those present that the experiments mentioned had probably taken place in a concentration camp.'

The defendant Mrugowsky, to Rose's surprise, approached him after the protest had been made and said he was of the same opinion. But Mrugowsky was at that time one of the links in the chain of command responsible for the Buchenwald experiments. Under cross-examination by the prosecution he made the following statements:

[PROT. p. 5500.]

'*Prosecuting Counsel*: After these expressions of disapproval and by the time it was plain to everyone present that concentration camp inmates had been used, did anyone make any attempt to stop further experiments being carried out at Buchenwald?

Professor Mrugowsky: I can't say that anyone did, in my presence. No one approached me. But I heard from Herr Rose that many of his listeners had discussed the question of admissibility with him. He mentions the fact, incidentally, in the affidavit he gave me, which is in my file here. I don't know whether any objection was lodged with any competent authority, represented in this case by Grawitz or by Ding himself. But it is possible that the matter was discussed with Ding. For Ding was very worried for some days after the meeting.

Q. So no one present interfered with what Ding was doing or made any attempt to stop his work, with the result that on the 27 August 1943 Ding started a further series of experiments in which fifty-three persons perished. But no one bothered about it, I suppose? Is that so?

A. I don't quite know what Counsel means to imply by "stop". If anyone intends to stop anything he must be in a position to do so. For my part, if I hear of a murder committed by anyone in some other city, it doesn't follow that I approve it because I was never in a position to stop it, since it had been committed before I heard of it. Nor would I be able to stop the man committing more murders. All I can do is not to commit any murders myself. Not one of those present at the meeting was in a position to exercise any influence on the course of events. And I must ask you to believe me when I say that neither Himmler nor Grawitz would have allowed any-one to have any voice in the decisions they reached. It was not possible in Germany for people to get an immediate favourable hearing for expressions of opinion. For when any of the responsible higher authorities had once determined upon a certain course of action, he never cancelled the orders he had given. I had a very great deal of rather regrettable experience myself in that way in my relations with my chief Grawitz.

Q. We shall not discuss any further the opportunities Mrug-owsky had to intervene. It is perfectly obvious from the orders given, the reports in the diary and the whole of the evidence in the case that he could have intervened if he had wished.'

Rose's attitude was also supported by others at the meeting. Professor Höring, a witness for the defence, stated:

[PROT. pp. 6168 f. and 6158 f.]

'Professor Rose pointed out in somewhat pungent language that such procedure was a departure from that which had been customary and approved for decades in research on immuniza-tion. He said the matter was extremely serious and that hygienists should stand by their traditional principles. He spoke for rather a long time, pretty sharply. ... At any rate it is certain that everyone present was made clearly aware that something, one might almost say, sensational had occurred. Accordingly, even after the meeting was over and also during the following days small groups continued to discuss the affair, as I well remember.

Defence Counsel: Well, what happened after Professor Rose had finished speaking? I mean, during the subsequent discussion?

A. The lecturer, Dr Ding, replied to Professor Rose and defended the experiments. He admitted that they had been carried out on human beings but said that all the subjects without exception were criminals sentenced to death. Rose retorted once more that this fact made no difference to his criticism of the proceedings. For the question at issue, he said, was one of principle. Further discussion was then ruled out, rather suddenly, by Professor Schreiber.

Prosecuting Counsel: Were you surprised by Professor Rose's protest?

A. It was a surprise to me, certainly.

Q. Would you have considered it possible that Professor Rose would later on have sent vaccines for testing at Buchenwald?

A. No.

Q. You were sure, then, that Rose regarded these experiments at Buchenwald as, more or less, scientific murder?

A. I certainly was.'

Nevertheless, the prosecution, after prolonged examination of the witnesses and the reading of original letters signed by Rose himself, were able to prove that he had been responsible, seven months after the incident with Dr Ding-Schuler, for a series of experiments at Buchenwald which caused six deaths. The incriminating letter read as follows:

[DOC. 1186.]*

'Oberstarzt Professor Rose,

O.U., 2 December, 1943

To Standartenfuehrer Dr Mrugowsky,
    Head of the Hygiene Institute of the Waffen SS
    Berlin-Zehlendorf 6
    Spanische Allee 10
Dear Herr Mrugowsky,

At present I have at my disposal a number of samples of a new murine virus typhus vaccine which was prepared from mice livers and proved in animal experiments to be quanti-

tatively a thousand times more effective than the vaccine prepared from mice lungs. In order to decide whether this first-rate
murine vaccine should be used for protective vaccination of
human beings against lice typhus, it would be desirable to
know if this vaccine showed in yours and Ding's experimental
arrangement at Buchenwald an effect similar to that of the
classic virus vaccines. Would you be able to have such an
experimental series carried out? Unfortunately, I could not
reach you over the phone. Considering the slowness of postal
communications I would be grateful for an answer by telephone. My numbers, all of which go through the same switch-
board, are: Berlin 278313; Rapid Exchange Berlin 90, Zossen
559; Luftwaffe Exchange 72, there you ask for RLM, L In 14.
    With best regards,

                                        Heil Hitler!
                                        Yours,
                                        Rose'

    The following letter shows what was subsequently arranged.

[DOC. 1188.]

'Reichsführer SS and Chief of Police
SS Administration Head Office
Group D. Concentration Camps
Telephone Sammel 3171   Oranienburg, near
Dictation Reference: Berlin
Group D III/Az.87/2.44 Dr Lg K.   14 February 1944
In reply quote without fail: Secret
Geh. Tgb.Nr.21/44 Ko.   Z.d.A.
Subject: Test of Typhus Vaccine.
Ref. Letter of 26.1.44. Tgb. Nr.82/44.Dr Mru Schm.
Enc. None.
To   Stamp.
Reich Physician SS and   Received 21 February 1944
Police   C 4   D
From Head Hygienist
Berlin-Zehlendorf, Spanische Allee 10
Copy to Reich Physician SS and Police.
    The approval requested for testing the protective effect
of a Danish vaccine on thirty prisoners is granted by SS

I

Obergruppenführer and Waffen SS General Pohl, Head of the SS Central Office, on condition that experiments are limited to gipsies.

Thirty suitable gipsies will accordingly be transferred shortly to the Typhus Research Institute at Buchenwald.

(*Signed*) CALLING

Chief of Medical Serice, SS Administration

Head Office and Director of Group D III,

SS Standartenführer.

Copy sent on 21.2.44
to SS-Staf. Dr Mrugowsky.'

Dr Ding-Schuler's station diary for the period 8 March to 13 June 1944 reports the performance of the experiments.

[DOC. 265.]*

'8 March to 18 March 1944: At the suggestion of Colonel of the air corps, Professor Rose, the vaccine "Kopenhagen", produced from mouse liver by the National Serum Institute in Kopenhagen, was tested for its protective effect on humans. Twenty persons were vaccinated for immunization by intramuscular injection ... Ten persons were provided for control and comparison, four of these thirty persons dropped out, owing to illness contracted meanwhile, before artificial infection started.

16 April 1944: The remaining experimental persons were infected on 16 April by subcutaneous injection of 1/20 c.c. typhus sick fresh blood. The following fell sick out of seventeen persons immunized: nine medium, eight seriously. Of the nine persons for control: two medium, seven seriously.

13 June 1944: Chart and case history completed and sent to Berlin. Six deaths (three "Kopenhagen") (three control).'

After the prosecution's witnesses had testified, Rose stated under cross-examination:

[PROT. p. 6568.]

'I was of course aware that earlier experiments of the kind had been performed, though I had declared myself in principle against them. The establishments in question accordingly existed in Germany. They were sanctioned and protected by the State. I therefore found myself in the position at this time of, let us say, a lawyer who disapproves in principle of capital punishment and the death sentence. Such a man would take every opportunity to advocate his views whenever he was able to discuss the question with Government officials or at public meetings of jurists. If he is not successful in his advocacy, he still remains a lawyer among lawyers and may even be obliged under certain circumstances himself to pronounce sentence of death, though he may be in principle against such an institution. Personally, I was not driven to such extremities. I merely associated with certain people whom I assumed to have been somehow professionally involved in organizations to which I objected in principle and which I wished to be abolished.'

At a later hearing Rose added, in reply to his defence counsel:

[PROT. p. 6579 f.]

'Well, the result of this experiment of course appears in Ding's diary and it showed that the vaccine in question seemed to be in all respects superior to the lung vaccine which had been used on animals but proved to be inapplicable to human beings. Such is the statement in Ding's diary and such was the result of his experiment. So as the practical result of one experiment, the Ipsen vaccine which I had urgently recommended for use in September 1943 was not taken into regular use. That was a very important decision. For if the Ipsen vaccine had been employed, it would naturally have been applied to a considerable extent in serious cases, since it was two and a half times as effective as the lung vaccines we were using. It is, of course, impossible to say for certain today how many people would have died as a result of the use of this unserviceable vaccine which I had recommended. But there can be no doubt that the figure would have been very substantially higher than actually occurred. My responsibility as hygienist for so many deaths in consequence of the use of a vaccine which I had recommended but which was really unserviceable would have been much heavier. For the figures would have been, furthermore, considerably higher than those due to the share of responsibility which can be attributed to me in law for having consented to the experiment and allowed it to be performed on persons duly designated by the public authorities concerned, as is clear from the papers submitted by the prosecution.'

Judgment dealt explicitly with these observations by Rose concerning the 'due designation' of subjects by the State authorities.

[Judgment p. 194 ff.]*

'Doubtless at the outset of the experimental programme launched in the concentration camps, Rose may have voiced some vigorous opposition. In the end, however, he overcame what scruples he had and knowingly took an active and consenting part in the programme. He attempts to justify his actions on the ground that a State may validly order experiments to be carried out on persons condemned to death without regard to the fact that such persons may refuse to consent to submit themselves as experimental subjects. This defence entirely misses the point of the dominant issue. As we have pointed out in the case of Gebhardt, whatever may be the condition of the law with reference to medical experiments conducted by or through a state upon its own citizens, such a thing will not be sanctioned in international law when practised upon citizens or subjects of an occupied territory.

We have indulged every presumption in favour of the defendant, but his position lacks substance in the face of the overwhelming evidence against him. His own consciousness of turpitude is clearly disclosed by the statement made by him, at the close of a vigorous cross-examination, in the following language:

"It was known to me that such experiments had earlier been carried out, although I basically objected to these experiments. This institution had been set up in Germany and was approved by the state and covered by the state. At that moment I was in a position which perhaps corresponds to a lawyer who is, perhaps, a basic opponent of execution or death sentence. On occasion when he is dealing with leading members of the government, or with lawyers during public congresses or meetings, he will do everything in his power to maintain his opinion on the subject and have it put into effect. If, however, he does not succeed, he stays in his profession and in his environment in spite of this. Under circumstances he may perhaps even be forced to pronounce such a death sentence himself, although he is basically an opponent of that set-up."

The Tribunal finds that the defendant Rose was a principal in, accessory to, ordered, abetted, took a consenting part in, and was connected with plans and enterprises involving medical experiments on non-German nationals without their consent, in the course of which murders, brutalities, cruelties, tortures, atrocities, and other inhuman acts were committed. To the extent that these crimes were not war crimes they were crimes against humanity.'

It was also proved that in 1942, and accordingly before the incident at the meeting just referred to, Rose had suggested another series of experiments which took place, like the series he had objected to, at Buchenwald. This additional series involved four deaths. He was sentenced to life imprisonment.

The motive for these experiments suggested by Rose was quite different from the circumstances which had occasioned the tests on human beings described above. In the latter case it was a question of blocking the ravages of an epidemic which had broken out in the course of the war. In the 1942 case considerations of the more effective use of a new weapon were involved. The State itself, therefore, not individual doctors, gave the first impetus to the start of these last experiments. In order to enable the reader to acquire a thorough understanding of the scientific and legal background, we quote some further passages from the record of Rose's replies to his defence counsel, in which he was given ample opportunity to justify his behaviour. They are followed by an extract from the 'Closing Brief' of his Defence Counsel which is concerned to stress the 'conflicting obligations' to which his client was exposed.

[PROT. p. 6266 ff.]

'*Professor Rose:* You have put a crucial question in inquiring what my motives were throughout this complicated affair.

General Taylor also referred to this demand in his opening speech. I quote from p. 55 of the German record: "It is our duty to make crystal-clear the ideas and motives which determined the conduct of the accused. . . ."

I agree with Prosecuting Counsel that this is one of the most important elements in the trial and I should therefore like to reply in detail to the question. In so doing I shall not only state what I myself thought on the subject but also what is known to me personally of the motives which influenced such of the scientists involved as are now dead and so unable to answer for themselves.

You have asked why I protested against experiments on criminals sentenced to death. I knew, of course, that such experiments had already been made. But my attitude in the matter was much affected by a number of considerations which I clearly recognized. In the first place the phrase "criminals sentenced to death" arises in the last analysis from a purely emotional reaction. For jurists and many others who are accustomed to think conventionally the problem may appear rather a simple one. If a man is legally sentenced to death, the matter is necessarily settled so far as they are concerned. The jurist studies the legal principle and in so doing has to bear a heavy responsibility for his decision. But when he has decided the affair is at an end for him and the sentence must be carried out. I, however, am not a jurist. I have a rather different approach to the matter. I have been around enough to know how extraordinarily precarious and relative legal judgments may be.

They not only vary from country to country and from nation to nation. They may undergo complete change in a very short time within a single country. This may happen even in ordinary times of peace. But it is still more liable to occur in periods politically disturbed and affected by war, when people are often punished for "crimes" which thousands of others regard as deeds of special heroism.

Secondly, as I told Ding when he declared that criminals under sentence of death were the subjects of his experiments, the question was one of professional principle for me as a hygienist and immunization research worker. I have already explained our normal proceeding in making new vaccines available. Their tolerance was always finally tested on human beings for the simple reason that no conclusion could be drawn from animal experiment, though there were of course some exceptions, such as that described in Herr Bieling's affidavit, when human beings were actually infected in order to test the protective efficacy of a vaccine.[1] But these cases remained exceptional and so far as I could see at that time they took place exclusively abroad. As a hygienist and immunization research worker I did not want the practice introduced into Germany, where I felt it would create a bad precedent. Naturally I did not underestimate the special current emergency in connection with these typhus vaccines. But I shall return to this point when I come to discuss the technical aspect of the experiments.

I am here concerned with their moral aspect. I was afraid that once a start had been made with this method of testing typhus vaccines we should very soon be asked to apply it to other vaccines in connection with different problems. As a technician in this field I am only too well aware what a tremendous advantage it would be to research if human beings could be made available for experiment whenever required. But however deeply convinced I might be intellectually of such an advantage to science, I was equally deeply opposed to it emotionally. I was guided by the well known axiom, *Principiis non obsta*.[2] If one does not resist such developments as soon as they arise, it will be impossible ever to control them. That was my second point.

Thirdly, a purely practical reflection occurred to me. Since 1921 I have studied experimental medicine in the most diverse countries and am well aware of the prejudices against my profession and the very subject of physiology. Very large sections of the public abused us as unfeeling tormentors of animals, simply because the science of immunization and physiology had to experiment to a great extent on living animals or give up work

1. In this affidavit [Doc. Rose 23] certain foreign influenza vaccine tests are described. They comprised the artificial infection of immunized subjects and unvaccinated checking personnel with living influenza virus. But they differed from the Buchenwald experiments, as is stated in the affidavit, in being 'clearly explained to the scientific world', in being applied to volunteers and in being 'in complete accord with the views of responsible physicians'.

2. The quotation should read *Principiis obsta*, 'Resist the first attack'. The misquotation exactly describes the position!

altogether. Well, I thought, if ever that prejudice is reinforced by one far greater against tests on human beings, my profession will be called upon to bear a very much heavier burden.

My fourth point was psychological.

Mr McHaney, the Prosecuting Counsel, stated in his discussion of Professor Hippke's attitude to the supercooling experiments—I quote:

"As soon as Hippke learned that the subjects were to be criminals under sentence of death, he felt that all was well and he need have no scruples."

In my opinion this statement by Mr McHaney shows a complete misunderstanding of the psychological factors which played a decisive part in the consideration of this problem. I have already suggested that the legal attitude may be different. A jurist bears a heavy professional responsibility in pronouncing the death sentence, and also when, as Prosecuting Counsel, he proposes it. But once the sentence has been pronounced the matter is settled so far as he is concerned and he exclaims *Fiat Justitia!* A fanatical scientist, too, who cares for nothing but science, may come to the same conclusion, that sentence of death has been passed and it no longer matters whether the condemned man is hanged or perishes under medical experiment. But those who are neither jurists nor scientific fanatics are influenced by different and very important considerations. I had seen the advanced state of the disease in checking personnel at Buchenwald who had not been infected and it made a permanent impression on me.

I happened to have spoken to Holzlöhner after his lecture at Nuremberg on supercooling. The story was not clear to me in detail after his speech and I therefore asked him to give me an account of the whole experiment. His reply showed me what a tremendous psychological burden the conduct of these tests had laid upon a doctor like Professor Holzlöhner. For even a man sentenced to death still remains a human being, capable of suffering. . . .

My fifth consideration was one of which it might perhaps be said that it was merely professional egotism and had little to do with professional morality. All the same, it did operate as one of the motives influencing me. It is generally recognized, after all, that only the most important experiments are carried out on human beings. Many scientists would avoid being involved in such tests, even when officially sanctioned, simply because they did not feel that they would have the strength of mind to carry them out. As a result, there is always a risk of the most vital research falling into the hands of cold fanatics, not the most satisfactory representatives of our profession. This reflection is admittedly of little moral account. But it naturally played its part in forming the final decision. The problem of fanaticism in medical research is an old one, as is proved by a reference to Moll's book, cited by Leibbrand, one of the witnesses for the prosecution. I quote from p. 757:

> "If a medical man is particularly devoted to research, he is more or less inclined to take that point of view in his attitude to his patients, too ready, in fact, to use them in helping him to solve a scientific problem, so that he tends to neglect their personal interests. This conflict between professional duty and the promotion of scientific knowledge has already been discussed in French literature, where a doctor is described who sacrifices his patients solely for the benefit of the science he idolizes."

So fanaticism in research is by no means a novelty, for these words were written in 1900.

I was concerned above all with the considerations that weighed with doctors in their treatment of such problems of experiment, including that of fanatical research, with its inherent risk to professional obligation. The whole question is illustrated, for doctors who have to make these experiments, by a well known historical episode. On the introduction to Europe of the oriental system of inoculation for smallpox, i.e. variolation, not vaccination, King George I ordered the process to be tested on six criminals sentenced to death. Maitland, the Embassy doctor charged with the experiment, refused to carry it out. He was not troubled by any moral scruples about the fate of the subjects, but by the purely personal reflection that he might be regarded as the executioner's assistant if the test had a fatal outcome. His refusal was therefore motivated solely by fear for his own reputation. He had no desire to infringe upon the executioner's domain.

In speaking just now of research fanatics I did not of course mean to imply that any doctor who agrees to experiment on human beings must be supposed a cold, unfeeling fanatic of this kind. That would be entirely wrong, for I am personally acquainted with very many research scientists of different nationalities who have performed experiments on both voluntary and involuntary subjects. So I have a pretty clear idea of the psychological strain to which men so engaged are exposed and what heavy burdens they assume in undertaking the task.

I am bound to represent this aspect of the tests in question to the Prosecution and the Tribunal. For their members are in the fortunate position, as jurists, of never having been confronted with such psychological strains, though of course their own profession also bears a heavy responsibility. There would not be much point in my instancing cases from the course of the present trial. For it would be difficult to draw an impartial picture of the true state of affairs from the experiences of these people. I shall therefore take an example which has a special claim to consideration as being the scientific basis and direct forerunner of the proceeding for which I am here made responsible. I refer to the first experiment in connection with the development of vaccination with live bacteria, actually plague bacteria. If you consult the relative papers at a later stage, you will find that these tests were performed on criminals sentenced to death and not, moreover, volunteers. You will be able to follow in detail how the scientists in charge proceeded step by step, gradually increasing very small quantities of live bacteria until in the course of the experiment he reached the quantity required for vaccination. He ended his series of tests with the words: "Surprising as it may appear, such a considerable quantity of live plague bacteria did not cause any seriously undesirable effects." He added that he did not regard as such the fact that his subject's fever temperature reached 40° C. (104° F.). The layman may suppose such remarks to have been cynical. But anyone experienced in this field will realize what bitter anxiety and apprehension that scientist endured for weeks and months on end, in case his theory should be proved false and his subjects should catch the plague and die of it. Today his experiment, carried out forty years ago, has been transfigured and justified by its brilliant success. For it laid the foundation of modern protective vaccination against plague, with its use of live, non-virulent plague bacteria. The same man conducted a further series of experiments, also on criminals sentenced to death, though this time the subjects had to sign a statement that they agreed to the tests. I refer to the experiments initiated in order to discover the cause of beri-beri fever. For this purpose the disease had to be induced artificially, by a low diet. This process succeeded. A detailed account exists of the development of the symptoms of this serious disease over a period of many weeks. They included paralysis, painful neuritis and grave cardiac disorders which finally led to the death of one of the subjects. The body was dissected half an hour after life became extinct. Those unacquainted with beri-beri can only imagine with difficulty the mental strain borne by the doctor who was obliged, week after week, to observe and attend this subject and note in minute detail the whole progress of a disease he had himself induced. The experiment was successful in the sense that typical symptoms of beri-beri were produced in a considerable number of subjects. But it failed scientifically. Since the course of the experiment showed definitely asymmetrical features, the factor which really causes the disease could not be identified. So even the consolation of having been justified by success was denied to the doctors who conducted the test, to the Government officials who reported it and finally to the subjects themselves. The resultant distress of mind, the embitterment, of the doctor concerned can never be understood by a layman. The question at once arises for what possible reason anyone can voluntarily undertake such a burden at the bidding of a Government Department. To suggest that it might be ambition or sheer fanaticism in research is too easy an answer. In this particular case I know the real reason, for I know the man and the conditions under which he worked. His true motive was simply duty, his feeling of responsibility for the millions of natives whose health was in his care. They were dying annually by hundreds of thousands of this terrible scourge of the plague, languishing by hundreds of thousands in the agonies of beri-beri. The consciousness of an obligation to help these people and at the same time of the impossibility of doing so in the current state of scientific knowledge induced him to search for new methods, shoulder the crushing burdens involved and encourage others to undertake similar ordeals.

The experiments I have just mentioned were carried out by Professor Richard P. Strong, while Public Health Officer at Manila. He was later appointed Professor at Harvard University, Boston, and Chairman of the American Society for Tropical Medicine. I hope that Prosecuting Counsel will not attempt to dismiss the work of a man whom I greatly honour with the words applied by the Prosecution to my own: "There are criminals everywhere." For I must ask the Court to believe that Strong was a man with an extremely high sense of duty and of deep moral sensibility. If Prosecuting Counsel will not take my word for it, he is at liberty to consult his expert, Professor Alexander, who is a Boston doctor and therefore certain to know Strong even better than I do. And I must also ask the Court to believe that the morality and motives of most of the German doctors who resolved to take charge of or participate in such experiments were not separated by such a vast abyss, after all, from those which inspired their foreign colleagues in the same situation.

We are accompanied here in the dock by three dead German professors, President Gildemeister, Eppinger of Vienna and Holzlöhner of Kiel. Being dead, they are far more exposed than ourselves to public disparagement and to criticism here in Court. For we at least have the opportunity to defend ourselves. It is for that very reason that I feel compelled today to give evidence on their behalf, though while they were actually at work I openly opposed them. Two of them, Gildemeister and Holzlöhner, informed me personally that they were so exclusively guided in their activities by a sense of their medical duty to prevent sickness and distress, that they took up their share of the work in no light spirit, but as a heavy burden. That was exactly how Gildemeister argued against me at our interview. I have no such verbal testimony from Eppinger, as I never met him. But I am sufficiently acquainted with his character to include him with the others.

I may perhaps be allowed to add that obviously I have no intention of putting Rascher and Ding in this category. If I do not say so, I run the risk of being accused of some such attitude after I have finished my account of the matter. Accordingly, I shall now mention the last of the various motives which led me to protest even against experiments on criminals sentenced to death. I objected to this dreadful burden, which I myself regarded as intolerable, being laid upon our profession in addition to all that it had already to bear. We hygienists spend our lives in contact with human misery and disease. We are sent to places which others abandon. We risk our lives as a matter of course. We never mention this fact among ourselves. I don't know how many doctors and their assistants have perished at the Robert Koch Institute during its existence of more than fifty years as the result of infections which they have administered to their own persons in the laboratories. Undoubtedly more than twenty died in this way. No memorial tablets were put up for them. Their sacrifices were passed over in silence, as our professional ethics require. I hope therefore that my desire to retain at least my honour will be understood. I should like to explain finally, in concluding this survey of the ethical aspect of the matter, what is implied for the doctor in charge of a potentially fatal experiment by the voluntary participation of the subject. I am by no means so one-sided a scientist as not to see that the question is legally of much importance. Speaking as a doctor, I may stress the fact that in a certain clearly defined category of experiments, including the typhus tests at Buchenwald, the yellow fever tests in Cuba and Holzlöhner's supercooling tests, medical men in general and I myself would consider it immoral to employ voluntary subjects. For the psychological strain then borne by the physician in charge would be unacceptable. He has no right to acquiesce in an offer of suicide. Such experiments are in my view only admissible when the sovereign power of the State nominates subjects who have forfeited their lives by committing crimes against the community. I stated years ago in public that I myself condemned such a system. That has already been admitted as a fact by the Prosecution and it is not the first time that I have called attention to it in Court. I am also anxious, in the interests of my profession as a whole, that such bitterly distasteful work should never again be forced upon us by the demands of society and the State authorities. I know that this is only my personal view and that at all times and in all countries the matter has been judged otherwise, so that doctors of high moral standing have repeatedly believed that they were doing their duty in carrying out such experiments. In the many cases where I have had to discuss this matter I have laid emphasis on all these points, lending priority to one or another as circumstances might suggest. But they might all be resumed, in practical terms, though I have just spent half an hour in recapitulating them here, in the one retort I involuntarily made to Gildemeister when he first told me what was to be done. I said: "If this system becomes the fashion, we might as well hand over all our immunization data to executioners and set up a special school for them here in the Institute." It is this purely emotional reaction which is the decisive factor in the problem. In my account of it I have stressed the psychological burden borne by the physician who has to carry out such tests. I have said little about their victims for the simple reason that their sufferings initiate the whole problem with which the doctor is faced and he is in closer contact with them than anyone else. It is so obvious that any decent physician would sympathize with the suffering of his patient that I would not have mentioned the fact at all if I did not realize that such an omission might well lead to the distortion of my evidence later.'

Rose went on to comment on a book cited by one of the prosecution's experts, Moll's *Ärtzliche Ethik*.[1]

'. . . Moll, however, does not refer in any way to the question which lies at the root of the present trial, viz. whether the State has any right either to force certain individuals to undergo medical tests or to appoint doctors to carry them out.

There is only one sentence at most which might have some bearing on the point. Moll remarks on p. 500 that the medical research scientist has no such executive authority as is claimed by the State. The observation amounts to a denial of the doctor's right to perform experiments on his own initiative, while clearly admitting that he may do so with State authority. Throughout Moll's extremely long book he repeatedly condemns experiments on the patient and in particular those on persons with no hope of recovery, which were so frequent in the last century that they were described in a special technical phrase as "*corpus vile*" experiments. Even modern literature

1. Stuttgart, 1902, Enke-Verlag.

contains a few references to them. We have seen from the documentary evidence submitted by Dr Servatius in this court that the Military Government itself clearly recognizes such experiments as still permissible.[1] Only in a single instance does Moll approve a State-authorized experiment on a human being. This was the well known experiment carried out by the American doctor Arning, in connection with leprosy research, on a murderer condemned to death. And even here Moll admits that opinions may differ as to whether a doctor may honourably perform such an experiment. The author always writes, accordingly, from the standpoint of professional medical ethics, not from that of the subject of experiment. On the question of the latter's voluntary consent Moll, too, arrives at the conclusion that in such circumstances there is no moral obligation to recognize the right to freedom of choice. He says so on p. 538 of the work cited by Leibbrand. Moll, moreover, queries in general terms the validity of the statements regarding voluntary participation which often accompany published material dealing with medical research. He proves that such statements of consent must always be intrinsically false, owing to the incapacity of the subject himself to judge of the matter, the influence of the doctor's authority and the fear of the consequences of a refusal. But the decisive point here is that Moll is concerned only with experiment on patients, not on subjects nominated by the State. To that extent Leibbrand's quotation from the book really missed fire altogether in relation to the present trial. Moll was, of course, aware of the existence of State-authorized experiment. For long before his time criminals, foundlings and soldiers had been given protective inoculations against smallpox. He treats exhaustively of the transmission of venereal disease to patients and refers in this connection to the experiments carried out at the orders of the French Government. He must also have known of the experiments by Huffgen with anti-plague vaccines in the Bombay gaols. All these events were prior to the publication of Moll's book. But as he raises no objection to them, I can only assume that he approved State-authorized experiment. He continually stresses that the physician has no executive power, which is the privilege of the State only. . . .'

1. Doc. KB 93 is quoted in the penultimate chapter.

Rose's further statements were concerned with the magnitude of the typhus epidemic of that time, the conflict of specialist opinion on the subject and the impossibility of determination, in war conditions, of the most effective vaccine through statistical research on epidemiology. He continued:

'I have already stated that my protest against Ding's lecture was not universally supported. The minutes of that meeting contain a sentence which has escaped the notice of the Prosecution. But to those present it clearly referred to the experiments and proved that they had been discussed. The sentence, on p. 11, runs: "Experiments of this kind are necessary." The phrase comes from the debate and in fact shows that those who had listened to Ding's exposition believed that criminals under sentence of death were his subjects. Otherwise no one at a public meeting would ever so expressly have approved such experiments, least of all the man who uttered the words in question. For he had spent his life in the service of humanity and his international reputation rendered it out of the question that he should ever have spoken out openly in favour of inhuman action.

Until May 1945 no authority was in any position to distribute even a provisional report on the value of the vaccines tested, let alone to publish any material relating to it. In all medical literature throughout the world I have yet to see any serviceable publication, apart from Ding's work, dealing with the matter. It is quite possible, of course, since I have now been in custody for two years, that something has meanwhile appeared. The practical difficulties in the way of epidemiological assessment of vaccination processes have naturally long been familiar. Consequently, Dr Conti, Chief of the Medical Service, was called upon to decide whether he should simply allow mass production and utilization of an unknown vaccine or, in view of the magnitude and imminence of the danger of epidemic, seek State sanction for experiments on human beings, in order to determine the efficacy of the vaccines proposed.[1]

1. Rose had already mentioned 10,000 typhus infections and 1,300 deaths from typhus in the Army during the month of February 1942 alone. A report by the President of the Westphalian Labour Board [No. 5222] refers to thousands of deaths daily in camps for Russian prisoners of war over a limited period.

Conti decided on the latter alternative, which involved risking and in some cases sacrificing the lives of a number of duly nominated persons so as to obtain data upon which the lives of thousands of others depended. The Government of the day made itself responsible for the project, as it had of course also assumed responsibility for the sacrifice of hundreds of thousands of lives in the interests of much less important objectives. On purely rational grounds the result justified Conti's decision. The Buchenwald experiments provided four principal data. They proved that faith in the protective effect of Weigl's vaccine, though it seemed to be supported by prolonged observation, was an error. They proved that under the conditions prevailing at Buchenwald the serviceable vaccines, though they could not prevent infection, were practically certain to prevent death. They proved that the objections raised against the biological value of yolk of egg vaccines as compared with the louse vaccine were invalid, and that on the contrary yolk of egg and the lungs of rabbits, mice and dogs were all equally protective. We first learned this fact from the Buchenwald experiments and it cleared the way for mass production of typhus vaccines. Fourthly, it was also the Buchenwald experiments which warned us in time against the use of certain other vaccines. These included that of Otto and Wohlrab, and that of Cox, a mixture of Prowazek's Rickettsia and Rickettsia murina taken from egg cultures. Secondly, the Behring Works vaccines, manufactured in accordance with Otto's process but structurally different, and finally Ipsen's mouse-liver vaccine were proved unserviceable. At least tens of thousands of doses of the Behring Works vaccine were at that time being administered and consequently represented a serious danger to health. If it had not been for the Buchenwald experiments the vaccines which they proved unserviceable would have been put into mass production. For they were all very much easier and cheaper to manufacture than the serviceable vaccines. One thing is therefore at any rate certain. At least the subjects of these experiments did not suffer or die in vain. There was only one choice in the matter. Either duly selected persons had to be sacrificed or else affairs could be allowed to take their course and innumerable people would die, though they would not of course be selected in an office

K

of the Criminal Records Department but would meet their fate
by blind chance. We know today how many of the subjects of
experiment perished. But we cannot, naturally, prove how
many lives were saved through these experiments. The very
individual who owes his life to them is unaware of the fact.
Such a man may well be one of the chief representatives of
those who today accuse the doctors who undertook the exacting
task I have described.'

The following is an extract from the Closing Brief of Rose's
Defence Counsel.

[Closing Brief Rose p. 87 ff.]

'Current international law recognizes the principle of self-
preservation. It is agreed in theory and practice that transgression of the ordinances and prohibitions of international law is
permissible if such transgression is necessary for the preservation
of life and property in the face of danger and there is no other
way of eliminating the risk.

This conception is basically the same as that of national
emergency, except that the preliminary conditions for appeal
to international law are somewhat less stringent than those
required if national emergency is to be declared.

The instances usually adduced in the literature on this
subject relate almost wholly to infringements of the territorial
sovereignty of another State as a measure of defence against a
threat to national integrity. But it is nowhere maintained that
the principle of self-preservation must be restricted to such cases.
And in particular there is no ground for not conceding this
right in the circumstances of an epidemic.

In the present instance recognition of the right to self-
preservation appears all the more justified since the elimination
of the typhus epidemic from the further course of the last war
was not only in the interests of Germany but also in those of
her adversaries, including their civil populations, their armies
and especially their prisoners of war in German hands. For
the epidemic had already attacked the latter and might easily
spread to international dimensions. Accordingly, there is no
place here for the objection, incidentally refuted by Professor
Ivy, the Prosecution's expert witness, that the needs of war are

no excuse for the transgression of law.[1] For the effort to control
the typhus epidemic was not merely a military measure in the
interests of Germany. It aimed at the elimination of an international peril which had arisen during the war.

The idea that the right to self-preservation may also be
exercised in order to eliminate emergencies due to natural
catastrophe is expressly approved by Oppenheim in his out-
standing work on international law.[2]

... The defendant Rose could not have been expected to
look on passively while the catastrophe ran its natural course.
We must remember that it was his duty, as a prominent
hygienist, to do all in his power to eliminate the danger he had
recognized. The duty, however, to go to the rescue of the hundreds of thousands of persons menaced by typhus had to be
reconciled with the duty to behave strictly in accordance with
the principles of medical ethics. There can be no doubt that
Rose was most painfully afflicted by this conflict of duties and
that he weighed up their contrasting demands with the greatest
earnestness and care. That he did so is guaranteed by his
character as described by the most various authorities both in
Germany and abroad. In deciding to concentrate upon the first
of these duties he showed that he considered it supreme at that
particular moment. One of the chief circumstances influencing
his decision was the fact that he had done most of his research,
and the most important part of it, not in Germany, but abroad.
He knew, therefore, that medical experiments involving danger
to human life had also been carried out in foreign countries on
voluntary subjects. He was furthermore aware that the genuine
consent of these people was in many cases open to the gravest
doubt and that a large number of them had been criminals
sentenced to death.'[3]

1. So far as the editors are aware Professor Ivy merely stated that the
'necessities of war' constituted a basis for experiment but did not permit
encroachment upon rights. (See p. 59.)

2. Oppenheim, *International Law*, 6th Edn, 1947, p. 256, note 2.

3. Of the great quantity of documentary evidence submitted to the
Court on the subject of non-German experiments on human beings the
following items, dealing with protectively vaccinated subjects and with
checking personnel not so vaccinated, may be cited:

(*a*) Blanc et Baltazard, Action de la bile sur le virus du typhus murin,
Comptes Rendus de la Société de Biologie 124/1937/I/S. 428 f.

It was Dr Ding-Schuler who performed the experiments at Buchenwald. Witnesses agreed that ambition was a conspicuous element in his character. He was personally acquainted with Grawitz, the senior SS and police physician, and Genzken, head of the Health Department of the Waffen SS. It was the former who usually gave him the orders authorizing him to conduct the experiments, as Grawitz alone controlled medical research in the SS, Genzken being only responsible for the SS medical services. The defendant Mrugowsky issued from his own sphere of activity, the Institute of Hygiene of the Waffen SS, important suggestions for the organization of the tests, though he himself may have experienced some conscientious scruples in principle about putting them into effect.

The following letter was included among the documents before the Court.

[DOC. 1198.]

'Chief Hygienist to the Reich SS and Police Physician, Berlin-Zehlendorf.

Dear Mrugowsky,

I write to inform you that the Reichsführer SS has today consented to the following series of experiments proposed by you:

1. Specific therapy in cases of typhus.
2. Tolerance of serum containing carbolic acid.

I agree to both series being carried out in the Typhus and Virus Research Department of the Waffen SS Institute of Hygiene at Weimar-Buchenwald and beg you to keep me

---

(b) A. Yersin et J. J. Vassal, Une maladie rappelant le typhus exanthematique observé en Indochine, Bulletin Soc. Path. exot. 1908, S. 156.

(c) Edm. Sergent und Mitarbeiter, Transmission à l'homme au singe du typhus exanthematique . . . C. R. Ac. Sci. 158, 965 (1914).

(d) Otero, Agente patogene del tifo exantematico, Gazeta med. del Mexico, Appendice 1908.

(e) Sparrow, Recherches exper. sur le typhus exanthematique C. R. Soc. Biol. 91, 1341, 1924/89, 1349, 1923.

(f) Hamdi, Über die Ergebnisse der Immunisierungsversuche gegen Typhus exant. Zeitschr. für Hygiene 1916, 82.

(g) Veintemillas, Schutzimpfung von Menschen gegen das mexikanische Hoden-Fleckfieber (Doc. NO. 3964).

(h) Heilbrunn, Infektionsversuche am Menschen, 1937, Würzburg (Inauguraldissertation) und weitere a. a. O.

informed of the results obtained, if possible by submitting interim reports.

Heil Hitler!

(*Signed*) GRAWITZ.

Accordingly, Dr Ding-Schuler made the following entry, dated the 13 November 1944, in his station diary:

[DOC. 265.]*

'13 November '44:

THERAPEUTIC EXPERIMENT WITH TYPHUS VACCINE

By order of the senior hygienist of the Waffen SS of 12 August 1944, it is to be determined whether the course of typhus can be tempered by the intravenous or intramuscular injection of typhus vaccine.

For the experimental series twenty persons were considered, of these, ten for intravenous injection (Series A), ten for intramuscular injection (Series B) and, in addition, five persons for control.

On 13 November 1944, the twenty-five experimental persons were infected by subcutaneous injection of 1/10 c.c. each fresh typhus-infected blood. All persons fell sick as follows: Series A—ten serious; Series B—one medium, nine serious; Control—five serious.

22 December 1944:

The experimental series was concluded.

2 January 1945:

Chart and case history completed.

Nineteen deaths (nine Series A; six Series B; four Control).

DR SCHULER'

On the 29 September 1944 an article in manuscript by Dr Ding-Schuler dealing with another 'therapy experiment' was received in Berlin. The article was entitled 'TyphusTreatment with Acridin Derivatives' and was intended for the *Zeitschrift für Hygiene und Infektionskrankheiten*, in which periodical a previous paper by Ding-Schuler had appeared. The September essay discussed the effects of two new preparations by I.G. Farben Höchst, acridin-granulat and rutenol. It contained the following passage.

[DOC. 582.]

'In April/May 1943, thirty-nine persons arrived for treatment at the clinical centre attached to the Typhus and Virus Research Department of the Waffen SS Institute of Hygiene. They had been serologically and clinically certified to be suffering from typhus. Indubitably severe symptoms had been observed, during the epidemic, in the central nervous system, circulation and skin eruptions. A fatal outcome was expected in over 50 per cent of cases. As strict measures had been taken for quarantine the date of infection could be established in many instances. This fact is of particular importance for the determination of the period of incubation ... and the application of specific treatment. It was possible to arrange for a very early administration of remedies in these last cases, thus enabling precise assessment of efficacy to be reached.'

Further paragraphs read:

'Eight of the fifteen patients vomited after rutenol up to seven times a day. Mortality at 53·3 per cent was extraordinarily high. There was no apparent relation between tolerance and the proportion of deaths. Four patients digested the rutenol and were cured. Three also digested it but died ... of the eight who vomited three survived and five succumbed.'

'Mortality in the third group of typhus patients who were not treated with rutenol or nitroacridin during the epidemic was only 2 per cent higher, standing at 56 per cent.'

The digestibility of acridin was noted in these terms:

'Digestibility was far less than in the case of rutenol. ... Mortality was again very high at 53·3 per cent.'

The station diary has the following entry for 24 April 1943, a date within the period referred to in the publication.*

'24 April 1943: Therapeutic experiments Acridine-Granulate (A–GR2) and Rutenol (R–2) to carry out the therapeutic experiments Acridine Granulate and Rutenol, thirty persons (fifteen each) and nine persons for control were infected by intravenous injection of 2 c.c. each of fresh blood of a typhus sick person. All experimental persons got very serious typhus.'

On 1 June 1943 the following entry appears:

'Preparation of case histories and charts.

Series of experiments terminated.

Twenty-one deaths (eight A–Gr subjects, eight Rutenol and five checking).'

This entry proves that there was no question of an epidemic but solely of an artificial infection of persons undergoing experiment.

Table 2 summarizes the therapy tests performed as noted in the diary.

TABLE 2

TYPHUS THERAPY EXPERIMENTS

Subjects artificially infected		Deaths	
Therapy test with	*No special therapy (Checking personnel)*	*Therapy subjects*	*Checking personnel*
Acridin 20 Methylene Blue 20 }	7	1 *Infection partially ineffective*	—
Rutenol 15 Acridin-Granulate 15 }	9	8 8	— 5
Typhus vaccine intravenous 10 intramuscular 10 }	5	9 6	4
Totals 90	21	32	9

There was a third group of persons, not hitherto mentioned, whom Ding-Schuler treated with 'Matelska', his strain of Rickettsia-Prowazek virus, from the Robert Koch Institute.

They were used as 'passage' subjects. The term was explained in Dr Kogon's evidence on the 7 January 1947.

[PROT. p. 1202.]*

'A third category of the experimental persons was used to maintain the typhus cultures. Those were the so-called passage persons, amounting to three to five persons per month. They were merely infected for the purpose of ensuring a constant supply of fresh blood containing typhus. Very nearly all those persons died. I do not think I am exaggerating if I say that 95 per cent of these cases were fatal.'

The methods by which people were selected for these series of experiments were described by Dr Kogon as follows in reply to questions in court.

[PROT. p. 1197.]

'The choice of subjects was not always the same at different times. To begin with the camp staff were invited to report voluntarily. They were told that the tests would do them no harm, and that they would receive a substantial addition to their diet. After one or two experiments it was found impossible to obtain any more volunteers. Dr Ding then requested the camp doctor or the camp managers to supply him with suitable subjects. He gave them no special directions. The managers chose any prisoners they pleased, criminals, political offenders, homosexuals and other so-called antisocial elements. Intrigues among the prisoners themselves influenced the selection, so that some persons were subjected to experiment when there was no particular reason why they should have been. Some time in the autumn of 1943 the three camp managers declined to take any further responsibility for the selection of subjects. Even Dr Ding himself was no longer satisfied with verbal instructions from Mrugowsky to proceed with the tests. He demanded written authority. Accordingly, he suggested to Mrugowsky that Himmler himself should nominate subjects. SS Gruppen-führer Nebe of the Berlin Criminal Police Department after-wards obtained instructions from Himmler, which I have seen, to the effect that only persons under sentence of at least ten years penal servitude should in future be used.'

The prosecution asked whether the persons selected for experiment were exclusively prisoners under sentence of death. Dr Kogon answered:

[PROT. p. 1197.]

'I do not know a single case in which a person judicially sentenced to death underwent test at the Experimental Centre in Block 46. In the case of four Russian prisoners of war it was stated that they had been condemned to be shot. But this was not a judicial sentence. They belonged to a certain category of Russian prisoners of war some 9,500 of whom were either shot, hanged or strangled at Buchenwald.'

The proof that final ruling as to the choice of subjects was not obtained until 1944 appears from a teleprinted message containing Himmler's actual order.

[DOC. 1189.]

'Chief of Security Police.

I agree to the use of professional criminals for tests of the typhus vaccine. But of such criminals only such are to be selected as have been sentenced to at least ten years' imprisonment, not such as merely have ten previous convictions. SS Gruppenführer Nebe will supervise the provision of such prisoners. I do not wish the doctor to choose them on his own authority without counter-check.

(*Signed*) HIMMLER

Reich Security Head Office, Section V
Berlin, 29 February 1944

Director of the Waffen SS Institute of Hygiene,
SS Standartenführer Mrugowsky,
   Berlin-Zehlendorf, Spanische Allee 10.
For information to SS Standartenführer Dr Ding,
   Buchenwald/Weimar.
I enclose for information the above decision by the Reichsführer SS concerning the inquiry as to the provision of subjects for typhus vaccine tests. In conformity with our discussion

Criminal Investigation Councillor Otto, official representative of Section V of the Reich Security Head Office, will arrive at the Buchenwald concentration camp on the 2 March 1944 with the necessary documents and will then undertake, in collaboration with Dr Ding, the selection of subjects as ordered by the Reichsführer SS. I assume that you have acquainted our colleague Dr Ding with the situation by telephone as we arranged.

(*Signed*) NEBE.   Certified (*Signature*)
Criminal Investigation Department
Secretary.'

The results were stated by Rose in his evidence as quoted above.

B. The experiments with typhus vaccine in the Natzweiler concentration camp, including Schirmeck, in Alsace, were carried on from the autumn of 1943 until the capture of the camp in the autumn of 1944. The series was begun by the Professor of Hygiene at Strasbourg University, Dr Eugen Haagen. The Buchenwald tests had been mainly organized by a study group of SS members only. Haagen was commissioned from the sources given below, which we take from a letter addressed to him on the 10 July 1944 by Hirt, Professor of Anatomy at Strasbourg.

[DOC. 129.]

'The Reichsführer SS would be glad if your announcement could contain the following passage:

"The investigations were carried out on the instructions and with the support of the Director of the Medical Service of the Air Force, with the support of the Reich Research Council and under the patronage of the Reichsführer SS personally, as well as that of the SS Administration Head Office and the Waffen SS Institute for the Practical Advancement of Military Science." '

Haagen's typhus experiments were not, like those at Buchenwald, undertaken with a view to checking the efficacy of current vaccines. They were concerned with ascertaining the digestibility of a new vaccine developed by himself and establishing its effect in the countering of infection.

He commented as follows on the employment of a 'living vaccine'.[1]

[PROT. p. 9577 f. and 9585 f.]*

'There are various vaccines available. Now, to get down to the crux of the matter, I must say that the typhus vaccines which are made from dead typhus virus do not provide absolute protection against the disease. They may lead to a milder form of the disease, but the infection itself is not prevented. Dead typhus vaccine, in other words, has no absolute anti-infectious effect, which, however, is the main point of any vaccine.

We developed a live vaccine, not on the basis of our own experiences and research, but we made use of the experiences of others. I should like to mention primarily the work of the French typhus research scientists, Blanc, Baltasard, and assistants Laigret and Lecolle. When vaccinating, a vaccine must be used which gives anti-infectious protection, and in general, in the case of virus diseases, successful vaccination is also achieved only with live virus. Let me mention the examples of smallpox, influenza and yellow fever. In all these cases the vaccines are made from a live virus, but it is true that this virus is mutated, that is, it is no longer pathogenic to human beings. Its pathogenic characteristics have been suppressed and have disappeared but the virus retains its anti-infectious efficacy. This change is accomplished in two ways, either by passing the virus through an animal—this is frequently done—which sometimes effects mutation in the virus and sometimes weakens the virus. . .

Our work was limited to the development of a live vaccine, and this work was based on the great experiences of foreign scientists, especially the French scientist Blanc; the technical side was always carried out in animal experiments. . . .

We did succeed in developing such a vaccine from a so-called murine typhus virus strain, that is, from rat typhus. The weakening was brought about through animal experiments, through cultivation in chicken eggs, and thirdly through a conservation process.

1. Haagen appeared as a witness at Nuremberg. His trial took place at Strasbourg.

Q. Was this vaccine then tested for its effectiveness and if so, how?

A. Yes. The vaccine was tested for its effectiveness. First, of course, by animal experiments for its immunizing qualities. After this quality had been proved, the first vaccinations were undertaken in order to test the effectiveness and the tolerance on human beings. This was done on volunteers . . . of whom I myself was the first, followed by members of my Institute and a number of students from the University.'

Haagen stated in evidence that 'the first practical protective inoculations were administered in May 1943 at the security camp of Schirmeck, part of the Natzweiler concentration camp. These inoculations were administered to patients in special danger.' [PROT. p. 9587.]

In accordance with the request of the commandant of the Natzweiler camp the subjects were inmates of the so-called 'East Block'. Twenty-eight inoculations were given. Haagen said they had no serious after-effects.

His argument was, in brief, that it had not been necessary for him to test the efficacy of his vaccine by subsequently infecting the subjects with typhus. A serological reaction, the Weil-Felix, was sufficient for the purpose. A rather long discussion of the meaning of the word 'after-infection', which appeared in Haagen's original notes, ensued. The view that the word implied artificial infection with typhus after protective inoculation was denied by Haagen, who said he used it as a technical term with a specialized meaning in the context of virus research. In this sense 'after-infection' referred to inoculation with a 'living vaccine', i.e. a substance virulent but not causing disease in human beings, after a first vaccination with agents in which life had been destroyed. In such cases the first vaccination was intended to weaken reactions which might follow upon the second or 'after' inoculation, known as the 'after-infection'. It was agreed by other experts in hygiene who gave evidence that this account of the meaning of the term might be regarded as correct.

It turned out later that the prosecution had some ground for the belief that Haagen's chief motive in his inoculations at Schirmeck and Natzweiler was not to provide 'protection' but to undertake experiments on prisoners with a vaccine which had not yet been proved practically effective and which he felt it would be too dangerous to test by any other methods. It also seemed that he might have intended to follow up such checks of the digestibility of his vaccine by artificially infecting subjects with typhus, as had been done at Buchenwald, so as to test, in addition, the efficacy of the substance in actually countering infection.

Under examination by the prosecution he stated:

[PROT. p. 9740 ff.]

'*Q*. Is it not a fact that you did not carry out any "after-infection" tests with your murine vaccine because you had been obliged to take prisoners indicated by the SS and that body had not given you permission to experiment on the twenty-eight persons you had actually vaccinated?

A. No. There can be no question of any such thing. There were no experiments of the kind referred to in this trial. It was a matter of protective vaccination.'

And again, at a later stage:

'*Q*. Did you not give it as your expert opinion to the Tribunal that the protective vaccination of twenty-eight persons with the murine vaccine had made a real contribution to the control of a potential typhus epidemic at Schirmeck?

A. I don't think my statement took that particular form.

Q. All the same, I can't quite understand how you could suppose that the vaccination of twenty-eight people at Schirmeck and 200 or, as I think you said, eighty in Natzweiler would have any appreciable effect on the expected typhus epidemic. There were some 12,000 prisoners at Natzweiler, were there not, Professor?

A. I don't know anything about that. There were certainly a great many. But, as I explained yesterday, I had to work, so to speak, slowly at first, since I could not produce any great quantity of vaccine with the laboratory resources at my disposal.'

The subjects were not volunteers, as both Haagen himself and other witnesses admitted.

In a letter to Rose dated the 4 October 1943 he wrote, *inter alia*:

[DOC. 2874.]

'I have already given you the figures of the first successful inoculations of human beings. Serum strength was considerably higher, even after a single inoculation, than after three inoculations with vaccines in which life had been destroyed. Unfortunately I have been unable so far to undertake infection tests on those vaccinated. I applied to the SS Ancestral Heritage Community for suitable subjects but received no reply. We are now commencing further inoculation of human beings. I will inform you later of the result. I believe that we shall then be in a position to suggest that as a first step our new vaccine might be taken into use in the absence of infection tests. . . . If we can obtain people through the SS for experimental inoculation, we could take the opportunity to test the efficacy of the liver vaccine also against infection. I would then propose that our own material might be used at the same time as the Ipsen tests.'

At this stage of Haagen's examination he tried to justify his use of the word 'experiments' as equivalent to 'comparative investigation'. [PROT. p. 9792.]

A number of witnesses agreed that in May 1943 experiments were carried out at Schirmeck on twenty-five Poles who arrived all together at the camp. (See the evidence of Dr Hirtz, a pharmacist on duty, as a prisoner, in the sick bay.) [PROT. p. 1312.]

The following extract from Hirtz's testimony vividly depicts the treatment of prisoners and subjects for experiment at that time.

[PROT. p. 1314 and 1316.]

'*Dr Hirtz:* I had to take the Poles' temperature three times a day. After some thirty-eight to forty-eight hours temperatures began to rise, reaching 39° and 40° C. (104° F.) and more. The patients' reactions differed as was only to be expected from the differences in their physique. Some were young, a few being still robust, while others were older and showed visible signs of prolonged detention in the camp. On the second or third day, in the morning, I found two of them dead in bed, already cold. The fever lasted about seven or eight days. Towards the end of the period marked symptoms of agitation, anxiety and defective verbal articulation appeared.

Prosecuting Counsel: You say that on the third day after the injection two of the Poles died as a result of the experiments. Did you yourself see the bodies?

A. I did indeed. I sewed them up myself in paper bags and they were incinerated in the Natzweiler crematorium.'

Haagen countered this evidence by saying that 'no one ever died of typhus after two days' incubation'. The extent to which reactions to inoculation might have caused the death of the prisoners was not made clear at the hearing. Nevertheless, the diary of the experiments kept by Haagen's female technical assistant shows that when blood samples were taken on the 6 July 1943 in order to check serological reaction 'the other two were no longer available'. [DOC. 3852.]

This diary also proves that, contrary to Haagen's evidence, further inoculations took place at Schirmeck after May 1943. Dr Gräfe, Haagen's assistant, pacified the remonstrances of the technical staff during the first experiments in May by remarking that 'the tests would not be performed on the prisoners, but only on Poles,' who could not really, he added, 'be regarded as human beings.' [PROT. p. 1376 and 1767.]

In the summer of 1943 Haagen transferred his experimental activity to the camp at Natzweiler in order to undertake, as he stated in evidence, further 'protective inoculations' there, this time with a recently developed pedicular vaccine, which he said was virulent but not liable to cause disease in human beings.

It is not quite certain from the documentary testimony available why Professor Hirt of Strasbourg now became concerned in the organization of the new series of experiments. The following correspondence clearly refutes Haagen's claim that the object was the protective inoculation of the inmates of the camp at Natzweiler. On the 15 November 1943 he addressed a letter stamped 'secret' to Hirt.

[DOC. 121.]*

'On 13 November 1943, an inspection was made of the prisoners that were furnished to me in order to determine their suitability for the tests which have been planned for the typhus vaccines. Of the 100 prisoners that have been selected in their former camp, eighteen died during transport. Only twelve prisoners are in such a condition that they can be used for these experiments, provided their strength can first be restored. This should take about two to three months. The remaining prisoners are in such a condition that they cannot be used at all for these purposes.

I might point out that the experiments are for the purpose of testing a new vaccine. Such experiments only lead to fruitful results when they are carried out with normally nourished subjects whose physical powers are comparable to those of the soldiers. Therefore, experiments with the present group of prisoners cannot yield usable results, particularly since a large part of them are apparently afflicted with maladies which make them unsuitable for these experiments. A long period of rest and of good nourishment would not alter this fact.

I request, therefore, that you send me 100 prisoners, between 20 to 40 years of age, who are healthy and who are so constituted physically that they furnish comparable material.'

The dispatch of prisoners mentioned was obviously arranged by Hirt with the support of the 'Institute for Practical Research on Military Science'. The fact appears from a letter dated 30 September 1943 written by the defendant Wolfram Sievers.

[DOC. 120.]

'I acknowledge receipt of your application of the 16 August 1943. I am quite prepared to be of assistance and have accordingly requested the authority concerned to put the persons you mention at your disposal.'

In connection with the same affair Haagen also wrote to Rose.

[DOC. 1059.]

'Dear Herr Rose,

I enclose the report anticipated a few days ago regarding

our experiments with dried typhus vaccine. As I intend to publish the results obtained to date I wrote out my report at once
in MS. After you have glanced through it I should be glad if
you would submit it to the competent authority for permission
to publish in the *Bacteriological News*.

Some time ago I had 100 persons put at my disposal in a
concentration camp here for protective vaccination and after-
infection. Unfortunately the subjects were in so wasted a condition that eighteen of them died on the way here. The rest
were also in such a pitiable state that they could not be utilized
for inoculation purposes. I have now again requested the SS
Head Office to send me a further 100 subjects, who must,
however, be in normal health and adequately nourished, so
that experiments may be made on persons in a condition
physically approaching that of our troops.'

Rose's answer shows that he had long since overcome his
earlier scruples.

[DOC. 122.]*

'Dear Herr Haagen,
Many thanks for your letter of 8 December. I regard it as
unnecessary to make a renewed special request to the SS Main
Office in addition to the request you have already made. I request that, in procuring persons for vaccination in your experiment, you requisition a corresponding number of persons for
vaccination with the Copenhagen vaccine. This has the advantage, as also appeared in the Buchenwald experiments, that
the testing of various vaccines simultaneously gives a clearer
idea of their value than the testing of one vaccine alone.'

Haagen's protest resulted in his being sent some ninety fresh
subjects from Auschwitz, only recently released from the Army
and SS and taken into custody. He divided them into two
groups. Forty were vaccinated by scarification and forty by
intramuscular injection. The experiments were carried out in
the winter of 1943–44. According to Haagen's evidence the
immunizing effect of his new vaccine was more marked. But
the reactions to inoculation were more vigorous, including high
fever, headaches and so on. 'There were no symptoms whatever
of typhus.' [PROT. p. 9616 f.]

L

The witness Nales, a fomer Dutch political prisoner, stated in court that more than twenty-nine deaths had occurred as a result of this series of experiments by Haagen. In proof of his testimony he produced a copy, made by himself and others in the camp, of the original list of the dead. The names of those who died during Haagen's experiments had not been entered in the original lists because the prisoners in question had not been registered on their arrival at the camp but immediately segregated. [PROT. p. 10588 ff. and 10622 ff.]

Haagen was not able to reply to this statement, as it was made after his own examination. But he had already commented on similar testimony by the witness Edith Schmdit, a technical assistant at the Strasbourg Institute of Hygiene. She had declared that about fifty of the checking personnel had died. Haagen answered [Prot. p. 1381] that they had succumbed to a typhus epidemic in the camp which lasted until the summer of 1944. He had himself, he said, 'no time' for protective inoculation against the epidemic at that period. [PROT. p. 9769.]

In two letters dated 9 May and 27 June 1944 Haagen again applied for prisoners, 200 this time, for use in testing his vaccine. It is clear from the second letter that he intended the artificial infection with typhus of persons who had not been immunized, i.e. to conduct the same sort of experiments as had been undertaken at Buchenwald.

[DOC. 123.]*

'Main Office SS
     through Professor Dr Hirt,
     Anatomical Institute of the Reich University Strasbourg.

I enclose herewith a carbon copy of a paper on our experiments with a dry typhus vaccine. The paper was sent to the Chief of the Luftwaffe Medical Service as a manuscript, with the request for permission to publish it. It constitutes a report concerning further experiments with a typhus vaccine which has not been made sterile by chemical agents or by heating. As may be seen from the results, it has been possible to produce a vaccine which provides not only an antitoxic immunity but also a definite anti-infection immunity which is of particularly practical significance. However, it is clearly pointed out that vaccination is followed by a rather long fever reaction and, therefore, its introduction cannot yet be recommended. Further tests are now in progress to alter the vaccine so that, without losing its antigenic property, it will produce so weak a reaction that no general indisposition will result. These tests will be made by reducing the dose or by storing the vaccine for a longer interval.

To carry out this research, experimental subjects will again be needed. I, therefore, again request that subjects be furnished to me for this purpose. In order to obtain results which are accurate and which can be statistically evaluated, I ask that 200 persons be furnished to me for inoculation. I may point out that they must be in a physical condition similar to that of members of the armed forces.

It is highly desirable that I again be permitted to carry out these experiments at camp Natzweiler.

PROFESSOR DR E. HAAGEN'

[DOC. 127.]

'Professor Hirt,
    Anatomical Institute of the Reich University of Strasbourg.
    Subject: Tests of dried typhus vaccine.

With reference to and in completion of my report of the 9 May 1944 I write to inform you that no such prolonged reactions to the vaccinations themselves are to be expected as were observed in the previous experiments. Consequently no considerable loss of working time should occur.

But in the case of the infections with virulent typhus agents to be undertaken later with a view to testing the vaccination protection obtained we must count on some of the subjects falling ill, especially those in the parallel group of unvaccinated persons. These after-infections will be necessary in order to establish beyond doubt the efficacy of the dry vaccines against infection. On this occasion 150 subjects will be protectively vaccinated and fifty exposed to the checking infections.

I should like again to stress the need for vaccination experiments to be carried out only on persons in a physical condition comparable with that of the troops.

Heil Hitler!

PROFESSOR E. HAAGEN,
Chief Medical Officer.'

Even in the face of these documents Haagen continued to assert that the inoculations had been merely planned, never carried out. But two further documents, a record of experiments [Doc. 3852] and a letter [Doc. 131] dated 29 August 1944 from the Luftwaffe Health Department inquiring 'whether it is to be assumed that the present epidemic of typhus at Natzweiler has any connection with the current tests of a vaccine' suggest that Haagen was continuing his experiments throughout the summer of 1944. His examination also revealed that all the experiments were performed on persons against their will. [PROT. p. 9671.]

Haagen admitted, moreover, that he had inoculated twenty women at Schirmeck with an influenza vaccine developed by himself. In this case too the number of persons 'protectively vaccinated' contrasts fantastically with the number imprisoned in the camp at the time and with Haagen's excuse that 'epidemics are always to be feared in a camp.' [PROT. p. 9707].

CHAPTER FOUR

EPIDEMIC HEPATITIS VIRUS RESEARCH

The unusually high incidence of *hepatitis epidemica*, especially during the Russian campaign, did not often lead to fatal results. But the percentage of casualties due to this cause which adversely affected the 'fighting power' of the troops rendered it urgent to make a special study of the aetiology of the disease. Professor Gutzeit, hospital consultant to the Army Medical Service, was appointed on the clinical side of the investigation and Dr Dohmen as bacteriologist. Haagen and others also took an interest in the problem at the same time.

Gutzeit stated in court, as a witness, that he devoted himself to this work on account of the great quantity of material for study which reached the Army Medical Service Academy from all the fronts. He started investigations at his hospital in Breslau. Dr Dohmen, a member of the Academy, conducted research independently in Professor Gildemeister's laboratory in the Robert Koch Institute, 'using the normal, generally accepted methods of experiment on animals'. Dohmen's work succeeded. He discovered the agent of the disease, a virus.

Both Haagen and Grawitz approached Dohmen with a request that he should make over his cultures to the senior SS physician, as the SS wished to perform experiments of its own. Dohmen refused in each case. He intended to retain control over the cultures himself and continue his work alone. But in order to avoid the possibility of future disputes with Grawitz and accusations of sabotage he finally:

[AFFIDAVIT by Professor Gutzeit, DOC. Handloser 12.]

'declared himself ready to work at the Sachsenhausen concentration camp. As a result of our experiments on ourselves and on our assistants and medical students, we were sure that we had found the virus. No serious consequences had followed from the experiments on ourselves. Nor were any anticipated from clinical observation of the many thousands of cases of jaundice.

Dohmen only pretended to work at Sachsenhausen in

compliance with the demands of Grawitz and was obliged to
conceal what he did do in order to evade such compliance.'
(Grawitz eventually requested Dohmen to conduct experiments on human beings by artificial infection.) 'Dohmen
informed me that he paid a number of visits there at longer or
shorter intervals, examining and treating the prisoners allotted
to him, just as he had in the Army hospitals he had visited to
examine actual or suspected cases of jaundice, testing them for
duodenal ulcers, analysing blood and urine, and injecting
vitamins and so on. He did not carry out any infections. In the
talks I had with him he gave me no information about the
other work at Sachsenhausen. Nor did he mention experiments
on human beings in the lectures he gave at the Vienna congress
of specialists in internal disease in the autumn of 1943 and at
the conference on hepatitis in June 1944.'

No clinical or experimental records were available in support
of Gutzeit's statements. But that experiments on human beings
were demanded to elucidate the problem is proved by a letter
dated the 1 June 1943 from Grawitz to Himmler.

[DOC. 010.]*

'The General Commissioner of the Fuehrer, SS Brigade-
fuehrer Professor Dr Brandt, has approached me with the request
to help him obtain prisoners to be used in connection with his
research on the causes of Epidemic Jaundice which has been
furthered to a large degree by his efforts. . . . In order to enlarge
our knowledge, so far based only on inoculation of animals with
germs taken from human beings, it would now be necessary to
reverse the procedure and inoculate human beings with germs
cultivated in animals. Casualties must be anticipated.

The therapeutic and above all the prophylactic deductions
to be made will naturally depend to a large extent on this
experimental proceeding.

Eight prisoners under sentence of death, as young as possible,
will be required for treatment at the prisoners' hospital in
Sachsenhausen concentration camp.

I respectfully request your decision, as to whether (1) I may
order the experiments to be initiated on the above lines, (2) the
experiments are to be conducted by Dr Dohmen himself in the
prisoners' hospital at Sachsenhausen.

Although Dr Dohmen does not belong to the SS (he is a SA Führer and Party Member) I would in this case, by way of exception, recommend him, in the interests of continuity of the experimental series and accordingly in those of the accuracy of the results to be obtained.

The practical importance of the matter for our troops, especially those in southern Russia, arises from the fact that of late years the disease in question has reached very high proportions both in our own Waffen SS and in the Army, to the extent that 60 per cent of companies have gone sick for periods up to six weeks.

On the other hand early and appropriate treatment of the disease has in general relatively good prospects. If prophylaxis by vaccination should prove possible, it would be a matter of considerable tactical importance. GRAWITZ'[1]

Himmler consented in a letter of the 16 June 1943.

[DOC. 011.]*

'I approve that eight criminals condemned in Auschwitz (eight Jews of the Polish Resistance Movement condemned to death) should be used for these experiments.'

No witnesses or evidence of the experiments were available.[2]

1. Professor Haagen declared, with reference to this letter 'that not a single specialist, not even Dr Dohmen himself, participated in this affair at all. For every doctor who has ever had anything to do with hepatitis knows that the communication or infection quota is not big enough to permit useful results being obtained from the experimental infection of only eight subjects. Nor, as I have already stated, did I ever learn of any deaths from these hepatitis experiments. Consequently they cannot be described as having been dangerous to life.' [Prot. p. 9550]

2. The Military Tribunal of the Soviet Zone of Occupation, dealing with former commandants and administrative staff of the Sachsenhausen concentration camp, sat from the 31 October 1947 to the following day under the chairmanship of Colonel Mayorov. It sentenced Dr Heinz Baumkötter, Senior Physician of the camp, to imprisonment for life with compulsory labour. Judgment mentioned among a number of experiments performed on prisoners by Baumkötter the infection with jaundice in 1944 of six girl prisoners between the ages of 8 and 14. The object was to test a new treatment of the disease. (Documented Report of the Sachsenhausen Trial, SWA Verlag, Berlin, 1948.)

No suggestion could be traced of any connection between these experiments and the projects described above. The editors could not obtain access to any further records.

At the conference on hepatitis in June 1944, mentioned in Gutzeit's evidence, Surgeon-General Schreiber, the authority on contagious diseases serving on the National Research Council, dealt with the question of co-ordinating the investigation of this malady.

[DOC. Handloser 12.]

'Several groups of doctors were formed to study the problem.'
One of the groups referred to consisted of Gutzeit, Haagen and Dohmen.

In connection with their common professional activities Gutzeit wrote to Haagen on the 24 June 1944 that he was trying

[DOC. 124.]

'to render it possible to conduct the crucial experiment on a human subject ... but certain precautionary measures to which I cannot refer in writing will have to be undertaken.'

Gutzeit stated in his evidence and also in his affidavit that he [Doc. 125] had made arrangements in his hospital for ... 'the crucial experiment on a human subject, in the same way as before, medical students having agreed to undergo the perfectly safe test in question.'[1] [PROT. p. 2738.]

Gutzeit meant by his 'certain precautions' 'facilities for isolation'. But he added that the experiments were never carried out and that he had 'at no time used concentration camp prisoners in tests of any kind.'

1. Earlier experiments on human beings at the Breslau hospital are noted in a publication by that establishment in the *Munich Medical Weekly* for 1942, p. 76 ff. The article is by D. H. Voegt, Assistant Physician at the clinic, and is entitled 'Aetiology of Hepatitis Epidemica'. Incidentally, it illustrates very clearly how the question whether the subjects were volunteers or not was left vague. In describing the first series of the experiments the voluntary participation of the subjects was emphasized. When it came to the second, with six subjects, no reference was made to this condition. In the last experiment 'a woman aged 30 with a slight tubercular prominence of the lymphatic gland on the left of the neck ... drank 100 c.c. of urine from patient B. in a bowl of soup and ... (somewhat later) another 25 c.c. from case Sch.' The 'tubercular lymphatic gland prominence flared up' soon after the first application.

Haagen's similar intention to perform experiments on human beings is clear from his answer to Gutzeit. [DOC. 125.]

In another letter he wrote that such experiments 'would best be carried out here in Strasbourg or close by.' [DOC. 126.]

In reply to the prosecution he explained that he did not mean that such experiments should be undertaken at the Natzweiler camp near Strasbourg, on prisoners, but on members of the student body at Freiburg or Heidelberg. [PROT. p. 9715.]

He added that these plans also came to nothing.

A number of other scientists with whom Haagen worked declared, in support of his own statement to that effect, that they merely provided him with specimens taken from diseased persons or else examined mouse-liver on his behalf. [PROT. p. 9544 f.]

A further document shows the organization of hepatitis experiments at the Buchenwald camp. [DOC. 1303.]

On the 29 January 1945, at Schreiber's request, Mrugowsky, the 'Senior Hygienist on the staff of the leading SS physician' approached Grawitz. He asked for 'effective permission' for an experiment on twenty prisoners with a new hepatitis virus produced at Leipzig. The experiments 'were required in order to prove the efficacy of the virus.' Dr Ding-Schuler of the Buchenwald camp was sent a copy of the letter 'for information'.

The defendant Mrugowsky, when questioned about this letter, alleged that 'nothing came of it' because meanwhile the war ended. [PROT. p. 5466.]

The extensive and prolonged experiments undertaken by Professor Claus Schilling at the Dachau concentration camp in connection with malaria were only marginally considered at the Nuremberg trial. For Schilling had by then already been condemned to death and executed as a result of proceedings taken against those in charge of the Dachau camp.

Documentary evidence of the nature of these experiments was not available to the editors.

CHAPTER FIVE

SULPHONAMIDE TESTS

THESE experiments were performed in the Ravensbrück concentration camp for women, about eight miles from the orthopaedic sanatorium of Hohenlychen. The head physician of that establishment, Professor Karl Gebhardt, in his capacity as consultant surgeon of the Waffen SS, was responsible for the execution of the work.

There were two main courses open to the accused in their defence. They could try to deny their influence upon or knowledge of the events and in so doing endeavour to take refuge behind the orders they had to carry out, thus weakening their personal responsibility to that of a functionary. Or else they could seek to prove that the experiments were 'legal' in two senses, one moral, in so far as the subjects had already been condemned to death by law, and the other in so far as 'public emergency' had required the most expeditious assembly possible of data relating to this or that problem. In this connection they could say that they had been dealing with a scientific question raised on adequate grounds and that every precaution dictated by humane feeling had been taken to safeguard the subjects, so far as circumstances allowed.

The defendant Gebhardt made vigorous use of all these arguments in Court. It was of advantage to him that the origins and the true motivation of the Ravensbrück experiments could no longer be ascertained documentarily. The prosecution could rely only on the evidence of participants. Surviving eyewitnesses reconstructed events which had occurred on the spot. It was also possible to derive from the facts which came out in Gebhardt's testimony some idea of the circumstances preceding the experiments and thus to deduce the factor which eventually set them going.

According to Gebhardt three things happened in May 1942 which caused Himmler to order a rapid solution of the problem of sulphonamides by means of experiments on human beings. In the first place SS Gruppenführer Nebe, chief of the Criminal

Investigation Department, reported at a conference that there had been a serious loss of confidence in Army surgeons on the part of troops on active service and wounded men. The SS had experienced heavy casualties in the eastern theatre owing both to 'the destructive power of hostile armaments and the unalterably conservative methods of doctors in the field'. The resentment was notably increased by the scattering over the German lines of leaflets by the enemy announcing the supply to Allied soldiers of sulphonamides and penicillin, which the German troops soon came to talk of as:

[PROT. p. 4040.]

'miraculous remedies which guaranteed the sick or wounded man against infection from the start.'

It was also at this time that Himmler had informed Hitler of his first inspection, together with the SS General Wolff, of an experiment by Rascher on a human subject. Hitler had then decided that

[PROT. p. 4045.]

'in principle, when the well-being of the nation is at stake, experiment on human subjects is permissible . . . and that the persons of those detained in concentration camps or prisons ought not to remain completely unaffected by the war while German soldiers are being subjected to almost unbearable strain and our native land, women and children are being engulfed under a rain of incendiary bombs.'

After Nebe had spoken Grawitz gave Himmler an exhaustive account of the positive results of research and therapy tests at hospitals both in Germany and abroad. He thus encouraged Himmler's constant search for expedients to bolster up his shaky position as 'redeemer of the SS'. This conversation caused Gebhardt, who was present, to change his opinion as a hospital surgeon about the sulphonamides.

He felt it intolerable that their immediate surgical employment in the treatment of wounds should be held up by hesitation about their effects. Moreover, from the point of view of the Medical Service the introduction of sulphonamides appeared likely to compensate for the shortcomings of the doctors in the field.

There is no documentary evidence in connection with the conference between Himmler, Grawitz, Nebe and Gebhardt. The latter gave its date as between the 22 and 25 May. Two days later, on the 27th, Reinhard Heydrich, SS Obergruppen-führer, Chief of the Security Service and Deputy Protector of Bohemia and Moravia, was assassinated. This event was of the greatest possible importance for Gebhardt personally in con-nection with the sulphonamides question. The influence of Heydrich's death on the subsequent performance of experi-ments on human beings at Ravensbrück can hardly be over-estimated.

Gebhardt, in reply to his Defence Counsel, described as follows what happened after the assassination.

[PROT. p. 4050 ff.]

'I arrived by air too late. The operation had already been carried out by two leading Prague surgeons. All I could do was to supervise the subsequent treatment. In the extraordinary excitement and nervous tension which prevailed and was not diminished by daily personal telephone calls from Hitler and Himmler in person asking for information very many sugges-tions were naturally made. I was practically ordered to call in Privy Councillor Sauerbruch, my old teacher, or the Führer's own doctor, Morell, who wanted to intervene in his own fashion with his own remedies. I did not hesitate to take personal res-ponsibility and state my own view, as to which I had no doubts. The two gentlemen from Prague had already operated and done everything professionally necessary to deal with the severe wound, the bullet having ripped open the abdomen and thoracic cavity. They had made a first-rate job of the operation and also administered sulphonamide. I consider that if any-thing endangers a patient it is nervous tension at the bedside and the appearance of too many doctors. I refused, in reply to direct demands, to call in any other doctor, not even Morell or Sauerbruch. Heydrich died in fourteen days. Then I had to see to his family affairs. The situation at that time is scarcely imaginable today. I was summoned by Hitler, who did not,

however, receive me. He sent me on to Himmler. My talk with
him gave me no trouble. I was simply told that in Hitler's
opinion Heydrich's death represented a defeat such as we had
never hitherto experienced.'

Professor Morell, Hitler's personal physician, was said to
have

[DOC. 2734.]

'remarked at table, in a very quiet and authoritative tone: "If
he had been given my own modern sulphonamide, perhaps a
good many things would have turned out differently."

The discussion was soon over. It was resolved that tests of
the efficacy of the sulphonamides should at once be begun
under Grawitz's direction. The latter was himself enjoined to
justify his work clinically. His final position and future re-
habilitation would depend on the result of the experiments.
Gebhardt immediately consulted him in the matter. His
situation has to be taken into account in order to appreciate
Gebhardt's phrase of a "voluntary influence" on the tests. He
stated, with reference to their conversation, that "Grawitz at
first sympathized with me for having been so thoroughly
squashed, and said he would make a point of putting things
right again."

Gebhardt then actually contrived that the conduct of the
experiments would be left to himself, alleging that he did so
because he desired their performance to be scientifically
irreproachable.

The only documents available concerning the first series of
experiments and naming the doctors directly participating,
are reproduced below.

[DOC. 2734.]*

'To the Reich Leader SS H. Himmler,
Berlin.

Reich Leader:

Attached please find a provisional report by SS Brigadeführer Professor Dr Gebhardt on his clinical-surgical

experiments at Ravensbrück concentration camp, furthermore a concluding provisional report on experiments on the biochemical treatment of sepsis as performed at Dachau concentration camp.

(*Signature*) GRAWITZ
(Handwritten)

Settled, after conversation, with RF, SS. Obersturmführer F. Fischer has been given new instructions for Ravensbrück and Dachau.

(*Signature*) GEBHARDT'

'Professor Dr K. Gebhardt,
SS Brigadeführer and Brigadier General of the Waffen SS.
To the Reichsarzt SS Gruppenführer Grawitz.

PROVISIONAL REPORT ON CLINICAL EXPERIMENTS AT RAVENSBRÜCK CONCENTRATION CAMP FOR WOMEN

By order of the Reich Leader SS, I started on 20 July 1942 at Ravensbrück concentration camp for women on a series of clinical experiments with the aim of analysing the sickness known as gas gangrene, which does not take a uniform course, and of testing the efficacy of the known therapeutic medicaments.

In addition, the simple infections of injuries which occur as concomitant symptoms in war surgery had also to be studied, and a new chemotherapeutic treatment apart from the known surgical measures had to be tried out.

* * *

I appointed SS Obersturmführer Dr Fischer as co-worker. SS Oberführer Dr Blumenreuther put the complete surgical instruments and medicaments at my disposal. SS Standartenführer Mrugowsky put his laboratory and co-workers at my disposal.

SS Obersturmführer Dr Lolling, Chief of Office IIID at Oranienburg, assigned as co-workers: SS Obersturmführer Dr

Schiedlausky[1] garrison-physician at Ravensbrück concentration camp for women, SS Untersturmführer Dr Rosenthal[1] and Fräulein Dr Oberheuser, both camp physicians at Ravensbrück concentration camp for women.

* * *

The question was to define firstly, by way of a preliminary experiment, the mode of infection, making use of the known results from experiments upon animals. In these questions I was advised by SS leaders of the Hygienic Institute of the Waffen SS who had taken over the culture and dosage of the inoculation material.

The point was to implant the lymph cultures on the damaged muscle tissue, to isolate the latter from atmospheric and humoral oxygen supply, and to subject it to internal tissue pressure. The inoculation procedure was as follows: a longitudinal cut of ten centimetres over the musculus peroneus longus; after incision into the fascia the muscle was tied up with the forceps in an area the size of a five-mark piece; an anaemic peripheral zone was created by injection of 3 c.c. adrenalin and in the area of the damaged muscle the inoculation material (a gauze strip saturated with bacteria) was imbedded under the fascia, subcutaneous adipose tissue, and skin sutured in layers.

In the first series of experiments (preliminary experiments), three selected prisoners of as much the same constitution as possible were used. They were inoculated as follows:

The first: Aerobic mixculture (staphylococci, streptococci, bact. comm. try. à 5 Mil).

The second: Para Oedema Malignum, sarc, flav. 4·5 mh.

The third: Bact. Fraenkel and earth. Stimulus 4·5 mg.

The experiment was concluded after ten days. After an initial local swelling in the inoculation area and an increase in temperature up to 39°, the inflammation died down, the wound having broken open on the fourth day. There was no danger to the life of any of the prisoners. We succeeded in producing locally the symptoms of gas gangrene in the third prisoner.

1. Sentenced to death at Hamburg in the trial of fifteen former members of the staff of the Ravensbrück concentration camp.

After twenty days the prisoners were released again to their working blocks.

The course of the preliminary series of experiments had proved that we were not successful in producing the same symptoms as of clinical gas gangrene. In a conference with the Hygiene Institute of the Waffen SS the nature of the infection and the conditions for the germs were not considered to be equivalent to the natural conditions in war surgery and consequently the experimental arrangements were changed.

Bacteria coli were added to the aerobe culture and the germ number was increased to twenty millions. Bacteria coli and dextrose were added to the mixture of para oedema malignum.

Bacteria coli were added to the gas gangrene culture by Fraenkel, and while doubling the number of germs, earth was administered to produce a similar environment. Six selected youthful prisoners were inoculated two by two with the above mixture of bacteria in the subsequent first experimental series. One of them remained untreated for control purposes, the other one was powdered with cataxyn wound powder immediately after the inoculation. The first change of dressing took place three days afterwards, the following each second day. Those who remained without treatment were covered with sterile layers, those treated with cataxyn (indicated in the graphs as TK-cases) were continuously powdered with cataxyn. The aerobe cultures in both cases showed local abscesses which could be easily treated surgically.

The para oedema malignum inoculation produced a local inflamation with central suppuration, small formation of necrosis in depth and moderate emphysema of the skin. The regional lymphatic glands were not affected.

Those prisoners who were infected with Fraenkel's gas gangrene, and who immediately received tetanus-antitoxin for the administered earth, produced by far the strongest inflammatory reaction: abscesses with deep necrosis in the area of the inoculation, emphysema of the skin with formation of blisters, and initial necrosis, with collateral oedema extending from above the joint of the knee to the lower third of the thigh and going as far as the back of the foot. The inflammatory appearances receded considerably after the opening of the injury on the first dressing day. The effect of the opening of the wound was particularly significant in the TK-cases which started inflammations in spite of simultaneous therapy. Greater pressure of the tissue due to oxygen, liberated by the medicament, was considered to be the reason for the accentuated local inflammation.

Comparing non-treated cases with the TK-cases, the final critical observation shows:

1. Immediate therapy does not prevent the occurrence either of an ordinary suppuration or of a "gangrene".

2. The cleaning of the wound is faster in TK-cases than in control cases.

3. The formation of fresh wound granulations occurs earlier with cataxyn.

4. The part played by the paranchymatic organs (liver, kidneys) is less important under the influence of cataxyn.

Since in this experiment definite gangrene could also be produced clinically speaking, though its picture did not in any way correspond to the one known in war surgery, after further consultation with the collaborators in the Hygiene Institute of the Waffen SS, the vaccine was changed by adding wood shavings. It is known from bacteriological literature that the virulence of the bacteria in the experimental animal can thereby be considerably increased.

The triple distribution was reserved for the second series of experiments now in progress. Three prisoners in each group were inoculated. One person was left without treatment as control, the second was treated with cataxyn as before, and with the third the Marfanilprontablin powder manufactured by I. G. Farben was employed, since this was strongly recommended by the Army Medical Inspectorate.[1] The powder was applied according to the Schmick procedure. This experiment is still in progress.

Even if as yet nothing definite can be said about this series of experiments it can already be stated that:

1. There is no decisive difference between cases which are treated and those which are not treated.

2. That opening the wound, in addition to immobilization,

---

1. No document proving any connection of the Army with these experiments was submitted. The phrase used in the Report refers to a General Army Order.

M

has proved the most effective means of controlling the inflammation.

3. The effect of the MP powder seems at least doubtful, since in the third TK-case the most definite gangrene observed up to now developed.

We are now investigating the problem as to why the gangrene in the present case did not fully develop. For this purpose, the injuring of the tissue and the exclusion of a muscle from the circulation of the blood were undertaken during a special operating session, and the large-scale necrosis resulting therefrom is to be inoculated with bacteria strain which has already had one human passage. For it is only when the really definite clinical picture of gas gangrene has appeared that conclusions may be drawn on therapy with chemotherapeutics in connection with surgical operations.

(*Signature*) GERHARDT.
SS Brigadeführer'

Gebhardt and Fischer agreed in their evidence that the first fifteen subjects were male prisoners from the Sachsenhausen concentration camp. But in another passage of the report mention is made of 'six specially selected young prisoners' of whom it is added that 'one remained untreated for checking purposes, while the other ...' These observations suggest that only the first three subjects were males, the rest being female.[1]

An interval occurred after the first series of experiments. Then a female subject was suddenly brought to Gebhardt's assistant for inoculation. Gebhardt stated in this connection:

[PROT. p. 4077.]

'I was seriously ill myself at the time. My conscientious assistant Fischer came to my bedside and said: "Chief, I have disobeyed your orders by not working any more today. The subject brought to me had been anaesthetized and was, contrary to my stipulations and instructions, a woman. I was told that directions had come from a high quarter to the effect that in view of the absence of risk and the data required, women could be used as subjects henceforth.'

1. Because the feminine singular of the German for 'one' and 'the other' is used. (*Translator's Note*).

Gebhardt declared in his evidence that he went straight to Grawitz and asked him for an explanation. But he did not consider the answer satisfactory. Thereupon, relying on his long-standing familiar relations with Himmler, he paid a visit to the latter who was himself visiting some relatives in the neighbourhood of Hohenlychen. Himmler was said to have been of the opinion that since the experiments proceeded 'quite harmlessly and gradually', in accordance with Gebhardt's instructions, they represented 'an excellent chance of reprieve' and should therefore be open to the Polish women under sentence of death.

The prosecution, however, saw no reason why these imprisoned female members of a Polish resistance movement should have expected execution. They had only been sent to Ravensbrück because the Governor had refused to confirm their sentence.

After Gebhardt had heard what Himmler had to say he gave in and ordered Fischer to continue the experiments on women.

There were thirty-six women in the second group of subjects. The organization of the tests was described by Dr Fischer as follows:

[PROT. p. 4345.]

'This group was divided in three sections of twelve persons each, so as to afford comparison of results. Two in each section were given no sulphonamide. The other ten were given it after inoculation, at different times. In all three groups the only uniform result was that inflammation did not occur when the sulphonamide was administered to the wound at the same time as the bacterial cultures. In the other cases local inflammation appeared which at times reached the dimensions of a boil about the size of a walnut. The swelling, accordingly, was absolutely restricted to a certain spot and did not affect in any way the rest of the body. But as stated above two in each section, that is to say six subjects, who had been injected with sulphonamide at the same time as with the bacterial cultures, developed no inflammation at all.'

Fischer stated that in the first of these three series only bacteria, in the second bacteria and tiny splinters of wood and in the third bacteria, splinters and glass were introduced into the wounds.

At this stage Grawitz visited the camp. Fischer referred to this visit as follows.

[DOC. 228.]*

'I explained to Dr Grawitz the details of the operations and their results. Dr Grawitz, before I could complete my report on the procedures used and the results obtained, brusquely interrupted me and observed that the conditions under which the experiments were performed did not sufficiently resemble conditions prevailing at the front. He asked me literally, "How many deaths have there been?" and when I reported that there had not been any, he stated that that confirmed his assumption that the experiments had not been carried out in accordance with his directions.

He said that the operations were mere flea bites and that since the purpose of the work was to determine the effectiveness of sulphonamide on bullet wounds it would be necessary to inflict actual bullet wounds on the patients. He ordered that the next series of experiments to be undertaken should be in accordance with these directions.'

Gebhardt and Fischer did not comply with the order to inflict wounds like those received in war. They took steps, however, to aggravate the conditions by applying ligatures to veins in the area of the shin to be inoculated. There were twenty-four subjects in this series, of whom twelve were exposed to mixed infection with gangrenous septic material. Fischer described the progress of infection as follows.

[PROT. p. 4346 f.]

'In this third group, in which altogether twenty-four subjects were tested, the symptoms of inflammation were definitely more severe. But they did not affect all the twenty-four subjects. At first there was no inflammation in the case of the four who had received, as before, the specific in combination with the cultures. Moreover, so far as I remember, and I can in fact recall a curve we showed, symptoms of inflammation were relatively insignificant in the case of the other eight. They were again boils of about the size of a walnut. In twelve of the subjects, however, inflammation was more severe, closely resembling gas gangrene. At any rate the slightest of them was highly intensive. Of those who were inoculated in isolation with agents which could live without air three subjects died in consequence of a spread of inflammation which we could not control even by surgical methods.'

Gebhardt stated the result of his experiments in the following affidavit:

Gebhardt Document

'All the recommended sulphonamide preparations were classified by their local and internal effects in differently composed doses, which were changed from time to time. Comparisons were made through the so-called "Check Cases", in which sulphonamide was not given but every therapeutic prophylactic measure was taken. The data obtained showed unmistakably the fact, extremely important for the care of wounded persons, that the sulphonamides are not suitable specifics for the prevention of the infection of wounds. In addition, we determined by clinical analogy what is still generally accepted today, viz. that the sulphonamides, like all other remedies, penicillin for instance, cannot be carried along the blood-vessels in an abscess owing to the latter's capsular membrane.

Dr Fischer, however, later discovered a tentative solution, of which nevertheless he made no practical tests at that time, after the deaths which had occurred, important as his idea was for medical science in general, in his suggestion that the sulphonamides might be carried by electrical current. The process is now known as iontonophoresis.'

According to Gebhardt's evidence, which was not contested, he arranged in 1945 for the subjects to be handed over to the Swedish Red Cross at the time when the SS was organizing the evacuation of the women in the camp at Ravensbrück as a result of the Russian advance. Four of the subjects who had been in the second and third groups appeared in Court, described the experiments and exhibited their scars.

These and other subjects and prisoners gave evidence and put in affidavits of what they had seen.

Dr Zophia Maczka, a Polish X-ray specialist and a political prisoner at Ravensbrück during the greater part of the war, presented a clinical account of the operations performed. She had been employed as an assistant in the X-ray Department of the sick bay. Her evidence was taken in the Seraphim Hospital at Stockholm, where she was working under Professor Lysholm. The following is an extract from her sworn statement.

[DOC. 861.]*

'Weronika Kraska was infected with tetanus. She died after a few days. Kazimiera Kurowska was infected with gas gangrene bacillus; she died after a few days. The following were infected with oedema malignum: Aniela Lefanowicz, Zofia Kiecol, Alfreda Prus, and Maria Kusmierczuk. The first three died after a few days; Maria Kusmierczuk survived the infection. She was lying ill for more than a year and became a cripple, but she is alive and is living evidence of the experiments.'

The way in which patients were ordinarily treated in the camp was also vividly illustrated by Dr Maczka, in her eye-witness's description of the situation of the survivors of these experiments.

[PROT. p. 1453.]

'If the girls survived and felt pain and their legs festered and they still did not die, they were occasionally bandaged at odd moments. Sometimes they had three days to wait, sometimes fourteen. There was an incredible stench of pus in the room. The girls went on waiting for help. There was no assistant staff at night. They had to help one another.'

The attitude of a doctor who thus interpreted his duties to his patient or 'subjects' agreed perfectly with the general style in which the camp was run.

Jadwiga Dzido, one of the subjects of experiment who appeared in Court, gave a further account of the ratio of power to helplessness which permits any such experimental treatment.

[PROT. p. 880.]*

'In 1942 great hunger and terror reigned in the camp. The

Germans were at the zenith of their power. You could see haughtiness and pride on the face of every SS woman. We were told every day that we were nothing but numbers, that we had to forget that we were human beings, that we had nobody to think of us, that we would never return to our country, that we were slaves, and that we had only to work. We were not allowed to smile, to cry, or to pray. We were not allowed to defend ourselves when we were beaten. There was no hope of going back to my country.'

The witness Wladislawa Karolewska gave her own impressions in Court of the course of the operations.

[PROT. p. 857 ff.]*

'On 22 July 1942, seventy-five prisoners from our transport that came from Lublin were summoned to the chief of the camp. We stood outside the camp office, and present were Kogel, Mandel, and one person whom I later recognized as Dr Fischer. We were afterwards sent back to the block and we were told to wait for further instructions. On the 25th July, all the women from the transport of Lublin were summoned by Mandel who told us that we were not allowed to work outside the camp. Also, five women from the transport that came from Warsaw were summoned with us at the same time. We were not allowed to work outside the camp. The next day seventy-five women were summoned again and we had to stand in front of the hospital in the camp. Present were Schiedlausky, Oberheuser, Rosenthal, Kogel, and the man whom I afterwards recognized as Dr Fischer.

On this day we did not know why we were called before the camp doctors and on the same day ten out of twenty-five girls were taken to the hospital, but we did not know why. Four of them came back and six stayed in the hospital. On the same day six of them came back to the block after having received some injection, but we did not know what kind of injection. On the 1st of August, those six girls were called to the hospital again; those girls who received injections were kept in the hospital, but we could not get in touch with them to hear from them why they were put in the hospital. A few days later, one of my comrades succeeded in getting close to the hospital and learned from one of the prisoners that all were in bed and that their legs were in casts. On the 14th of August, the same year, I was called to the hospital and my name was written on a piece of paper. I did not know why. Besides me, eight other girls were called to the hospital. We were called at a time when executions usually took place and I thought I was going to be executed because some girls had been shot down before. In the hospital we were put to bed and the ward in which we stayed was locked. We were not told what we were to do in the hospital and when one of my comrades put the question she got no answer but an ironical smile. Then a German nurse arrived and gave me an injection in my leg. After this injection I vomited and I was weak. Then I was put on a hospital cot and they brought me to the operating room. There, Dr Schiedlausky and Rosenthal gave me the second intravenous injection in my arm. A while before, I noticed Dr Fischer, who left the operating theatre and had operating gloves on. Then I lost consciousness and when I revived I noticed that I was in a proper hospital ward. I recovered consciousness for a while and I felt severe pain in my leg. Then I lost consciousness again. I regained consciousness in the morning, and then I noticed that my leg was in a cast from the ankle up to the knee and I felt very great pain in this leg and had a high temperature.

I noticed also that my leg was swollen from the toes up to the groin. The pain was increasing and the temperature, too, and the next day I noticed that some liquid was flowing from my leg. The third day I was put on a hospital trolley and taken to the dressing-room. Then I saw Dr Fischer again. He had on an operating gown and rubber gloves on his hands. A blanket was put over my eyes and I did not know what was done with my leg but I felt great pain and I had the impression that something must have been cut out of my leg. Those present were Schiedlausky, Rosenthal, and Oberheuser. After the dressing was changed I was again put in the regular hospital ward. Three days later I was again taken to the dressing-room, and the dressing was changed by Dr Fischer with the assistance of the same doctors, and I was also blindfolded. I was then sent back to the regular hospital ward. The next dressings were made by the camp doctors. Two weeks later we were all taken to the operating theatre again, and put on the operating tables. The bandage was removed, and that was the first time I saw my leg. The incision went so deep that I could see the bone. We were told then that there was a doctor from Hohenlychen, Dr Gebhardt, who would come and examine us. We were waiting for his arrival for three hours, lying on our tables. When he came, a sheet was put over our eyes, but they removed the sheet and I saw him for a short moment. Then we were taken back to our regular wards. On 8 September I went back to the block. I couldn't walk. The pus was draining from my leg; the leg was swollen up and I could not walk. In the block, I stayed in bed for one week; then I was called to the hospital again. I could not walk and I was carried by my comrades. In the hospital I met some of my comrades who were there after the operation. This time I was sure I was going to be executed because I saw an ambulance standing outside the office, which was used by the Germans to transport people intended for execution.

Then we were taken to the dressing-room where Dr Oberheuser and Dr Schiedlausky examined our legs. We were put to bed again, and on the same day, in the afternoon, I was taken to the operating theatre and the second operation was performed on my leg. I was put to sleep in the same way as before, having received an injection. This time I again saw Dr Fischer. I woke up in the regular hospital ward, and I felt a much greater pain and had a higher temperature.

The symptoms were the same. The leg was swollen and the pus flowed from my leg. After this operation, the dressings were changed by Dr Fischer every three days. More than ten days afterwards, we were again taken to the operating theatre and put on the table; and we were told that Dr Gebhardt was going to come to examine our legs. We waited for a long time. Then he arrived and examined our legs while we were blindfolded. This time other people arrived with Dr Gebhardt, but I don't know their names, and I don't remember their faces. Then we were carried on hospital cots back to our rooms. After this operation I felt still worse, and I could not move. While I was in the hospital, Dr Oberheuser treated me cruelly.'

The defendant Fischer declared in his evidence that he had taken Gebhardt's order as 'on the highest authority and a public duty'. [PROT. p. 4332.]

He explained his situation at that time in a way characteristic of his generation. The most important passages in his testimony are given below.

[PROT. p. 4324 ff.]

'I had never previously thought in any practical way about experiments on human beings. I knew, however, that in the history of medicine such experiments had been carried out. But I never studied such things and it was my resolve and my wish not to have anything to do with such a question or the problems it involved. I knew that some people and doctors considered themselves entitled, as free individuals, to regard such tests as necessary even in normal times . . . and I knew that when one believes that medicine should be subdivided in some way and is not very keen on the clinical side, which in the last analysis derives from the ancient priest-doctor, and does no more than observe the invalid and his symptoms at the bedside . . . such doctors who, entirely on their own initiative, in normal times, choose to experiment on human beings, are those who turn to the domain of natural science, feel themselves morally justified in doing so and are regarded by humanity as so justified, because . . . in the view of a natural science applied to human biology the ultimate and decisive proof of a theory can only be obtained by observation of a human subject. But none of these questions had any practical significance for me. I would say that they were a theme of my academic colleagues at Medical School and I had occasionally reflected on the topic by way of rounding off my complete picture. But I had utterly forgotten it later and never dreamed that it could ever constitute an actual problem for me.

Q. The matter has also been discussed in this courtroom by Professor Leibbrand and Dr Rostock.[1] They declared that they themselves would not have carried out such experiments. What is your own basic attitude to the point?

A. My chief feeling was envy of Professor Rostock at being able to give such a reply. I think he is lucky to be able to say such a thing as a successful surgeon. I always used to believe

1. Professor Leibbrand had expressed his views on medical ethics while acting as the prosecution's expert.

that I might be able to make some such remark myself, some day. For it never occurred to me personally to regard such experiments as necessary or if I had I would never, as a man in a position to make his own decisions and draw his own conclusions, have put such tests into practice. In short, therefore, I would say that I quite consciously still regard these problems in that way and that my attitude in the present connection only differs in so far as I did not consider the question in those days as one for me personally but as one characteristic of the war and the times and only arising in the conditions they promoted.

Q. Well, we have heard what Professors Leibbrand and Rostock think in 1947. What were your views of the situation in 1942?

A. The situation in 1942 was so different from the peaceful circumstances of 1947 that I find it difficult to recall precisely and in detail. I cannot describe, or only inadequately, either the public or private conditions of that time without going into their origins. I was born just before the First World War and my schooldays corresponded with the period that followed it. We were always told by the masters at school that Germany could expect nothing but poverty and hopelessness after having lost the war, since at a decisive hour in her history she had fallen a victim to her old hereditary maladies of particularism and disunity.

Whatever the political views of the individual teacher and the various Parties might be, they were all unanimous in believing that matters could only be improved by hard work in the first place and secondly by united effort and the acceptance by individual citizens of that discipline and commitment which were the essential integrating preliminaries for the creation of better conditions, Such were the beliefs with which all the political parties approached us young people. The differences between them, with which we didn't concern ourselves, really only characterized the margins of this central programme. But, despite the general desire for unity, order and the creation of an obedient and disciplined nation, disunity grew steadily. At last, in 1933, to the surprise of many and to something like the surprise of all, Hitler assumed power. However various personal reactions to the event might be, the facts that German life was again mobilized, that public order was once more emphasized and that the economic problem of unemployment was solved, obviously combined to form a convincing argument for acceptance of the change and so induced many to adopt a patient and benevolent attitude even to the National Socialist Party. We did not all believe at that time that war would come. But we were certain that if it did the economic restrictions under which Germany of necessity laboured would render the risk of defeat most serious. The only counterpoise to such a depressing outlook then appeared to be the moral strength imparted by unity. On the outbreak of war the situation changed radically. I should like to point out once again that hostilities were not welcomed by anyone, politically active or not. I myself belonged to a group deliberately inactive in that sense. But our case was now altered. We could no longer see ourselves as independent of the national destiny. The external propaganda which reached us, I mean that of the National Socialists, implied that we were like the crew of a ship in a storm, when no one aboard was entitled or even able to register a protest, since every individual's fate was bound up with that of all and the only question was whether the ship would go down or whether the common effort would succeed in bringing it safe to land. I am sure that it was this argument which at bottom persuaded many who had till then been lukewarm or hostile to take an active part in national policy or at least to drop their passive attitude and render loyal, unquestioning, obedience to the Führer, no longer as a Party leader and exponent of a political system, but as Head of the German Reich and supreme commander in war. Thus the whole position in 1942, as we all recognized, had become that of a life and death struggle, a circumstance which I notice that no witness in this Court has yet indicated. . . . We did not regard ourselves as anything but German citizens of a State depending for its organization on unqualified and absolute obedience to orders given from above. We could only do our duty as responsible people and our duty as subordinates by such compliance with instructions.

I should like also to refer to another typical feature of the situation.

I mentioned in relation to experiences on active service how spiritually and morally binding this law of war became, simply because we found that in obedience to and fulfilment of it our friends, and soldiers both known and unknown to us, laid down their lives. I discovered, in attempting to account philosophically for this situation, that it cannot be understood by the individual, since it arises in an order of magnitude beyond the grasp of one mind, on the level, that is, of the State. Thus the situation before 1942 was characterized by the recognition of the individual that he must comply with the orders of the State wherever he might happen to receive them, without being entitled to demand an explanation of any particular measure required and without expecting that his acquiescence in it as a measure would be needed. These feelings were not only prevalent in the comparatively narrow field of military life. This kind of martial law, formerly strictly confined to its own domain, was now extended to people behind the lines. This extension of military conditions led automatically to the field of private response to the duties demanded by war. Consequently, in such non-military activities as, for instance, the mobilization of labour, all regulations dealing with the individual were abolished, overlaid or reinforced by new arrangements quite incomprehensible to minds of a pacific cast. It was announced that everyone, even women, must work. Confusion arose, accordingly, in many walks of life, when individuals were no longer able to determine at what points the rights of a citizen in peacetime could still be justified and where the demands of war overrode them. I know, too, that at this time certain scientists were allotted tasks, for instance the preparation of chemical warfare or work on increasing the effect of explosives, which were certainly not in the interests of any individual but obviously had destructive aims in view. In such cases also the person charged with the assignment was not in a position to decline it or even to declare it permissible or otherwise.'

Fischer added elsewhere, in replying to questions about his feelings and experiences during the Russian campaign:

[PROT. p. 4315 ff.]

'It was then that I really experienced war for the first time and found that it did not in the least resemble the statements in books. The period was a most difficult one, as we had to live

under rules quite different from those of peace. Since not everyone has experienced war in his own person and many at least
of those who have did not reflect on what happened to them,
those who were deeply impressed by the circumstances later
became isolated and risked misunderstanding of their feelings.
I should have been lucky if my generation had been spared
that experience. But it was forced upon us. Such was the
tragedy to which my generation was exposed. It would not be
right to complain of it, because I should then be complaining
of having been born a German. . . .

We saw daily that men we knew and who—which was another
strange thing—did not hate the enemy, nevertheless obeyed
orders and in carrying them out performed actions or received
wounds or died. Yet we knew they had received no prior
recognition and were no more bound to do what they did than
anyone else. They acted simply because they did not refuse to
comply with the law of the land. This was a real shock to those
desirous of analysing the circumstances intellectually, for they
realized that war had its own moral imperative, not only a
variation of that of peace but actually a direct reversal of it.
If the individual in times of peace stood at the centre of things
and the State in a sense represented merely an organization to
protect him, there could be no other explanation, except for
an anarchist, but that in war the State occupied the centre,
overriding the individual, who was thrust into a secondary
position without being able to do anything about it. One might
remember that there were philosophical grounds for such a
view, in Hegel for instance, who regarded history as in fact
the fulfilment of the Divine Will and the State as representing
both the highest moral standard, actually authorized by God,
and at the same time the instrument by which history was
made. Two imperatives were therefore simultaneously opposed.
neither having any similarity to the other but on the contrary
both being in many respects mutually antagonistic. Both were
rooted in ethical principle. Neither could be denied justification.
For even the second imperative was clearly vindicated and
established by the daily suffering, anxiety and death experienced by soldiers. I intended at that time to give myself,
later on, the opportunity I longed for to evade such terrible
experiences for the future. I could not see my way clear to do

so at the time, for I did not wish to abandon my comrades in the field. But I meant, at a later date, after the war was over, to speak to young people against the institution of war. For I believed it to be the root of all evil and I thought I would be able to convince an audience if I did not address them from a comfortable armchair but as one who in his time had endured with courage the realities of battle. It was already clear to me at that time that it would be a particularly tragic situation if a man had to act at a moment when the law of peace and the law of war were simultaneously present to his mind and he had to consider the differences and contradictions of the two imperatives, both founded on moral principles and claims.'

Fischer observed with reference to the care of the wounded:

[PROT. p. 4321 f.]

'At these two main casualty stations there were four surgeons, who were responsible, or chiefly so, for medical and surgical attention. I think this fact is in itself a matter for reflection and that it goes far to provide an explanation. But as soon as one realizes that there was a frankly inadequate ratio in that war between the destructive power of the weapons used and the unalterable constant of the individual doctor's capacity, one has the real answer to the question so repeatedly put, though it was hoped to solve the problem by reorganization.

In this distressing and difficult situation the news of the effect of the sulphonamides made a special impression. For if we were not simply to fold our hands in despair and watch these people, our own men and enemy prisoners, being left to their fate, we would have to find resources to counteract the technical progress of destructive weapons.'

Towards the end of the hearing Fischer was asked by his Defence Counsel:

[PROT. p. 4372 f.]

'Q. You have been present at this trial for some months now. You have heard Prosecuting Counsel and have yourself described the share you took in these experiments. I ask you now to tell the Court your final impressions of this whole affair, as represented by the speech of Prosecuting Counsel and your own account of the tests, so far as you yourself are concerned.

A. First and foremost I regret that fate compelled me to transgress, as a doctor, the fundamental principle of '*nihil nocere*'. I also regret that people have come forward to bear witness that I did not help but rather inflicted injuries on them. I am particularly sorry that they should have been women. But I have learned that any action one performs and subsequently considers has to be judged with reference to the motives and circumstances that gave rise to it. My own basic motive for the conduct which has brought me before this Court was solely my desire to help the wounded. Such help was urgently needed at that exceptionally difficult time, when millions lay wounded. I acted in obedience to orders like any other member of the great mass of the German armed forces. My belief and confidence in the legality of the established authorities representing the State and the Führer protected and justified me, so I supposed at the time, and relieved me, as I was then expressly told, of individual responsibility. In those days, when my country was fighting for its life and the final result of the conflict was imminent, I considered, since I was not a member of any resistance movement, that the State had the right to embark upon measures the objects of which were beyond the understanding of individuals. Loyalty to the State appeared to me at that period, when some 1,500 soldiers were falling daily on active service and several hundred people were dying daily behind the lines as a result of war conditions, to be the supreme moral duty. I believed we were offering reasonable chances of survival to the subjects of our experiment, who were living under German law and could not otherwise escape the death penalty. I was sure that I myself would welcome such an opportunity if I were in the same situation. This experiment did not take place in 1947, but in 1942, in wartime, and actually at the most critical point of the war. I was not then a doctor in civil life, free to take his own decisions. I was and felt myself to be, of necessity, for that was impressed upon me, a medical expert bound to act in exactly the same way as a soldier under discipline. That order, uncongenial to me personally, was given me by an authority of immense power, the State as represented by Hitler and reinforced by a medical authority of international reputation. The authority in question, Professor Gebhardt, with whose professional work I was well acquainted, inspired me with confidence. I felt that if he had decided upon such experiments as necessary, they must really be so. And he himself pointed out to me that situations sometimes arose in the lives of individuals and countries when it would be the duty of the former to suppress personal scruples because public interest demanded it. I could not then suppose, and I still cannot, that any other motives induced soldiers on active service to perform under discipline actions which as free individuals they would never have attempted to carry out, and which were contrary to their most intimate personal feelings. I consider that the situations are identical and it was in such a situation that I found myself, one in which a member of the armed forces is obliged to discharge a torpedo at a ship or ordered to bomb the residential quarter of an open city. Nor can I believe that when people do such things they are simply obeying their own individual instincts. I am sure, on the contrary, that they have to subdue their personal feelings and that they suppose themselves to be legally justified in their acts on the ground that in battle the word of command is law and also because both sentiment and reflection convince them that they are acting in a higher sense ethically by contributing to the victory of the nation to which they belong.

As to the more marginal questions of what may or may not be permissible I did not then consider that a subordinate could be expected to enter upon them. I thought they concerned only the State authorities and the specialists employed.

I found during the war that such ideas of discipline and indeed discipline in general were by no means a specifically German invention. For they were also the bases of military organization in the countries with which we were at war. I was not in a position to judge at that time how far their systems differed from our own. But these two great authorities, the State with its soldierly conception of duty and structure and Gebhardt with his medical eminence, were the driving forces which faced me with the alternative of either disobeying or obeying orders in wartime. In this dilemma I considered disobedience, rebellion in war, as the more reprehensible of the two decisions open to me.'

N

After the close of the experiments concerned with the artificial production of gas gangrene Gebhardt and Fischer sent in a report for consideration at the 'Third Eastern Meeting of Consultant Specialists, held from the 24 to the 26 May 1943 at the Army Medical Academy in Berlin'. The report was entitled 'Special Tests of the Effects of Sulphonamides.'

The meeting was being organized by Professor Schreiber of the Army Medical Service, who in this case joined Grawitz of the SS in a preliminary examination of the data provided by Gebhardt and Fischer. Gebhardt alleged that he had originally wished to entitle the report 'Tests on Human Beings of the Effects of Sulphonamides' and to describe the experiments quite frankly, since he believed that they were perfectly legal and was anxious for them to be approved by the specialists attending the meeting. But he was ordered to change the title to that given above. A passage in Gebhardt's evidence proves that the organizing authorities felt considerable doubt whether the report should be submitted to the conference at all.

[PROT. p. 4134.]

'I can only indicate the nature of the discussion between Grawitz and myself and suppose that he described it in the same terms to Schreiber. Grawitz was at that time against publication, unless suitably camouflaged, of the experiments, on account of the attention which they had already attracted abroad. For my part I continued to maintain the attitude I had adopted at the start. Our dispute was concentrated on the wording to be employed. I forget whether the phrase "Special Experiments" was suggested by myself, by Grawitz or by Schreiber. In the end I agreed to its use. . . .'

Some two hundred Army medical experts attended the meeting. The report, before being read by Fischer, was introduced by Gebhardt. He said that the experiments had been carried out by order of the Government and that the subjects were all persons sentenced to death and reprieved by the fact of their selection for the tests. But he did not reveal either that they were political offenders or that they were women. Nor did he mention the place where the experiments had been performed.

Fischer's lecture specified the number of subjects, the groups into which they were divided and all the details of procedure, adding that in three cases death had occurred.

The subsequent discussion extended to all the lectures which had been given that day. No criticism was heard of the experiments on human beings as performed by Gebhardt and Fischer.

The latter recited from memory in an affidavit [Doc. 228] the names of some of the most eminent doctors present at the conference.

After the reading of this document in court Mr McHaney, for the prosecution, commented:

[PROT. p. 986.]

'This affidavit proves beyond doubt that knowledge of the criminal experiments reached leading representatives of the medical profession in Germany.... They were people who had the authority and the duty to take steps to prevent such things happening.'

This statement was made before the facts of the case had been more clearly recognized as a result of the evidence given by the accused under examination. But could those present at the conference, unless further details had been made known to them privately, for instance, through Gebhardt, who considered himself, by his own account, perfectly innocent, have been aware that the experiments described had been indisputably criminal in the legal sense? The answer to this question must be in the negative. But after what Gebhardt and Fischer had publicly announced—the latter's statements had been precise enough to render the facts obvious—could the audience have realized that the proceedings reported had been contrary, from a medical standpoint, to the hitherto accepted usages of German clinical practice and professional responsibility? Should they not have found such an aberration, at the very least, 'reprehensible'? Undoubtedly they should have made such a judgment. To that extent the prosecution was justified in maintaining that it was their duty 'to prevent such things happening.'

Objections were heard to this opinion. But on what grounds was the silence at the conference defended at this later date?

An affidavit of one of the participants reads:

[DOC. Handloser 52.]

'In the speech in question people were mentioned who had been sentenced to death. So far as I remember, nothing was said about the experiments having been carried out on concentration camp prisoners against their will. My personal opinion is that such experiments on healthy persons with a view to provoking in them symptoms of disease on which therapeutic measures might be tested are impermissible by the principles of medical ethics and therefore to be condemned without qualification.'

A similar declaration was made by one of the accused under examination in Court.

The best impression of the atmosphere of the meeting was given by one of those present in an affidavit dated the 18 June 1947.[1]

'... I am perfectly certain that it was impossible for any of the speakers to take up the question of the persons treated in the experiments.

The Medical Service officers present ... would not have been able, at a meeting almost wholly composed of members of their own Service, to criticize measures taken by SS doctors, for considerations of inter-Service tact alone would have precluded such a step. As Professor Gebhardt had taken full responsibility, as Lieutenant-General of the SS, for the experiments, criticism of the choice of subjects to be experimented on would have been tantamount, in the circumstances then prevailing, to criticism of the SS. I don't think there is any need for me to refer here to the consequences which would have followed for any such critics. ...

Any objection raised with reference to the subjects of the experiment or any disapproval of the system of their selection would have been, if expressed at this meeting, an unparalleled insult, a demonstration which, moreover, could not have been

1. The reluctance of many of the participants even now to criticize their own behaviour at the time is evident from the attacks made upon the editors of the present work in the *Göttinger Universitäts-Zeitung* for 1947 and 1948.

kept secret, owing to the large number of those present, and would probably soon have been broadcast from foreign transmitters. A charge of treason would then instantly have followed. After the meeting I talked to a number of my colleagues and expressed my opinion, with which they agreed, that the experiments could not at the time have been expected to provide any positive result and that they must therefore be regarded as having been unnecessary. The cruelty of the tests was also unanimously emphasized by all those with whom I spoke. But not a single one of them made the slightest suggestion that it would have been the duty of the lecturers to give expression to this view in their accounts of the matter. Almost all those who attended the meeting were well-known scientists. Those who were not university professors were independent directors of departments in large hospitals or active Medical Service officers of very high rank. My frank opinion today is that it would have been the duty of every one of them—and there were over 200 present—to protest against the experiments described.'[1]

It is only too shockingly clear from this statement how in the course of a long war military habits of mind, innumerable considerations of a private nature and the ever-present threat of force could combine to suppress, even among doctors, ordinary humane feeling. Respect for others could only be expressed at very great risk. It did not seem to be anybody's business to extend it to 'candidates for death' in Himmler's realm.

1. This affidavit was not submitted at the trial but in another connection.

CHAPTER SIX

EXPERIMENTS IN BONE
TRANSPLANTATION

A further group of experiments carried out on female prisoners in the Ravensbrück concentration camp were concerned with the regeneration and transplantation of bone.

Dr Maczka, the witness mentioned above, described these experiments from the standpoint of an X-ray expert in her affidavit.

[DOC. 861.]*

'The bone experiments were checked by X-ray photographs. As ward attendant I had to do all the X-ray photographs. In this way I was given the opportunity of gaining an insight in this matter. The following were carried out: (a) bone breaking, (b) bone transplantation, and (c) bone grafting.

(a) On the operating table, the bones of the lower part of both legs were broken into several pieces with a hammer, later they were joined with clips (for instance Janina Marczewska) or without clips (for instance Leonarda Bien) and were put into a plaster cast. This was removed after several days and the legs remained without plaster casts until they healed.

(b) The transplantations were carried out in the usual way, except that whole pieces of the fibula were cut out, sometimes with periosteum, sometimes without periosteum. The most typical operation of this kind was carried out on Krystyna Dabska.

(c) Bone grafting. These operations were customary in the school of Professor Gebhardt. During the preparatory operation two bone splints were put on the tibia of both legs; during the second operation such bone splints were cut out together with the attached bones and were taken to Hohenlychen. As a supplement to the bone splint operations such operations were also carried out on two prisoners in protective custody who suffered from deformation of bones of the osteomyelitis type.'

The defendant Gebhardt stated under examination that Dr Stumpfegger, Himmler's personal physician, previously an assistant surgeon at Ravensbrück, had performed 'six so-called splinter operations' on the same group of Polish women. These experiments were undertaken, Gebhardt declared, as the result of a 'special inquiry' and 'special approval' by Himmler, against Gebhardt's own professional judgment and without his collaboration, between the autumn of 1942 and the spring of 1943, in order to ascertain whether regeneration was caused by the periosteum or by the fluid expressed by the supporting tissue. Gebhardt asserted that the idea originated in research by the Russian Bogomoletz, of Kiev, whose work had come to the knowledge of Himmler and Stumpfegger. [PROT. p. 4116 ff.]

Details were given to the Court of a case of homoeoplastic transplantation of the shoulder-blade of a female prisoner at Ravensbrück to a private patient at Hohenlychen. Gebhardt stated in evidence that the transplantation was carried out by Stumpfegger on the basis of positive results he had obtained in splinter removal. The witness added that he had definitely advised Stumpfegger not to undertake any such therapeutic experiment, since it could not succeed and would cause serious injury to two persons. [PROT. p. 4123.]

Stumpfegger, however, according to Gebhardt, took a different view and the latter had therefore consented, in this one case, to an operation in which 'a therapeutic object might be attained with the least possible injury to others'. The patient at Hohenlychen was a youngish man who had lost a shoulder-blade and his collar-bone owing to a blood-vessel tumour, so that his arm was useless. The project was to transfer to the patient the shoulder-blade of a prisoner at Ravensbrück so that the question of the feasibility of bone transplantation from one human being to another could be decisively answered. Gebhardt enumerated the conditions under which he consented to the operation and announced its result as follows:

[PROT. p. 4124.]

'1. That no further bone transplantations are to be made in

consequence of this experiment if it does not succeed; 2. That no further plans are made for bone transplantation to the wounded; 3. That the shoulder-blade be then grafted into the body of the patient showing symptoms of cancer. The result proved that I was right. The patient's arm was saved. The transplanted shoulder-blade healed and functioned normally and up to 1945 there were no more signs of cancer. The subject survived. The woman or man——' he means the concentration camp prisoner—'with whom I am always being reproached, I don't know why, had the same chance of survival after being sentenced to death.'

The defendant Fischer had already—in November 1945—made the following sworn statement.

[DOC. 228.]

'As a disciple of Lexer, Gebhardt had for long been planning free heteroplastic transplantation of bones, i.e. the transplantation of the bone of one person to another person. Though some of his colleagues were not in agreement with the project he was determined to undertake such an operation in the case of his patient Ladisch, whose shoulder-joint (scapula, clavicle and head of humerus) had become displaced owing to a tumour.

My colleagues and I continued to advance objections to the operation on both medical and humane grounds until the evening on which it took place. But he insisted on our performing it. Dr Stumpfegger of the Medical Service, to whose field of research the operation pertained, was to remove the scapula (shoulder-joint) at Ravensbrück and had already made special arrangements there to do so. As, however, Professor Gebhardt needed Dr Stumpfegger for the eventual transplantation to Ladisch, I was instructed to proceed to Ravensbrück and perform the operation the same evening. I asked Dr Gebhardt and Schulze to give me a precise description of the technical means they wished me to employ. Next day I left for Ravensbrück. . . . The camp doctor assisted me with the operation and terminated it himself, as I had to return as soon as possible to Hohenlychen with the bone for transplantation. This step was taken to shorten the period between removal and transplantation. The bone was handed to Professor Gebhardt

at Hohenlychen and he transplanted it with the help of Drs
Schulze and Stumpfegger.'

Fischer's statement under examination in Court agreed more
closely with Gebhardt's. He said that he himself was told at
that time that 'a shoulder-blade would be taken from a shoulder
which was not functioning quite normally owing to a previous
amputation of the hand.' [PROT. p. 4358.]

The alarming extent of Fischer's submissiveness and narrow
specialist's outlook is clear from his own evidence.

[PROT. p. 4401.]

'*Q.* Was the prisoner whose shoulder-blade you removed a
man or a woman?

A. I can't quite remember.

Q. Do you recall the prisoner's name?

A. No.

Q. In your previous evidence, Dr Fischer, you have stated
that it was a man, while Dr Gebhardt has said that it was a
woman. Can you clear up this mystery at all for us?

A. Yes, to the extent that I was given no information at the
time, for reasons which I have also stated, regarding the person
in question. During the discussion that evening I gathered from
Stumpfegger that the shoulder-blade would be that of a male
prisoner whose hand had been amputated. . . .

Q. Well, Doctor, didn't you examine that man yourself?

A. No, I didn't.

Q. Did you talk to him?

A. No.

Q. Do you know whether he agreed to the removal of his
scapula?

A. No, I didn't know anything about that either. I have been
trying today to tell you in what peculiar circumstances I was
charged with the operation and how I got into the situation in
which I obtained the shoulder-blade.

Q. I know all about that, Doctor. Do you intend to tell me
that you could possibly perform an operation on anyone to
remove the scapula and yet not be in a position to say whether
the subject had one hand or one arm or not?

A. Certainly, it is quite possible.

Q. Good heavens, Doctor! You were attending that person, were you not?

A. Yes.

Q. And yet you can't tell us whether the patient had one arm or not?

A. I would ask Counsel to note that in operations the subject is completely covered except for the area of operation.

Q. I should have thought it possible, even with a covering, to be aware that there was no arm under the blanket or whatever the covering might be.

A. No. That is not the case.

Q. Well, do you know what happened to the man afterwards?

A. The patient in question was transferred to the care of Dr Stumpfegger.

Q. Did you ever see him again?

A. Counsel will please note that at the beginning of January I went to Berlin in compliance with orders and did not see the patient again.'

Dr Maczka agreed with another witness, a woman doctor who had also been a prisoner at Ravensbrück, that the shoulder-blade was removed from an insane female inmate of the camp, who was given a fatal injection of evipan immediately after the operation. [DOC. 875 and 861; PROT. p. 1466.]

In addition to these experiments others concerned with nerve and muscle regeneration, as well as a further amputation and certain experiments carried out by the camp doctors in the air-raid shelter were mentioned. The nature and extent of these tests did not come to light.

If prisoners reached a physical condition in which early death seemed probable, they were quite often given fatal injections. Dr Herta Oberheuser confessed in an affidavit:

[DOC. 487.]

'I have myself dispensed five or six such injections.'

Another of the camp doctors, Rosenthal, stated:

[DOC. 858.]

'I saw Dr Oberheuser give prisoners benzine injections on a

few occasions. She used a 10 c.c. syringe on the vein of the arm. The effect was that of acute heart-failure. The patients reared up and then suddenly collapsed. From three to five minutes elapsed between injection and death. The patients were fully conscious until the last moment. The process of injection took some fifteen to thirty seconds. Dr Oberheuser told me that the prisoners to whom she administered these petroleum ether injections all had serious diseases which were incurable.

I have myself administered overdoses of morphine to about twenty or thirty desperately sick patients in order to give them an easier death.'

The Court sentenced Professor Karl Gebhardt to death, Dr Fischer to life imprisonment and Dr Oberheuser to twenty years.

Judgment recapitulated and refuted the arguments of the defence, in particular that based on the legal position of the subjects as of foreign nationality.

[Judgment p. 108, 113 f.]*

'It is claimed by Dr Gebhardt that all of the non-German experimental subjects were selected from inmates of concentration camps, former members of the Polish Resistance Movement, who had previously been condemned to death and were in any event marked for legal execution. This is not recognized as a valid defence to the charge of the indictment.

The Polish women who were used in the experiments had not given their consent to become experimental subjects. That fact was known to Gebhardt. The evidence conclusively shows that they had been confined at Ravensbrück without so much as a semblance of trial. That fact could have been known to Gebhardt had he made the slightest inquiry of them concerning their status. Moreover, assuming for the moment that they had been condemned to death for acts considered hostile to the German forces in the occupied territory of Poland, these persons still were entitled to the protection of the laws of civilized nations. While under certain specific conditions the rules of land warfare may recognize the validity of an execution of spies, war rebels, or other resistance workers, it does not under any circumstances countenance the infliction of death or other punishment by maiming or torture.

We do not see how the principle of superior orders can be used in refutation of the charges brought by the Indictment. This axiom would never be regarded as applicable to a case in which the recipient of the order was free to accept or reject it. Such were the circumstances in Gebhardt's case. The evidence proves beyond doubt that he was not ordered to carry out the experiments but on the contrary sought the opportunity to do so. This fact is particularly clear in the case of the sulphonamide experiments.

In reality Gebhardt took them from Grawitz's control in order to prove that certain surgical measures recommended by Gebhardt himself in May 1942 at Heydrich's death-bed in Prague were superior both scientifically and medically to the treatment proposed by Hitler's personal physician Dr Morell. The principle invoked is therefore inapplicable. But even if it were, the existence of such orders could only be taken into consideration under Regulation 10 of the Supervisory Council as mitigating circumstances.

A further argument featured by the defence tries to rely on the disputed notion that in the general interest of the alleviation of human suffering a State may legally arrange for the performance of medical experiments on prisoners under sentence of death without their consent, even if such experiments may involve the severe suffering or death of the subject. Whatever the law of a State in relation to its own citizens may be, it is clear that such legislation cannot be extended to apply to foreigners exposed under the worst form of slavery to experiments carried out against their will in conditions of the greatest cruelty and absurdity.'

CHAPTER SEVEN

PHLEGMON EXPERIMENTS

During 1942 and 1943, at the same time as the experiments on human beings referred to above were being undertaken, similar operations were performed at Dachau, in which phlegmon was artificially induced, the object being to compare the effects of therapeutic treatment by the methods of allopathy and biochemistry respectively.

According to the witness Stöhr the head physician, Dr Wolter, chose as subjects Catholic priests of various nations and monks occupying the clerical block of the camp, after a series of experiments with ten German prisoners had been carried out. The artificial infections were given in the operation theatre of the camp hospital. Heinrich Stöhr, a political prisoner employed as a male nurse, was present at this proceeding. He stated that it was conducted by a camp doctor, Pape, and 'attended by Sturmbannführer Dr Schütz and the biochemist Dr Kiesewetter.' [PROT. p. 625.]

At the same time as artificial infection was thus induced, patients already suffering from autogenous phlegmon, 'the characteristic camp disease', were experimentally treated by allopathy and biochemical methods.

Stöhr stated:

[PROT. p. 624.]*

'Three similar cases were observed. One of these cases was given allopathic treatment; another biochemical, and the third one received only ordinary surgical treatment. That is, the third one received no drugs whatsoever, and the wound was treated in an ordinary way with bandages and so on. These were the directives of the physicians who were there. We saw on many occasions that the patient was cured much faster who received no drugs or injections.

Experiments of that kind were conducted for many weeks,

and if I may as a layman make a judgment, I must say that
the physicians, according to my observations, were not satisfied
with these experiments.

In addition, I have to emphasize that not only wounds were
treated according to these methods, but internal diseases too.
They tried to find out whether biochemical treatment was
suitable for treating the thirst for water, which was so frequent
in the camp. We saw that the biochemical drugs had no
influence whatsoever as to the cause of this illness.'

The subjects of experiment were also treated with sulphonamides and by biochemical methods respectively, in two groups.

On the 29 August 1942 Grawitz sent a report to Himmler
which gives an idea of the extent of these tests.

[DOC. 409.]*
'Reich Leader.

With regard to previous results of biochemical treatment of
sepsis and other cases of illness, I beg to submit the following
provisional report.

1. The following forty cases were treated with biochemical
remedies in the SS Hospital Dachau in the time mentioned in
the report. Besides septic processes, such diseases were treated
where a decisive change for the better should be achieved by
means of biochemistry:

Phlegmonous-purulent processes	..	17
Sepsis		8
Furuncles and abscesses ..	..	2
Infected operational incisions	..	1
Malaria		5
Pleural empyema		3
Septic endocarditis		1
Nephrosis		1
Chronic sciatica		1
Gall-stones		1

According to the indications of the biochemistry applied to
the different cases, we used the following remedies:

Potassium phosphoricum	..	.. D6
Ferrum phosphoricum	..	D6 and D12
Silicea ..	..	.. D6

Sodium muraticum	..	.. D6
Calcium phosphoricum	..	.. D6
Sodium sulfuricum	..	.. D6
Magnesium phosphoricum	..	.. D6
Sodium phosphoricum	..	.. D6
Calcium fluoratum	..	.. D6

The cases of sepsis were mostly artificially provoked.

Up to now we found that the unfavourable course of the severe cases could scarcely be stopped by means of biochemical remedies. All sepsis cases died. The malaria cases were not influenced by it.

The cases of extended purulent processes, with development of abscesses, the pleural empyema, the septic endocarditis, the nephrosis, the chronic sciatica and the gall-stones showed no definite influence from biochemical treatment. Insofar as they were conducted with positive results, they took the same course as is customary, according to medical experience, when patients are restricted to staying in bed without receiving any special treatment.

The impression of a favourable effect on morbid cases of sickness by biochemical means appeared in five cases only, four of which were comparatively slight. The fifth case involved a 17-day-old child with severe furunculosis. In this case an improvement set in only a few days after treatment had been applied. However, an error occurred in the experimental procedure, for at the beginning of the treatment a sulphonamide preparation was used.

The strong formation of pus, clearly noticeable in a few cases, is perhaps due to the biochemical remedies applied. The doses of sugar, which were frequently given and mainly consisted of pure milk sugar in the form of biochemical tablets, probably promoted the effect. Experiments are being undertaken to elucidate this matter.

In a case of a joint mould the antiseptic potassium phosphoricum D6 was given as a prophylatic because the incision of the operation was greatly endangered by infection. In spite of that the temperature rose to 39° on the following day. Consequently, the biochemical treatment could not prevent appearance or breaking-out of an infection, although potassium phosphoricum D6 was given immediately and intensively.

It is also to be noted that very soon all the seriously ill cases flatly refused to take biochemical tablets, because it meant torture to them to take the tablets every five minutes, even at night.

Finally it must be said that from a total number of forty cases there are one positive case and four positive cases with certain reservations, against thirty-five failures, of which ten ended fatally.

The experiments in Dachau are being continued.

Besides the hitherto existing programme, special attention is directed to research on twin cases in similar conditions, of which one will receive an allopathical, the second a biochemical treatment.

2. In the concentration camp of Auschwitz, three typical cases of sepsis, which developed from phlegmons, were treated —according to prescription—with potassium phosphoricum D4. In none of these cases a therapeutical influence on the progress of the disease could be observed. All three cases ended fatally.

The experiments are being continued.

(*Signature*) GRAWITZ'

The following extracts from a case history with entries running uninterruptedly from 11 November 1942 to 18 January 1943 was found at Grawitz's private residence. He had 'taken an extraordinarily keen interest in the unbroken maintenance of the experiments'. [DOC. 408.]

[DOC. 994.]

'*Diagnosis:* Artificial phlegmon of the left thigh and right upper arm.

Natorski, Stefan, *b.* 12 1 1909, Sch. P. 30 300.

Admission to sick bay, 10 11 1942.

Medical history: No recollection of childhood ailments. 1941, typhus.

Finding: 33-year-old patient in undernourished and weak physical condition, head and throat, no findings.

Thorax: No sign of any active specific lung affection. Heart, no findings.

Abdomen: soft, not sensitive to pressure. Limbs, no findings. *Temperature:* 35·8°. Pulse 60. Weight 51 kg. Height 1·63 m.

CASE HISTORY

11 11 42. At 6 p.m. patient given an injection of 1 c.c. 'Purolin' (pus) in which numerous chains of streptococci had been microscopically identified. Injection point at interior of left thigh adjoining position of abductor canal. Late in evening patient complains of severe headache and dragging pains in left thigh.

12 11 42. Swelling and sensitivity to pressure at injection point on left thigh.

13 11 42. Further swelling of left thigh, especially on inner side. Pains mainly on movement of left leg, occasional painful throbbing of left thigh even while at rest. Reddening of an area the size of a handsbreadth round injection point.

14 11 42. Same condition.

15 11 42. Whole of left thigh much swollen today, Sensitivity to pressure higher and pains more severe. Persistent headache.

16 11 42. Pea-sized purulent pustule formed at injection point on left thigh, where otherwise no change. Patient complains of severe throbbing pains.

17 11 42. Whole of left thigh still much swollen. Reddening at small isolated spots round injection point, where a pus-filled carbuncle about the size of a farthing appears. Sensitivity to pressure high all over interior of left thigh.

18 11 42. Condition unchanged.

19 11 42. No important visible change in left thigh. Some increase of swelling towards the knee. Patient complains of severe throbbing pains in that area. Left leg today put to rest in splints. A perforation of the interior of the left thigh released 14 c.c. of creamy pus, of which 3 c.c. were immediately injected intravenously into the patient's right arm.

20 11 42. Photograph taken. In front of the middle of the left thigh, to one side of the median vein, a hump-like lump, with maceration of the epidermis and reddening of an area the size of a large coin. Creamy pus being discharged from the original perforation. Whole of left thigh swollen. Patient etherized and an incision made in the centre of the inner area, the cut being cauterized. About 250 c.c. of yellow, creamy pus

o

were discharged. A counter-incision was made on the back of the left thigh. The two cuts were connected by rubber draining tubes and the flow of pus thus facilitated. Finally drying bandages and splints were applied.

22 11 42. Swelling of left thigh slightly less. The incision cuts were discharging a brownish pus, mixed with blood. Sensitivity to pressure in the left thigh occurred only near the cuts. The lower half of the right arm, especially the inside, was slightly reddened, swollen and sensitive to pressure.

Therapy: Leg bath, rivanol washing, drainage. Dry bandaging, splints.

23 11 42. Further slight decrease in swelling of left thigh. Copious discharge of yellowish-brown pus and blood-clots from incision cuts. Necrotic shreds of tissue also came away.

Right upper arm still swollen in its lower half, slightly reddened and painful on pressure.

Therapy: As yesterday . . . .

28 11 42. No important visible changes in left thigh. Moderate discharge of yellowish-brown pus from incision cuts. At the lower end of the upper arm, in the flexion area, a swelling was observed almost the size of a hen's egg, the skin being reddened. Slight fluctuation of the swelling was noticeable

Ethyl chloride was administered and an incision made. A copious flow of creamy pus was discharged. Finally a strip of iodoform gauze and a rubber draining tube were applied, followed by dry-bandaging. The entire left arm was kept at rest.

Therapy: Left thigh wounds washed with rivanol, draidiazol-sympatol subcutaneously.

29 11 42. Left thigh still rather swollen. Slight brownish pus discharged from incision wounds. Swelling on right upper arm somewhat less. Copious discharge of thick, reddish-brown pus from wound in that area. Surrounding epidermis excavated over about a handsbreadth.

Therapy: Left thigh wound-washing with rivanol, drainage, dry-bandaging, splints. Right upper arm swabbing, dry-bandaging, splints. Internal as yesterday. . . .

18 1 43. The patient's condition has continued to improve substantially during the last few days. He does not complain at all now. He will be allowed to leave the sick bay today.

SUMMARY

In this case a complete abscess formed in the left thigh after purolin injection. An abscess also appeared in the right upper arm after intravenous purolin injection. Both ulcers were opened. Widespread and deep necrosis occurred in the left thigh. Blood-vessels were broken. Much bleeding resulted. Ligature applied to the saphena magna vein stopped the bleeding. The wounds suppurated for a few weeks. The patient was given fair-sized doses of albucid and tibatin internally. Cleaning of the incision cuts took a relatively short time in comparison with that spent with patients biochemically treated. The patient made a good recovery and is now fit for work again.

Sulphonamides administered during the whole course of treatment comprised 124 grams of tibatin given intravenously and 336 grams of albucid orally.'

An extract from the evidence of the witness Stöhr gives some idea of the risks of the experimental infection.

[PROT. p. 626.]*

'*Q*. You have told us that they had one group, the first group, of ten Germans. How many died in that group?

A. I believe that the first group consisted of ten people of whom, as far as I remember, seven died.

Q. Now, you have told us of a second group of forty clergymen. How many died in that group?

A. I have seen a list of the survivors, and according to that list, twelve clergymen, or rather monks, must have died.'

On the 12 September 1942 SS Standartenführer Dr Theodor Laue, one of those responsible for the parallel experiments in therapy by allopathy and biochemical methods, wrote to Rudolf Brandt, Himmler's personal consultant:

[DOC. 409.]

'I was particularly gratified to find that as a direct consequence of certain failures recently experienced at Dachau Gruppenführer Dr Grawitz now intends to concentrate on the purely scientific side, so as to drive a wedge once and for all into the tradition of mineral salt therapy. I believe that his plans can only meet with general satisfaction, as no better field for their realization can be found than at Dachau. Since the key to the lock has now been discovered, in other words the collaboration of a physician experienced in that direction——' This was Dr Kiesewetter, a biochemist— 'I am sure that success will not be long delayed.'

The members of the SS who have been mentioned in connection with these experiments are all dead or missing. Of the accused only Gebhardt, who knew of the experiments, stated in his evidence that he had protested against them to Himmler. But he added that the latter, in his eagerness 'to dig up old popular remedies out of the rubbish heap' and as an opponent of academic medicine, had been convinced of the propriety and urgency of the tests in question. [PROT. p. 4149 ff.]

CHAPTER EIGHT

MUSTARD GAS AND PHOSGEN
EXPERIMENTS

MUSTARD GAS experiments were carried out at Sachsenhausen and Natzweiler-Struthof between September 1939 and April 1945. The object was to discover the best remedies for the wounds inflicted by this gas. The organization of the experiments and the names of the persons involved were revealed in documentary and oral evidence by eyewitnesses.

The prosecution based its indictment on Doc. 198, a preliminary report by one Dr Sonntag on eight cases of 'Oil O' injuries and their treatment with the specifics 'H' or 'F 1001' at the Sachsenhausen concentration camp on the 22 December 1939. The following is an extract from the report:

[DOC. 198.]

'In order to obtain a comparatively good chance of forming a judgment from a relatively small number of cases both arms of each subject were cauterized. "Oil O" was applied with the platinous compound to an area of skin about the size of a florin and allowed to dry by air for thirty minutes. A protective bandage was then placed over the arm. In cases 1 and 4 infection of the left arm was induced on the third day and in cases 7 and 8 on the fourth day by rubbing a mixture of strepto-, staphylo- and pneumococci into the parts under the abraded blisters or the scabs which came away when the bandage was changed.

The infections induced in cases 1, 4, 7 and 8 by mixtures of strepto- and pneumococci took somewhat different courses. In case 1 the symptoms were sepsis with high temperatures, shivering fits, swelling of the regional glands and enlargement of the spleen. In cases 4, 7 and 8 moderate temperatures were observed. In all cases the general condition was powerfully affected. Agents could not be identified in the blood. Smears were taken after two and four weeks. In all cases strepto- and staphylococci were found and in case 8 pneumococci as well.

The tendency of the infected cauterizations to heal was slower.'

There was no evidence of agreement by the subjects to the experiments.

Further experiments with mustard gas, of which fairly detailed documentary evidence exists, were carried out on prisoners at Natzweiler, supplementary to the experiments on animals, by the Professor of Anatomy at the university of Strasbourg, Dr August Hirt, and Dr Wimmer, faculty lecturer in medicine. The tests on human subjects can be traced back to a letter from Sievers, business manager of the 'Ancestral Heritage' Community for research and instruction.

In this letter he wrote, *inter alia*, to Professor Hirt:

[DOC. 703.]

'But above all the Reichsführer SS would like to hear more details from you at an early date about your mustard gas experiments. In connection with special secret experiments which we are carrying out just now at Dachau we are sure to be in a position to put at your disposal for the furtherance of these experiments unique facilities. Could you not some day write a brief secret report for the Reich Leader SS on your Lost' (Mustard gas) 'experiments?'

The Reichsführer duly received the secret report he desired. [Doc. 097.] It contained a summary by Hirt of the experiments he had undertaken at the request of the Army on officers of the Military Academy. Himmler accordingly, on the 14 July 1942, directed the Professor, who held the rank of SS Hauptsturm-führer, to proceed with research which was to include experiments in the concentration camp at Natzweiler. For Hirt had explained, at the close of his secret report, that the practical application of the vitamin prophylaxis and therapy devised by himself and also the therapeutic potentialities of the acrinidin dye trypaflavine could only be tested by 'direct experiment'.

A secret memorandum by the defendant Sievers, dated the 26 April 1942, proves that these plans for research by Hirt and some of the latter's other ideas, such as that for a collection of the skeletons of Jews, led to the foundation of the 'Institute for Practical Research on Military Science' within the 'Ancestral Heritage' Community.

[DOC. 2210.]

'Continuation of Lost experiments:
Hirt cannot leave Strasbourg at present, as he has no
colleagues there. He has to give no less than twenty-eight hours
a week to lecturing. He is very pleased with the prospect offered
of carrying out Lost experiments on human beings (prisoners).
We have agreed that he will draw up a programme of work for
the experiments at Dachau concentration camp, which will be
entrusted to the chief camp doctor, SS Hauptsturmführer Dr
Wolter.
Different types of subjects will be chosen, put on a diet of
vitamin A to begin with and then treated with Lost.
In order to combine these experiments with similar investigations (those of Rascher on insects and rats), which are no
doubt also proceeding in the "Ancestral Heritage" Community,
and thus to facilitate their execution from an organizational
and technical point of view, I suggest:
1. The foundation of an Institute for Practical Research on
Military Science in the "Ancestral Heritage" Community.
2. The appointment of SS Hauptsturmführer Professor Hirt
to active membership of the Institute and his nomination as
Director of its H (Hirt) Department.'
This document also calls attention to the need for human
subjects in connection with Hirt's studies in microscopic
fluorescence. For he intended to bring out 'a completely new
microscopic anatomy of living organs in fluorescent light',
based on his 'intravital microscopy'.
In an order dated the 7 July 1942 [Doc. 442] Himmler
directed the 'Ancestral Heritage' Community to set up 'an
Institute for practical research on military science'. It was to
combine and render economically feasible all the studies he
himself considered necessary and also likely to increase the
reputation of the SS institutions. The defendant Wolfram
Sievers, business manager of the 'Heritage', was put in charge
of the new Institute. He had in former times been a bookseller.
During the ensuing years he came under powerful attack, in
his latest capacity, by Grawitz and Gebhardt, the former's
chief clinical authority, in particular.
Himmler's instructions to Hirt to carry out research at

Natzweiler were brought to the knowledge of the SS officials concerned. A 'Heritage' memorandum of the 3 November 1942 contains the following passages:

[DOC. 098.]*

'We were further informed that prisoners, who are later to be experimented on, would have to be paid for by us while they are subjected to the experiment. For the prisoners in the L-experiment we propose that they are put on full diet (guards' diet), so that the experiments can be carried out under the same conditions as would prevail with the troops in an actual case. . . .

. . . I was very astonished to find that the prisoners participating in the experiment are to be charged for. If we only use ten for an experiment which may last ten months, they alone will cost us altogether nearly 4,000 marks.

When I think of our military research work conducted at the concentration camp Dachau, I must praise and call special attention to the generous and understanding way in which our work was furthered there and to the co-operation we were given. Payment for prisoners was never discussed. It seems as if at Natzweiler they are trying to make as much money as possible out of this matter. We are not conducting these experiments, as a matter of fact, for the sake of some fixed scientific idea, but to be of practical help to the armed forces and beyond that to the German people in a possible emergency. . . .

Provided that the prisoners who are to participate are given the required preliminary diet, I should say that the experiment might start on the 10 November 1942.'

The witness Ferdinand Holl, at that time a political prisoner, acted as chief orderly in 1942–43 of the Sick Bay Section which was put at the disposal of the 'Ancestral Heritage' Community as from October 1942. He gave the following details, in evidence, of the proceedings.

[PROT. p. 1081.]

'In the middle of October, as soon as the "Ancestral Heritage' Community was installed, certain prisoners who were still to some extent fit, that is, still looked fairly healthy, were selected by Professor Hirt and taken to two rooms, into each of which fifteen men were introduced. They were at first, for about fourteen days, put on SS diet. Then the experiments began.

The subjects were transferred to the Pathological Department where the first experiments with liquid gas took place. Before these people were selected Professor Hirt had told them that if they would report voluntarily for the tests he would raise the question of their release with Himmler. But by that time the inmates of the camp had already heard of other experiments which had been carried out in other camps and no one volunteered. Thereupon the subjects were simply ordered to participate. . . .

Hirt himself supervised the first experiments. Afterwards they were conducted by a German Air Force officer. The prisoners were stripped quite naked. They came into the laboratory one by one. There I had to hold their arms while they were given one drop of the liquid 10 cm. above the forearm. Then they had to go into the next room and stand for about an hour with their arms spread out. Some ten hours later or perhaps after a rather longer interval the burns made their appearance, covering the whole body. The body was scorched wherever the gas exhalations reached it. Some of the subjects were blinded. They suffered intense pain, so that one could hardly bear to be near them. They were photographed every day, photographs being taken of all the burns on them. The first fatalities occurred on about the fifth or sixth day. The corpses were at that time sent on to Strasbourg, as there was then no crematorium in the camp. The bodies were, however, sent back again and dissected in the "Ancestral Heritage" Community. The intestines, lungs and so on were found to be completely eaten away. During the next few days another seven people died. This treatment lasted about two months. Then those who were still to some extent capable of travelling were dispatched to another camp.'

This evidence was confirmed by another former political prisoner at Natzweiler, who added that Professor Bickenbach participated in these experiments. [PROT. p. 10568 f.]

The same statement was made in Court by the last commandant of the Bergen-Belsen camp, since executed, who had been commandant at Natzweiler until April 1944.

[DOC. 807.]

'Professor Bickenbach came several times to the camp at
Struthof for conferences with the camp doctors Krieger or
Blanke. I don't know whether they carried out any experiments.
But he did tell me one day that he had been ordered to carry
out certain experiments on the inmates. He did not tell me
what kind of experiments they were. He had been sworn to
secrecy by the SS authorities.

As I was making a general inspection of the camp one day
I saw ten inmates with bandages on their arms in one of the
wards. I was told (by Bickenbach) that experiments had been
performed on them. I asked him what kind of experiments they
were. But he refused to give me any information on the subject.
I don't know the number of fatalities which occurred in the
camp during my time there.'

It is clear from a 'Heritage' memorandum that Hirt and
Bickenbach had already 'made use, with . . . surprising success'
of the opportunities offered them to carry out phosgen experiments at Natzweiler. [DOC. 2210.]

According to Holl's testimony further sequences of experiments with liquid gas were conducted by Hirt.

[PROT. p. 1093 f.]

'There were the experiments in the gas-chamber. . . . The
gas was in small ampoules containing between 1 and 2 c.c.
. . . The prisoners were taken into the gas-chamber, which was
situated about 500 yards from the camp, two at a time. The
gas-chamber was then of course closed. Thereupon one of the
prisoners had to break the ampoules, so that both were obliged
to inhale the gas released. After this they were taken out of
the chamber, sometimes unconscious, and brought to the
"Ancestral Heritage" Community sick bay, where they were
given further treatment and the development of their condition
observed. . . . The consequences were about the same as those
of the liquid gas experiments. I was sometimes ordered to
administer oxygen for restoration of the breathing apparatus

to normal. But certain subjects whom no one took the trouble to revive actually died of suffocation. The signs of burning were exactly or very nearly the same as those in the first experiments. I have seen the lungs of some of the corpses which were immediately dissected in the "Ancestral Heritage" Community. They were about the size of half an apple, corroded and full of pus.'

Holl was asked at the same hearing how many persons were subjected to these experiments. He replied:

[PROT. p. 1094.]

'While I was there, which was until 1943, about a year therefore, in the place where these experiments were conducted, about 150 subjects were treated in this way in the separate series. . . . In the first experiments—there were four sets altogether—on an average seven or eight of the thirty subjects perished and the same number during the gas experiments. . . . These people died in the camp, of course. But as soon as those experimented on were capable in any degree of travelling they were taken to Auschwitz or Belsen or Lublin or some other large camp.'

In March 1944 Professor Karl Brandt, Reichskommissar for Public Health, transmitted an order by Hitler stressing the urgency of experiment with poison gases. The order was issued in the utmost secrecy, for 'very restricted distribution'.

'In accordance with instructions' Sievers then reported to Brandt, in April, on Hirt's experiments, enclosing a 'Proposal for the Treatment of Lost Gas Injuries' which had been prepared by Hirt and Wimmer for publication. From this document it is clear that examples of external and internal burns so produced, of all grades of severity, had been studied. [DOC. 099.]

Karl Brandt, when giving evidence on his own behalf, denied that he had ever been told of experiments on human beings, either reported by Sievers or later by Hirt when he visited the latter at Strasbourg. [PROT. p. 2372 f.]

A declaration on oath [Doc. Karl Brandt 12] affirms that action had been taken at Brandt's suggestion to procure animals for the purpose of testing the efficacy of manufactured poison gases, foreign currency having been made available in this connection for the purchase of anthropoid apes.

At the trial of Professor Otto Bickenbach for murder at Strasbourg he stated at the first hearing, when explaining the origin, organization and nature of his experiments with phosgen, that he had succeeded in discovering a prophylactic against phosgen poisoning, the drug in question being hexamethylentetramine (urotropin). He added that he had accordingly been ordered by Himmler in 1943 to test it on human beings. Bickenbach himself described the experiments as follows:

[DOC. 3848.]

'I may add that I had previously, though Himmler had forbidden me to do it, undertaken an experiment on myself in the gas-chamber at Fort Ney. I then carried out two series of tests, one on forty persons and the next on fourteen. I am not now quite sure of the actual numbers. They can be found in my reports, which are in the hands of the judicial authorities. There were no fatalities in the first series. Only one subject fell ill in consequence of the experiment. During the second series four people died. I ascribe their deaths to their defective physiological condition. Those experimented on showed symptoms of pulmonary oedema. I would emphasize that Hirt was not present at the first series, though he took part in the second, at which Letz was also present. I admit that the reports you have shown to me are my own, with the exception of those signed by Ruhl and Letz. I would add that I am not well acquainted with the work of Professor Hirt. I am aware, however, that he was looking for a remedy to counteract the effects of the common mustard gas, called Lost. I admit that experiments on human subjects are contrary to medical ethics. I nevertheless practised them because I was above all aware of the horrors of gas warfare and knew that the population of Germany was not protected against it. I therefore regarded it as my duty to do all I could to provide such protection so as to save the lives, if need arose, of thousands of Germans, in particular women and children. Secondly I had to consider Himmler's orders. I have always been assured that my discovery in this field represented the only reliable prophylactic. Professor Brandt himself told me so.'

In Bickenbach's extant reports to Karl Brandt the following paragraphs are appended to the description of experiments on animals:

[DOC. 1852.]*

'7th Report.

On the protective effect of hexamethylentetramine in phosgene poisoning.

Experiments were carried out on forty prisoners on the prophylactic effect of hexamethylentetramine in cases of phosgene poisoning. Twelve of those were protectively inoculated orally, twenty intravenously, and eight were used as controls. ... The experimental subjects were all persons of middle age, almost all in a weak and underfed condition. On principle, the healthier ones were used as controls, only control No. 39 (series J) and the orally protected experimental subject No. 37 (series A) had a localized cirrhotic productive tuberculosis of the lungs. With the others, no pulmonary disease could be found. In the first experiments up to 6 grams hexamethylentetramine were given orally, later, despite the much higher concentrations, 0·06 g. kg./body weight, orally as well as intravenously.

Experiment XV is characteristic of the test schedule and its results, and will therefore again be specially described. Of four test subjects, the first was protectively inoculated orally, the second intravenously, the third received an intravenous injection of hexamethylentetramine after the poisoning, in order once more to ascertain the effect of therapeutic treatment, the fourth was not treated at all. The four subjects were placed in the chamber in which a phial containing 2·7 grams of phosgene was smashed. The test subjects remained under this concentration for twenty-five minutes. The phosgene content was measured three times during the inhalation. The readings showed an average concentration of 91 mg. per cbm. The subject protected intravenously remained healthy, and did not show the least signs of difficulties or symptoms, the orally protected subject contracted a slight pulmonary oedema, subsequently broncho-pneumonia and pleurisy, from which he recovered. One control subject also survived his pulmonary oedema; the second died a few hours later, and the autopsy showed the characteristics of very serious pulmonary oedema.

Summary

The conclusions of the experiment are impaired by the varying constitutions and the general poor state of nutrition and physique of the experimental subjects, as well as by the different behaviour and the different volume of respiration of the experimental subjects under gas, which was here demonstrated for the first time.'

Four deaths and twelve cases of illness are noted in the report.

CHAPTER NINE

COLLECTION OF THE SKELETONS OF JEWS FOR STRASBOURG UNIVERSITY

THE former Professor of Anatomy at Strasbourg University, Dr August Hirt, gave a precise account, in a repcrt dated the 9 February 1942 addressed to Himmler, of his object in wishing to form a collection of the skeletons of Jews.

[DOC. 085.]*

'Enclosure:

Subject: Securing skulls of Jewish-Bolshevik Commissars for the purpose of scientific research at the Reich University of Strasbourg.

There exist extensive collections of skulls of almost all races and peoples. Of the Jewish race, however, only so very few specimens of skulls are at the disposal of science that a study of them does not permit precise conclusions. The war in the East now presents us with the opportunity to remedy this shortage. By procuring the skulls of the Jewish-Bolshevik Commissars, who personify a repulsive yet characteristic subhumanity, we have the opportunity of obtaining tangible scientific evidence.

The actual obtaining and collecting of these skulls without difficulty could be best accomplished by a directive issued to the Wehrmacht in the future to immediately turn over alive all Jewish-Bolshevik Commissars to the field police. The field police in turn is to be issued special directives to continually inform a certain office of the number and place of detention of these captured Jews and to guard them well until the arrival of a special deputy. This special deputy, commissioned with the collection of the material (a junior physician attached to the Wehrmacht or even the field police, or a medical student equipped with car and driver), is to take a prescribed series of photographs and anthropological measurements, and is to ascertain, insofar as is possible, the origin, date of birth, and other personal data of the prisoner. Following the subsequently

THE DEATH DOCTORS

induced death of the Jew, whose head must not be damaged, he will separate the head from the torso and will forward it to its point of destination in a preserving fluid in a well-sealed tin container especially made for this purpose.

On the basis of the photos, the measurements and other data on the head and, finally, the skull itself, comparative anatomical research, research on racial classification, pathological features of the skull formation, form and size of the brain, and many other things can begin. In accordance with its scope and tasks, the new Reich University of Strasbourg would be the most appropriate place for the collection of and research on the skulls thus acquired.'

The Reichsführer also showed the greatest interest in this plan of his Hauptsturmführer and gave him all the assistance in his power. It was in fact Hirt's suggestion to Himmler which caused the latter to assign, as proposed by Sievers, a new task of fundamental importance to the 'Ancestral Heritage' Research and Instruction Community, viz. the erection of the 'Institute for Practical Research on Military Science'.

It cannot be ascertained from the available documents whether the Jews mentioned in the following letter were the 'Jewish Bolshevist Commissars' referred to in Hirt's proposal or prisoners of longer standing in the camp at Auschwitz. It is only evident that the persons allotted to Hirt for his 'anthropological' investigations were transferred from Auschwitz to the Natzweiler-Struthof camps in the neighbourhood of Strasbourg.

[DOC. 087.]*

'To
Reich Security Main Office,
Office IV B 4
Attention: SS Obersturmbannführer Eichmann,
Berlin SW 11, Prinz Albert Strasse 8
Subject: Assembling of a skeleton collection.

With reference to your letter of the 25 September 1942, IV B 4 3576/42 g. 1488, and the personal talks which have taken place in the meantime on the above matter, you are informed that the co-worker in this office who was charged with the execution of the above-mentioned special task, SS Haupsturmführer Dr Bruno Beger, ended his work in the Auschwitz concentration camp on 15 June 1943 because of the existing danger of infectious diseases.

A total of 115 persons were worked on, seventy-nine of whom were Jews, two Poles, four Asiatics and thirty Jewesses. At present, these prisoners are separated according to sex and each group is accommodated in a hospital building of the Auschwitz concentration camp and are in quarantine.

For further processing of the selected persons an immediate transfer to the Natzweiler concentration camp is now imperative; this must be accelerated in view of the danger of infectious diseases in Auschwitz. Enclosed is a list containing the names of the selected persons.

It is requested that the necessary directives be issued.

Since with the transfer of the prisoners to Natzweiler the danger of spreading diseases exists, it is requested that an immediate shipment of disease-free and clean prisoners' clothing for eighty men and thirty women be ordered to be sent from Natzweiler to Auschwitz.

At the same time one must provide for the accommodation of the thirty women in the Natzweiler concentration camp for a short period.

(*Signature*) SIEVERS,
SS Standartenführer'

What then occurred at the camp was described by the former commandant, Joseph Kramer, under examination.

[DOC. 807.]

'I was a book-keeper in Augsburg before 1932. I then voluntarily joined the SS and was ordered to supervise concentration camp inmates. Before the outbreak of hostilities I acted as Lieutenant in various concentration camps, in particular at Estervegen, Sachsenhausen, Dachau, Mauthausen and Auschwitz. In August 1943 I was ordered by the camp authorities at Oranienburg, or rather by the administrative headquarters of the SS in Berlin, from which I received the order, to take on some eighty inmates from Auschwitz. The

P

letter accompanying the order instructed me to get into touch at once with Professor Hirt of the medical faculty of Strasbourg.

I proceeded to the Strasbourg Anatomical Institute, where he then was.

He told me he had heard of a convoy of inmates going from Auschwitz to Struthof and that these persons were to be given poison gas in the Struthof camp gas-chamber, whereafter their corpses were to be brought to the Anatomical Institute for disposal.

He then gave me a bottle containing about $\frac{1}{4}$ litre (rather less than half a pint) of salts. I believe they were salts of prussic acid. He told me about how much would be required to poison the inmates coming from Auschwitz whom I have already mentioned.

At the beginning of August 1943 I received the eighty inmates who were to be gassed with the stuff Hirt had handed me. One evening about nine o'clock I went to the gas-chamber in a small van with about fifteen women for a start. I told them they would have to go to the disinfection room, but did not tell them they were to be poisoned.

With the help of some SS men I stripped them completely and when they were quite naked pushed them into the gas-chamber.

As soon as the door was shut they began screaming. After it was closed I poured a certain amount of the salts through a pipe which was fitted above the peep-hole, to the right. Immediately afterwards I blocked up the opening of the pipe with a cork which was attached to it. There was a metal tube in the cork which conducted the salt and water to the interior of the chamber I have mentioned. I turned on the interior light by means of a switch fitted near the pipe and looked through the peep-hole to see what was happening in the room. I observed that the women went on breathing for about half a minute before they fell down. I switched on the flue ventilation and then opened the doors. The women were all lying dead on the floor. They were completely covered with precipitates. Next morning at about 5.30 I told the SS hospital orderlies to load the corpses into a small van, so that they could be taken to the Anatomical Institute, as Professor Hirt had instructed me.

A few days later I took a certain number of women to the

gas-chamber in the same way and they were gassed like the others.

A few days later I returned to the gas-chamber. I went there two or three times more till fifty or possibly fifty-five people had been killed with the salts which Hirt had given me.

(In reply to questions the witness stated) I didn't trouble myself about what Hirt was going to do with the bodies of the inmates whom I had poisoned. After what he had said at Struthof I didn't think I ought to ask him. I didn't trouble to ascertain the nationality of the murdered inmates. I believe they came from south-east Europe. But I don't know which country they came from.

(The witness was shown the album containing photographs of the gas-chamber.)

I recognize these photographs as being of the Struthof gas-chamber. It was built in the middle of 1943 for the purpose of poisoning the inmates intended for Professor Hirt.

Q. You have described the circumstances in which you killed these inmates by giving them gas. If the gas had not been effective, would you have shot them?

A. I would have tried to gas them a second time by giving them a further quantity of gas. I was not affected at all by what I did, because I had been ordered to kill those eighty inmates in that way, as I have already told you.

After all, I had been trained to obey orders.'

This evidence, including the time of year, was fully confirmed by the witness Henry Henrypierre, employed at the Anatomical Institute until Strasbourg was occupied by the Allies.

[PROT. p. 775.]

'In July 1943 a high-ranking SS officer called on Professor Hirt. The officer called three times in July. Hirt showed him over the ground floor of the Institute in my presence. A few days later Bong told me that we should have to prepare tanks for 120 corpses. Bong and I prepared six tanks. They were filled with 55 per cent artificial alcohol. The first consignment we received was one of thirty women. It was due at 5 a.m. but did not come till 7 a.m. When we asked the driver why he was late, he answered: "They gave us plenty to do." The thirty female corpses were unloaded by the driver and two assistants, as well

as by Bong and myself. The preservation process was begun
at once. The bodies were still warm when they arrived. Their
eyes were wide open and glazing. The eyeballs were bloodshot,
red and protuberant. There were also traces of blood about
noses and mouths. The discharge of other liquids was percep-
tible in some cases. There was no sign of rigor mortis.

I reflected at the time, though I said nothing, that they
must have been murdered, apparently by poison or suffocation.
For none of the bodies we had hitherto preserved showed any
such traces as were evident when these arrived. I therefore
jotted down on a piece of paper the prison numbers on their
left arms and kept the paper hidden on me. They were all five-
figure numbers.

A few days later we received a second consignment, consisting
of thirty men, in exactly the same condition as the first, still
warm, with wide open, bloodshot and glazing eyes, bleeding
from the mouth and nose and discharging other liquids. The
preservation of these thirty male corpses was also immediately
undertaken in the same way, except for one small detail. In
each case the left testicle was removed and sent to the Anatomical Laboratory, which was that of Professor Hirt himself.

Some time later we received a third and last consignment,
consisting of twenty-six men. They came in exactly the same
state as the previous lot. I should like to make that point clear
once again and it is no more than the truth.

After we had received the first consignment of women I came
across Hirt at the door of the Institute. I repeat word for word
what he said to me. "Peter, if you can't hold your trap, you'll
be given the same treatment." I should also like to mention
another strange thing he said. In conversation with Bong on
the ground floor of the Institute, some time before the bodies
arrived, he observed: "They'll die like flies." I gathered from
all this that there could be no doubt the people had been
murdered. So I had every reason to believe that those eighty-six
corpses we received had not died a natural death.'

The course of war operations brought Strasbourg more and
more obviously into the danger zone, thus increasing the risk
of the Allies discovering what had been going on. Hirt asked
Sievers for advice and he in his turn sought instructions from
Himmler.

[DOC. 088.]*

'According to the proposal of 9 February 1942 and your approval of 23 February 1942, Professor Dr Hirt has assembled a skeleton collection which has never been in existence before. Because of the vast amount of scientific research that is connected with this project, the job of reducing the corpses to skeletons has not yet been completed. Since it might require some time to process eighty corpses, Hirt requested a decision pertaining to the treatment of the collection stored in the morgue of the Anatomy, in case Strasbourg should be endangered. The collection can be defleshed and rendered unrecognizable. This, however, would mean that the whole work had been done for nothing—at least in part—and that this singular collection would be lost to science, since it would be impossible to make plaster casts afterwards. The skeleton collection as such is inconspicuous. The flesh parts could be declared as having been left by the French at the time we took over the Anatomy and would be turned over for cremating. Please advise me which of the following three proposals is to be carried out:

(1) The collection as a whole is to be preserved.
(2) The collection is to be dissolved in part.
(3) The collection is to be completely dissolved.'

A memorandum to the SS Standartenführer Dr Brandt, dated 16 October 1944, contains confirmation 'that the collection at Strasbourg has been completely dissolved in conformity with the directive given at the time.' [DOC. 091.]

The eyewitness Henry Henrypierre described in a report the attempt to obliterate the incriminating evidence.

[PROT. p. 757 f.]

'After these bodies had been chemically preserved, they were put into the tanks. They stayed there a whole year without being touched by anybody. In September 1944 the Allies moved on Belfort. Professor Hirt thereupon ordered Bong and Meier to cut the bodies up and have them incinerated in the crematorium.... After Bong and Meier had carried out these instructions in the room where the tanks were, I asked Bong, on the following day, whether he had cut all the bodies up. He answered: "No, we couldn't cut them all up, it was too much work for us. We left some of the bodies lying at the bottom of the tanks." Then I asked him: "Were the gold teeth left in all the bodies burnt?" He told me that such gold teeth as these Jews still possessed had been handed over by Meier to Professor Hirt.'

A letter dated the 20 January 1945 from Sievers to Hirt strikingly illustrates the type of contingency upon which subsequent knowledge of the real magnitude of the criminal measures taken by the Third Reich depended.

[DOC. 975.]

'. . . Both Paris and London are meanwhile taking a great interest in the Strasbourg Institute and are sorry they didn't find you there. You have probably already received or will shortly receive, through the Ministry of Education, a request by the Foreign Office for your comments on the matter. We can congratulate ourselves that we destroyed all the evidence in time. So far the opposite side hasn't been able to produce concrete data.'

Hirt has disappeared. He is supposed to be dead. Wolfram Sievers and Rudolf Brandt were charged with participation in these particular proceedings of Hirt's. Both the accused were at the same time indicted in connection with most of the experiments on human beings mentioned above, since Sievers as business manager of the 'Ancestral Heritage' Community and Brandt as Himmler's personal consultant contributed to the official regulation and technical feasibility of the experiments.

A number of credible witnesses supported Brandt's contention that ever since his twenty-fifth year, owing to his exceptional ability as a stenographer, he had been Himmler's chief clerk and since he was entirely under the latter's influence had merely passed on Himmler's orders in writing.

Brandt was sentenced to death on the following grounds.

[Judgment p. 138 f.]*

'An extremely persuasive and interesting brief on behalf of the defendant Rudolf Brandt, filed by his Attorney, has received careful attention by this Tribunal. Therein it is urged that Rudolf Brandt's position under Heinrich Himmler was one of such subordination, his personal character so essentially mild, and he was so dominated by his chief, that the full significance of the crimes in which he became engulfed came to him with a shock only when he went to trial. This plea is offered in mitigation of appalling offences in which the defendant Brandt is said to have played only an unassuming role.

If it be thought for even a moment that the part played by Rudolf Brandt was relatively unimportant when compared with the enormity of the charges proved by the evidence, let it be said that every Himmler must have his Brandt else the plans of a master criminal would never be put into execution.

The Tribunal, therefore, cannot accept the thesis.'

Wolfram Sievers, also a SS Standartenführer, alleged in his defence that he had belonged to a resistance group. He stated that it was only this group's aims, which included the removal of Himmler, that had caused him to remain in the 'Heritage' Community even after he had become involved, in his official administrative capacity, in all the experiments the Institute for Practical Research on Military Science had to promote at Himmler's orders.

Several witnesses confirmed these statements generally and also that it was the resistance group's wish for Sievers to remain at his post and in close contact with Himmler. Defence Counsel appealed to the general principles of self-protection in a state of emergency under a criminal system of government.

But Sievers, too, was sentenced to death. The grounds were as follows:

[Judgment p. 165, 179 f.]*

'Sievers received orders directly from Himmler on matters of research assignments for the "Ancestral Heritage" Community and he reported directly to Himmler on such experiments. Sievers devoted his efforts to obtaining the funds, materials, and equipment needed by the research workers. The materials obtained by Sievers included concentration camp inmates to be used as experimental subjects. When the experiments were under way, Sievers made certain that they were being performed in a satisfactory manner. In this connection, Sievers necessarily exercised his own independent judgment and had to familiarize himself with the details of such assignments.

Sievers offers two purported defences to the charges against him: (1) that he acted pursuant to superior orders; (2) that he was a member of a resistance movement.

The first defence is wholly without merit. There is nothing to show that in the commission of these ghastly crimes, Sievers acted entirely pursuant to orders. True, the basic policies or projects which he carried through were decided upon by his superiors, but in the execution of the details Sievers had an unlimited power of discretion. The defendant says that in his position he could not have refused an assignment. The fact remains that the record shows the case of several men who did, and who have lived to tell about it.

Sievers' second matter of defence is equally untenable. In support of the defence, Sievers offered evidence by which he hoped to prove that as early as 1933 he became a member of a secret resistance movement which plotted to overthrow the Nazi Government and to assassinate Hitler and Himmler; that as a leading member of the group, Sievers obtained the appointment as Reich Business Manager of the "Ancestral Heritage" Community so that he could be close to Himmler and observe his movements; that in this position he became enmeshed in the revolting crimes, the subject matter of the indictment; that he remained as business manager upon advice of his resistance leader to gain vital information which would hasten the day of the overthrow of the Nazi Government and the liberation of the helpless peoples coming under its domination.

Assuming all these things to be true, we cannot see how they may be used as a defence for Sievers. The fact remains that murders were committed with co-operation of the "Ancestral Heritage" Community upon countless thousands[1] of wretched concentration camp inmates who had not the slightest means of resistance. Sievers directed the programme by which these murders were committed.

It certainly is not the law that a resistance worker can commit no crime, and least of all, against the very people he is supposed to be protecting.'

1. The total number of subjects proved by statistics given in Court was about 2,000. The numbers concerned in other experiments were not ascertained.

CHAPTER TEN

EUTHANASIA PROGRAMME, 'DIRECT ELIMINATION' AND MASS STERILIZATION

HITLER's interest in 'eugenic' measures conformed with the National Socialist Party line of action.

As early as the 14 July 1933 the 'Law for the Prevention of Hereditarily Diseased Posterity' was promulgated. By March 1934 a comprehensive commentary on this law had been issued by Gütte, Rüdin and Ruttke.

Such was the initial phase of a development which led on the one hand to the compulsory 'mercy killing' of the incurably insane and on the other hand to the elimination during the war of races declared to be inferior, such as Poles, Russians, Jews and gipsies.

In this connection the idea of 'special treatment' is also conspicuous, giving rein, even more than 'mercy killing', to an impulse deliberately hostile to humane considerations.

Such activities on behalf of 'public health' and 'the security of the German people' may accordingly be divided into three main categories: (1) Euthanasia Programme for Incurable Invalids, (2) Direct Elimination, by Special Treatment, of Undesirable National Elements and Undesirable Invalids, (3) Experimental Work Preliminary to Mass Sterilization.

In the ensuing pages a special classification has been followed arising from the individual cases heard at Nuremberg.[1]

(i) EUTHANASIA OF THE MENTALLY AFFLICTED CONFINED IN SANATORIA AND NURSING HOMES

The chief defendant, Professor Karl Brandt, while giving evidence on his own behalf, referred to a speech on the problem

1. A comprehensive summary of the procedure involved in euthanasia, together with accounts of various German court proceedings in connection with the subject, was published under the title *Die Tötung Geisteskranker in Deutschland* ('Killing of the Insane in Germany') by Dr Alice Platen-Hallermund (Frankfurter Hefte Verlag, Frankfurt am Main, 1948). The careers of some of the doctors employed were also noted in this report.

of euthanasia by Gerhardt Wagner, leader of the medical delegation to the Party Meeting of 1935, on which occasion he showed a film purporting to illustrate the lives of the insane.[1]

According to Karl Brandt, Hitler told Dr Wagner in 1935 that

[PROT. p. 2413.]

'in the event of war he would "take up and deal with this question of euthanasia". For the Führer was of opinion that in wartime measures for the solution of such a problem could be put through most easily and with least friction, since the open opposition which must be expected from the Church could not then, in all the circumstances of war, exert so much influence as it would in times of peace. . . .'

Petitions to Hitler appear to have had a certain influence on the course of events. Thus in 1939, according to Brandt, the father of a deformed child requested permission for a 'mercy killing'. Brandt continued:

[PROT. p. 2410.]*

'Hitler turned this matter over to me and told me to go to Leipzig immediately—it was in Leipzig—to confirm the fact on the spot. It was a child who was born blind, an idiot—at least it

1. The prosecution mentioned as an example of 'corruption of the mind' *Question No. 95* in 'a mathematical textbook for German children'. 'If the building of a lunatic asylum costs six million marks and it costs 15,000 marks to build each dwelling on a housing estate, how many of the latter could be built for the price of one asylum?'

'*Question No. 97.* Daily maintenance of an insane person costs 4 marks, of a cripple 5·50 and of a criminal 3·50. In how many cases does an official earn daily only about 4 marks, a factory employee barely 3·50 and an unskilled labourer less than 2 as the head of a family?

(*a*) Illustrate these figures graphically. According to careful calculations there are some 300,000 insane persons, epileptics, etc., in Germany under treatment in institutions.

(*b*) Give the total yearly cost of such persons at the rate of 4 marks p.d.

(*c*) How many State marriage loans of 1,000 marks, not repayable, could be issued annually from the amount now spent on the insane, etc. ?'

(*Mathematics for Education in National Politics, with Examples drawn from history, geography and science.* Adolf Borner, 1935.)

seemed to be an idiot—and it lacked one leg and part of one arm. . . . The doctors were of the opinion that there was no justification for keeping such a child alive. It was pointed out that in maternity wards under certain circumstances it is quite natural for the doctors themselves to perform euthanasia in such a case without anything further being said about it.'

The problem of euthanasia in cases of deformity was formulated and discussed in general terms by the Senior Physician of the Reich, Conti, and Dr Linden, Cabinet Councillor at the Ministry of the Interior, who controlled all sanatoria and nursing homes.[1] On the conclusion of the Polish campaign Hitler told both Brandt and Philipp Bouhler, head of the Chancellery, 'that he now intended to bring about a definite solution of the problem of euthanasia'.[2] At the end of October 1939 Hitler signed a decree with effect retrospective to 1 September 1939.[3]

The decree stated:

[DOC. 630—PS.]*

'Reichsleiter Bouhler and Dr Brandt, M.D., are charged with the responsibility of enlarging the authority of certain physicians to be designated by name in such a manner that persons

1. Dr Conti was at the same time Secretary of State for Public Health and thus his own supervisor. In this last capacity even Dr Linden was subordinate to him.

2. As early as July 1939 'professors, psychiatrists and other experts were for the first time formally briefed at the Chancellery in Berlin. They were told by the then head of the SS, Viktor Brack, that all the insane persons in Germany were to be liquidated under plans which would be carried out by 'euthanasia'. The audience was invited to participate in the programme. They all agreed to do so, with the exception of Professor Ewald of Göttingen, who explicitly declined his services.' (From the Judgment of the Coblenz Court of Petty Sessions delivered on the 29 July 1948 in criminal proceedings against the medical staff of the sanatorium at Andernach.)

3. Karl Brandt stated in evidence that the decree was made retrospective in order to indicate 'that it applied to the methods by which euthanasia was to be operated during the war. After the war, so I understood, it . . . was to be formulated in different terms.' [PROT. p. 2498.]

who, according to human judgment, are incurable can, upon a most careful diagnosis of their condition of sickness, be accorded a mercy death.'

Brandt described Bouhler as an 'honest man' who had become interested in euthanasia and its application:

[PROT. p. 2417.]

'because he feared that in these circumstances, with a war on, certain District Leaders might now and then take a hand in the matter and initiate measures in their Districts without due guidance.'

The defendant Viktor Brack, Bouhler's chief clerk and official deputy, added to the above observation one of his own, while under examination, which illuminates the views of one another held in this particular case by Party leaders of the highest standing. He said that the fundamental reason why Bouhler took over the execution of Hitler's order and in so doing obtained the support of Göring, Himmler and Frick, the Minister of the Interior, was that he did not want the affair to fall into the hands of Conti and, through him, Bormann. For 'Conti was on Bormann's staff' and Bormann had declared 'that euthanasia . . . would be by no means restricted to the incurable insane' and Bouhler 'had feared from the very beginning that Bormann would misuse his authority'. [PROT. p. 7658.]

After the appointment of some ten to fifteen doctors as a result of the decree, Bouhler and his subordinate Brack, together with Dr Linden's department of the Ministry of the Interior and three camouflaged organizations, undertook execution of the euthanasia programme. The 'National Group for Study of Sanatoria and Nursing Homes' began with the collection of statistics of the patients by dispatching and working over questionnaires. The 'Foundation for the Care of Institutions in the Public Interest' dealt with finance and the 'Limited Company for the Transport of Invalids in the Public Interest' arranged the travelling required. Three mutually independent assessors each received a photostat of every patient's file from the first-named body. These, after being stamped by the assessors, were sent to the Chief Surveyors Professors Heyde and

Nitsche and also, according to the evidence of the witness Dr Mennecke, to other university professors, among whom he remembered Professor de Crinis.[1] [PROT. p. 1879.]

It was the Chief Surveyors who finally decided whether a patient should be sent to an institution for observation. These institutions were mainly for the purpose of collecting patients before their compulsory conveyance to such establishments for euthanasia as those of Hadamar in Hesse, Hartheim near Linz, Grafeneck in Württemberg, Brandenburg on the Havel and Sonnenstein near Pirna. Neither the patients themselves nor their relatives had any say in the matter.

The preliminaries to these proceedings came to light in the evidence of Dr Fritz Mennecke, formerly in charge of the observation institution at Eichberg, where he was eventually tried and sentenced to death. He described a conference in Berlin at the beginning of February 1940 in the following terms.

[PROT. p. 1871.]

'Some ten or twelve doctors whom I did not know had been invited to this conference as well as myself. We were told by Drs Hevelmann and Bohne and by Brack that the National Socialist Government had passed laws to permit the extinction of lives not worth living. At the meeting we were asked if we would be willing to act as medical assessors. We were most earnestly enjoined to treat the matter confidentially, as it was an official secret. Brack read a paper at the meeting. But I cannot now quite remember what it was about. I believe, however, that an assurance was given that no doctor who participated in the programme would be punished. The question of the work required of us was then discussed. It was to be the medical assessment of patients in Institutions, that is to say, insane persons. The other doctors present were all elderly people, including, as I afterwards learnt, some of high reputation. As

1. Heyde was arrested in November 1959. He had been living and conducting a practice at Flensburg for some years under the name of Dr Sawade. The Public Prosecutor General of Saxony announced in 1947 that Nitsche had been sentenced to death on the 7 July in that year.

they all unhesitatingly agreed to participate I followed their example and offered to act as an assessor.'[1]

The former Head Physician at the Eichberg establishment, Walter Schmidt, subsequently sentenced to imprisonment for life, stated in connection with this conference:

[PROT. p. 1858.]*

'The jurists in Berlin told us that this was a legal matter, that it was a Hitler decree or a law which had been duly approved; also that the jurists had discussed whether Hitler was authorized to issue such a decree and decided in the affirmative, and we were told that this was a matter which was a quite legal——

Q. Witness, a little slower.

A. That it was a legal task of the State which had already been planned in 1932 and which was also being planned in other countries and that we would not incriminate ourselves in any way, on the contrary, a sabotage of this order would be a criminal offence. The question of secrecy was also discussed in detail and it was stated that this was a kind of law now; that the patients were not to have knowledge of such a measure beforehand because otherwise they would be excited, and that was probably the main reason why this law could not be published. In addition at that time we were at war and those kinds of measures should be kept secret in the interior.

Q. Who were the people to be concerned by the Euthanasia Programme?

1. By way of contrast with this account of the 'unhesitating agreement' of the doctors at this conference, the Judgment of the Düsseldorf Assize Court, presided over by Dr Näke, mentions that at a Berlin conference in April 'vigorous protests were raised by some of those present'. During the interval after Brack's speech the doctors resolved to agree to further participation 'for the sole purpose of obtaining a precise understanding of the aims and plans involved and thus, in a position from which there was otherwise no escape, perhaps to find an opportunity to restrict in some way, or at least an indication of how such restriction might be achieved, the execution of the programme and so to rescue as many patients as possible.' This Judgment also described how certain successful protective measures had been taken by doctors in the Rhineland as a result of their discovery of the purpose for which the questionnaires had been sent out relating to all insane persons and of the recognition by these physicians of the nature of the steps contemplated for euthanasia.

[8 KLs 8/48 –S—1/48.]

A. The incurably sick. However, it was not quite clear to me where the limit was to be drawn.'

It was several times stated in Court that attempts were made to persuade Hitler to pass a law on this subject. Both Lammers and Brack were said to have composed drafts, the latter using the title: 'Law concerning the provision of final medical assistance in the case of incurable invalids.' [PROT. p. 7685.]

Brack stated in evidence that he 'had not been shocked' by Hitler's decree.

[PROT. p. 7683 f.]

'Nor was I in any position to judge whether Hitler distorted in any way a form of words which may have been prescribed for him. But I should like to have seen anyone raise any objection at that time to any paper signed by Adolf Hitler, whatever its outward form might have been. . . .

. . . the doctors and jurists, however, concerned in this matter, took the view that a law must be passed.

Their position was that a secret decree by Hitler would be known only to a small group of people, whereas euthanasia was not the business of any individual or of the Government but of the whole population. The proceedings could not therefore be kept from public knowledge indefinitely. The nation would above all require to know what preliminary conditions for a mercy killing would be regarded as essential and what security measures would be taken to prevent abuse of them. But people could only obtain such knowledge from a law which laid down certain specific regulations. This consideration, however, did not affect our unanimous recognition of the decree itself as legally valid.'[1]

Dr H. H. Lammers, formerly head of the Chancellery, noted in an affidavit that the drafting of a law 'which would first have

1. The question of the legal validity of Hitler's 'euthanasia' decree was discussed in detail by Criminal Court No. 4 of the Petty Sessions at Frankfurt am Main. (See the section on 'Direct Elimination'.) The Judgment of Criminal Court No. 3 of the Coblenz Petty Sessions in relation to the accused medical staff of the Intermediate Station at Scheuern refers to a statement by Brack that 'the German people, in the intoxication of victory, would swallow even that law'.

to be considered by all the Ministries' had been 'uncongenial to
Hitler on political grounds'. [DOC. Karl Brandt 17.]

In order to ensure the secrecy of the measures to be taken
only assessors and heads of institutions who were trusted
National Socialists and SS chiefs were employed.

A clear picture of the extent and nature of what was done
appears from the study of over a hundred documents available.

We may cite an extract from the affidavit of a nursing sister,
P. Kneissler.

[DOC. 470.]

'. . . In 1939 I was ordered by police headquarters to report
on the 4 January 1940 at the Ministry of the Interior in the
Columbus building. Our group, consisting of twenty-two or
twenty-three persons, was addressed by a certain Herr Blankenburg. He explained the importance of secrecy in connection
with the euthanasia programme and said that the Führer had
composed a law on the subject which would not be published
owing to the necessities of the war. He assured us that we
would not be forced in any way to promise our co-operation.
None of us had any objection to the programme and Blankenburg accordingly administered an oath to us. We were sworn
to silence and obedience and warned by Blankenburg that any
transgression of the oath would incur the death penalty. . . .
After the close of the meeting we travelled by omnibus to
Grafeneck Castle, where we were received by Dr Schumann,
Director of that Institution. Our work there did not begin until
March 1940, though the male staff started somewhat earlier.
One of my duties was to visit various Institutions in the com-
pany of Herr Schwenninger, who was also a member of the
Foundation for the Care of Institutions in the Public Interest.
We fetched patients from these places to Grafeneck. Herr
Schwenninger was in charge of our convoys and kept lists of the
names of patients who were to be transferred. . . . The patients
we transferred were not the worst cases. They were insane, but
very often in good physical condition. Each convoy carried
some seventy people and such transfers took place almost daily.
. . . On the arrival of the patients at Grafeneck they were taken

to the huts there and briefly examined by Drs Schumann and Baumhardt on the lines of the questionnaires. These two doctors gave the final decision whether a patient was to be gassed or not. In certain cases gassing was postponed. But the majority of the patients were killed within twenty-four hours of arriving at Grafeneck. I was there nearly a year and know of only a few cases in which patients were not gassed. As a rule they were given, before gassing, an injection of 2 c.c. of morphine and scopolamine. These injections were given by the doctor. The gassing was undertaken by certain picked men. Some of the corpses were dissected by Dr Hennecke. Some idiotic children between 6 and 13 years old were also included in the programme.

After Grafeneck was closed I went to Hadamar and remained there till 1943. At Hadamar the same work went on, except that patients were no longer gassed but poisoned with veronal, luminal and morphine combined with scopolamine. About seventy-five patients were killed daily.[1]

From Hadamar I was transferred to Irrsee, near Kaufbeuren, where I continued with this work. Dr Valentin Falklhauser[2] was the Director of that Institution. The patients there were killed either by injections or by tablets. This programme was carried on until the collapse of Germany.'

One of the questionnaires sent out is quoted below:

[DOC. 825.]*

'Registration Form 1   To be typewritten
Current No.
      Name of the Institution...........................
      At...
Surname and Christian name of the patient...............
At Birth..

1. It will be clear from later extracts that after the official termination of the compulsory liquidation of mainly insane persons certain institutions carried the practice further by poisoning sick and incapacitated foreign labourers with morphine and luminal.

2. The indictment of Dr Falklhauser was drawn up in the office of the Public Prosecutor General at Kempten in Allgaü.

Q

Date of Birth.......... Place.......... District......
Last place of residence.................. District......
Unmarried, married, widow, widower, divorced:..........
Religion.................... Race* ....
Previous profession............ Nationality:..............
Army service when? 1914–18 or from 1/9/39...............
War injury (even if no connection with mental disorder)
    Yes/No..............
How does war injury show itself and of what does it consist?
    ....
Address of next of kin:...............................
Regular visits and by whom (address)....................
Guardian or nurse (name, address)........................
Responsible for payment................................
Since when in Institution..............................
Whence and when handed over..........................
Since when ill..
If has been in other institutions, where and how long........
Twin? Yes/No...... Blood relations of unsound mind:....
Diagnosis..
Clinical description (previous history, course, condition: in any
    case ample data regarding mental conditions):............
    ....
Very restless? Yes/No...... Bedridden? Yes/No........
Incurable physical illness: Yes/No (which)...............
Schizophrenia: Fresh attack............ Final condition
    .... Good recovery............
Mental debility: Weak...... Imbecile...... Idiot......
Epilepsy: Psychological alteration........ Average frequency
    of the attacks...................
Therapeutics (insulin, cardiazol, malaria, permanent result
    .... Salvarsan, etc., when?)...... Yes/No........
Admitted by reason of par. 51, par. 42b German Penal Code,
    etc., through...
Crime...... Former punishable offences................
Manner of employment (detailed description of work)........
Permanent/Temporary employment, independent Worker?
    Yes/No...............

* German or of similar breed (of German blood), Jew, Jewish mixed
breed Grades I or II, Negro (mixed breed).

Value of work (if possible compared with average performance
of healthy person)....................................
This space to be left blank
..........Place Date....................
......................;....................
Signature of the head doctor or his
representative (doctors who are not
psychiatrists or neurologists, please
state same)

The following Instruction Leaflet was attached.[1]

[DOC. 825.]

'*Instruction Leaflet.*

To be noted in completing questionnaire.

All patients are to be reported who—

1. Suffer from the following diseases and can only be
employed on work of a mechanical character, such as sweeping,
etc., at the Institution:

Schizophrenia,

Epilepsy (if not organic, state war service injury or other
cause),

Senile maladies,

Paralysis and other syphilitic disabilities refractory to
therapy,

Imbecility however caused,

Encephalitis,

Huntington's chorea and other chronic diseases of the
nervous system; or

1. The Judgment of Criminal Court No. 3 of the Coblenz Petty Sessions
relating to the accused medical staff of the Intermediate Station at Scheuern
notes that the object of the questionnaires was by no means clear to most of
the directors and staffs of the institutions concerned. 'It was conjectured
that a military measure might be contemplated, such as the recruitment of
the mentally afflicted for the Army or for agriculture. In the efforts of the
staff to retain their patients so far as possible, the incapacity of the latter
for work was in many cases unsuspectingly exaggerated, so as not to deprive
the institution itself of capable workers.'

2. Have been continuously confined in Institutions for at least five years;

3. Are in custody as criminally insane, or

4. Are not German citizens or not of German or related stock according to their records of race and nationality.

The separate questionnaires to be completed for each patient must be given consecutive numbers.

Answers should be typewritten if possible.

Latest date for return.........................

INSTRUCTIONS

Diagnosis should be as precise as possible. In the case of traumatically induced conditions the nature of the trauma in question, e.g. war wounds or accidents at work, must be indicated.

Under the heading "exact description of employment" the work actually done by the patient in the Institution is to be stated. If a patient's work is described as "good" or "very good" reasons must be given why his release has not been considered. If patients on the higher categories of diet, etc., do no work, though they are physically capable of employment, the fact must be specially noted.

The names of patients brought to the Institution from evacuation areas are to be followed by the letter (V).[1]

If the number of Forms 1 sent herewith does not suffice, the additional number required should be demanded.

Forms are also to be completed for patients arriving at the Institution after the latest date for return, in which case all such forms are to be sent in together exactly one month after the date in question, in every year.'

The circulation of the questionnaires as revealed by the following documents incidentally throws light upon the organization behind the actual proceedings. The then Secretary of State for Public Health took personal charge of them in a notice sent to all the institutions concerned.

1. For *versetzt*, i.e. 'transferred'. (Translator's Note).

[DOC. 825.]*

'The Reich Minister of the Interior,
    Berlin NW 40, Koenigsplatz 6, 16 November 1939
    IV g 4178   39–5100
                              Telephone:
                              Dept. Z, I, II, V, VIII 11 00 27
                              Dept. II, IV, VI
                              (Unter den Linden 72); 12 00 34
                              Tel. Address: Reichsinnenminister.

To the Head of the Hospital for Mental Cases,
    Kaufbeuren,
        or his deputy in Kaufbeuren.
    With regard to the necessity for a systemized economic plan
for hospitals and nursing institutions, I request you to complete
the attached registration forms immediately in accordance with
the attached instruction leaflet and to return them to me. If
you yourself are not a doctor, the registration forms for the
individual patients are to be completed by the supervising
doctor. The completion of the questionnaires is, if possible, to
be done on a typewriter. In the column "Diagnosis" I request a
statement, as exact as possible, as well as a short description of
the condition, if feasible.
    In order to expedite the work, the registration forms for the
individual patients can be dispatched here in several parts. The
last consignment, however, must arrive in any case at this
Ministry at the latest by the 1 January 1940. I reserve for myself the right, should occasion arise, to institute further official
inquiries on the spot, through my representative.
                              per proxi: DR CONTI'

    The Court considered at length the questions whether Jews
and foreigners were also included in the programme and to
what extent euthanasia was adopted on purely humanitarian
and legally valid grounds. The prosecution's enquiries were
based on the references to Jews and non-Germans in the
questionnaires, though such people were not apparently
destined for euthanasia. Professor Karl Brandt, who had only
appointed certain doctors, not himself participated in the

measures, considered 'that such extensive proceedings were simultaneously designed to acquire data of another sort.' But Brack, Bouhler's chief agent in the matter, stated that the completion of the questionnaires was intended to 'camouflage' 'economic planning'. He said that at a centre in Berlin known as T 4 (i.e. Tiergartenstrasse No. 4) Jews, foreigners and conscripts for labour and military service were classified. In reply to questions by the presiding judge he affirmed that insane persons who had suffered war wounds and also Jews were exempted from euthanasia, the former on grounds of 'war psychology' and the latter because 'the Government at that time did not wish to extend this favour to them . . . the benefit of euthanasia, in Bouhler's phrase, should only be conferred on Germans.' [PROT. p. 7758.]

As against all these views the prosecution maintained that according to Item 1 of the leaflet (see Doc. 825) no patients who could be employed on any useful work about the institution need be reported. Consequently the sole decisive factor in the matter was the capacity to work. Lammers, in an affidavit, added a further, secondary motive. He said that at the first discussion on euthanasia to which he had been invited by Hitler at the end of September or the beginning of October 1939 the latter had explained 'that he considered it reasonable to do away with the useless lives of some of the mentally afflicted by putting them out of their misery through a merciful death, which would also have the practical advantage of releasing buildings, doctors and nursing staff, etc., for other services.' [DOC. Karl Brandt 17.]

The documents and lists of names surviving from that period leave no doubt that Jews were included in the actual execution of the euthanasia programme.

Action proceeded methodically, rapidly and unopposed. The following exchange of letters between Chief Surveyors and Assessors proves that the work was in full swing a month after Hitler's decree had been issued.

[DOC. 1130 and 1129.]

'Director of National Labour   Berlin W.9,
    Community of Sanatoria and   25 November 1940
    Convalescent Homes.
To Dr Pfannmüller, Chief Medical
    Councillor, Member of the Board of Assessors.
Subject: Dispatch of Forms Nos. 137, 901–138, 200.

I enclose 300 Forms completed by the Lüneburg Institutions.
Please proceed with assessment.
Franked label for return also herewith.

                PROFESSOR HEYDE

                Eglfing,
                29 November 1940
To
National Labour Community of Sanatoria and
Convalescent Homes.
For the attention of Party Member Professor Heyde, Berlin,
W.9.
    Subject: Dispatch of 300 Forms 107, Nos. 137, 901–138, 200,
    as per your letter of the 25 November 1940.

Dear Professor Heyde,
    I beg with great respect to return herewith 300 Forms 107
Nos. 137, 901–138, 200 duly assessed.

                (Signature)'

It is clear from both letters that it took the assessors at most
three days to get 300 cases ready. Correspondence from the
Eglfing-Haar Sanatorium shows that Dr Pfannmüller passed no
less than 2,109 questionnaires between the 14 November and the
1 December 1940. It is also evident that the assessors only dealt
with questionnaires addressed to other institutions. A voluntary
sworn statement by Ludwig Lehner, then a prisoner of war,
who had worked in 1939 on this affair at the Eglfing-Haar
Institution, indicates who actually decided whether a patient
should live or die.

[DOC. 863.]

'There were some fifteen to twenty-five children between the ages of 1 and 5 in separate cradles. Pfannmüller explained his views at this Station with particular thoroughness. I must have taken rather special note of the remarks summarized below, as being astonishingly frank, either through cynicism or boorishness.

"These creatures——' he meant the children just mentioned —"I consider, as a National Socialist, to be a mere burden on our population. We don't kill them——" or he may have said, "We don't do the job——"—"by poison, injections and so on, as then the foreign Press and certain people in Switzerland ——" he probably meant the Red Cross—"would only have a fresh pretext for worrying us. No! Our method is a much simpler and more natural one, as you see." With these words he pulled one of the children out of its cradle with the aid of a female nurse who was apparently regularly entrusted with this sort of work at the Station. He held up the child for our inspection as though it were a dead hare, at the same time making some such remark, with a knowing and cynical grin, as: "This one, for instance, will only last another two or three days." I shall never forget the look of that fat, grinning fellow with the whimpering little skeleton in his fleshy hand, surrounded by the other starving children. The murderer went on to say that it was not the practice to deprive the children suddenly of food but gradually to reduce their rations.'

Dr Pfannmüller was called in evidence. He described Lehner's report as 'probably the later invention of a malicious mind' and commented:

[PROT. p. 7393.]

'Even if the child in question had been regarded as suitable for euthanasia, I would never have come to any such decision on National Socialist grounds. For euthanasia and the work of the National Board had, in my view, nothing to do with National Socialism. They were just as legal as the regulations for prevention of transmission of hereditary disease and infection in marriage. These laws were passed during the National

Socialist régime. But the ideas from which they arose are centuries old.'

Asked about the great number of questionnaires he had passed within a period of fourteen days Pfannmüller answered that 'as a physician he was unable to follow that particular legal train of thought'. He added that 'the cases concerned might have been easy to dispose of'.[1] [PROT. p. 7475.]

One of the orders for transfer issued by Linden's office at the Ministry of the Interior is quoted below.

[DOC. 1133.]

'Ministry of the Interior.   Munich, 18 October 1940
To
    Dr Pfannmüller,
    Director of the Sanatorium and Convalescent Home at Eglfing-Haar.
    Subject: Removal of Sanatorium and Convalescent Home Patients.

The present situation renders necessary the removal of a large number of patients confined in sanatoria and convalescent homes. At the request of the National Defence Commissioner I hereby order the removal of 120 patients from your Institution. Removal will probably take place on the 24 October 1940. Details of the removal consequent upon my order will be discussed with you by the Limited Company for the Transport of Invalids in the Public Interest, Berlin, or its Conveyance Manager. Preparations are to be made at the embarkation point for the transfer. If there are no railway facilities close to your Institution, transport of the patients to the nearest railway

1. According to information received from the Munich (I) Public Prosecutor's office Pfannmüller had been charged on the 16 June 1948 with a number of murders but was medically certified unfit to plead. Meanwhile, three nurses formerly employed at the Eglfing-Haar Sanatorium were sentenced for being accessory to the killing of at least 120 children. The victims had been given fatal injections or doses of luminal tablets on Pfannmüller's instructions. In two cases he had acted in person. To this extent Lehner's evidence could be substantiated.
[Akt. Z. ib Js 1791/47.]

station is to be arranged. Proper measures must be taken with unruly patients to prepare them for a journey of several hours. So far as possible they must wear their own under- and outer-garments. All their private property is to be handed over, securely packed, at the same time. If they have no clothing of their own, under- and outer-garments will have to be lent them at the embarkation point. Their personal papers and medical history documents are to be deposited with the Conveyance Manager. Accountants at the embarkation point should be told that no further payments are to be made after the date of transfer until demanded by the receiving Institution. In the case of those patients subject to court orders this information must be passed to the judicial authorities concerned together with the documentary evidence. The relatives of those transferred will be immediately notified by the receiving Institution. If any relative meanwhile inquires for a patient at the embarkation point and the name of the receiving Institution is not yet known there, the answer must be that the patient has been transferred to another Institution at the orders of the National Defence Commissioner concerned, and that the Institution in question will soon be communicating with the relatives of patients so transferred.'

Three more orders in exactly the same terms as those sent to Eglfing-Haar appear in the files. Between October 1940 and January 1941, 440 patients were concerned. Lists of their names and the 'receipts' of the appropriate official of the 'Limited Company for the Transport of Invalids in the Public Interest' were also filed.

The former Chief Physician of the Eichberg 'Observation Station' stated in evidence [Prot. p. 1841] that his chief, Dr Mennecke, had said that on each occasion the patients sent to Hadamar very early in the morning by the Company's omnibus were dead by the evening.

Shortly after the 'transfers' the institutions concerned usually received some such note as the following:

[DOC. 1696—PS.]*

'I beg to inform you that all the female patients transferred from your Establishment on the 8th November 1940 died during that month at the Establishments of Grafeneck, Bernburg, Sonnenstein and Hartheim.'

The patients' relatives were informed by the Institutions in letters which always took the same form.

[DOC. 840.]

'Grafeneck Münzingen National Convalescent Home
6 August 1940

Frau B...... Sch......, Z......
My dear Frau Sch......,

We are sincerely sorry to tell you that your daughter F......
Sch......, who had to be transferred to this Institution in accordance with measures taken by the National Defence Commissioner, died suddenly and unexpectedly here, of a tumour of the brain, on the 5 August 1940. The life of the deceased had been a torment to her on account of her severe mental trouble. You should therefore feel that her death was a happy release. As this Institution is threatened by an epidemic at the present time, the police have ordered immediate cremation of the body. We would ask you to let us know to what cemetery we may arrange for the police to send the urn containing the mortal remains of the deceased. . . . Any inquiries should be addressed to this Institution in writing, visits being for the present forbidden as part of the police precautions against infection. . . .

(*Signed*) DR KOLLER.'

The defendant Brack stated in Court that he had attended one of the euthanasia operations. The gas-chamber used, he said, was a room of ordinary size and appearance which communicated with others at the Institution. On that occasion between twenty-five and thirty persons were introduced into the room, without clothing, and poisoned with carbon monoxide gas. [PROT. p. 7759 ff.]

Public Prosecutors in certain districts were struck by the frequency of these events and notifications of them in the Press. The Public Prosecutor General of Dresden, for instance, addressed the Ministry of Justice on the subject, enclosing, *inter alia*, a list of obituary notices from the *Leipzig Neueste Nachrichten*, nearly all in identical terms.

[DOC. 897.]

'We have received from Grafeneck in Württemberg the sad news, communicated to us after cremation, of the sudden death of our beloved only son B.S.'

At a conference of the Provincial Press held at Frankfurt am Main on the 30 April 1941 editors were informed:

[DOC. 844.]

'that obituary notices have recently appeared in the daily press of the district in terms which are no longer to be used, for example:

(*a*) Sanatoria and convalescent homes announce the following deaths. . . .

(*b*) As expected, we have received the news. . . .

(*c*) After a long period of suspense. . . .

The Public Prosecutor General of Stuttgart forwarded to the Minister of Justice three full accounts of 'cases of unnatural death in sanatoria and nursing homes'. The current proceedings were quashed by the Secretary of State, Freisler.

Those put to death by euthanasia were also the subject of pathological research on the brain. Professor Hallervorden, for instance, who had no connection with the euthanasia proceedings, received at his own request 600 specimens of brain from the euthanasia stations. They were placed at his disposal, he said, in batches of 150 to 250 at a time, by the 'Limited Company for the Transport of Invalids in the Public Interest'. [DOC. L 170.]

Dr Mennecke, moreover, admitted that Dr Carl Schneider of Heidelberg, now deceased, one of the prime movers of the euthanasia plan, had received such specimens. [PROT. p. 1900.]

The following extract may be cited from a report by the Ansbach district chairman.

[DOC. D 906.]

'The transfer of invalids from sanatoria and convalescent

homes to other parts of the country could not, of course, be kept a secret from the public. It also appears that the committees concerned worked with excessive speed and not invariably with due discrimination, so that many blunders were made. Consequently, it is impossible to prevent certain cases from becoming known and being generally discussed. Such instances as the following should naturally never have occurred: (1) A certain family received, by mistake, two urns.[1] (2) The cause of death was given in one notification as appendicitis. But the patient's appendix had been operationally removed ten years before. (3) In another case the cause of death was stated to be disease of the spinal cord. Relatives had visited the patient a week previously and found him in full physical health. Another family received notice of the death of a female relative, though the woman in question is still alive in the Institution and enjoying the best of bodily health.'

The following extracts from official communications to the Ministry of Justice complete the picture of the euthanasia operations. In December 1939 the Frankfurt am Main Provincial Court of Appeal informed the Minister:

[DOC. 844.]

'People living near sanatoria and convalescent homes, as well as in adjoining regions, sometimes quite distant, for example throughout the Rhineland, are continually discussing the question whether the lives of incurable invalids should be brought to an end. The vans which take patients from the Institutions they occupy to transit stations and thence to liquidation establishments are well-known to the population. I am told that whenever they pass the children call out: "There they go again for gassing." I hear that from one to three big omnibuses with blinds down go through Limburg every day on their way from Weilmünster to Hadamar, taking inmates to the Hadamar liquidation centre. The story goes that as soon as they arrive they are stripped naked, given a paper shirt and immediately taken to a gas-chamber, where they are poisoned

1. Brack alleged in evidence that this statement had been proved erroneous by subsequent investigation.
[Prot. p. 7733.]

with prussic acid and an auxiliary narcotic. The corpses are said to be transferred on a conveyor belt to an incineration chamber, where six are put into one furnace and the ashes then packed into six urns and sent to the relatives. The thick smoke of the incinerators is supposed to be visible every day over Hadamar. It is also common talk that in some cases the heads or other parts of the body are detached for anatomical investigation. The staff employed on the work of liquidation at these Institutions is obtained from other parts of the country and the local inhabitants will have nothing to do with them. These employees spend their evenings in the taverns, drinking pretty heavily. Apart from the stories told by the people about these "foreigners", there is much anxiety over the question whether certain elderly persons who have worked hard all their lives and may now in their old age be somewhat feeble-minded are possibly being liquidated with the rest. It is being suggested that even old peoples' homes will soon be cleared. There is a general feeling here, apparently, that proper legal measures should be taken to ensure that above all persons of advanced age and enfeebled mentality are not included in these proceedings.'

The following is an extract from one of the many communications from ecclesiastical authorities. It is a fifteen-page memorandum from Pastor Braune, Chairman of the Central Committee of the Home Mission of the German Evangelical Church.

[DOC. 823.]

'During the last few months it has been noticed in many parts of the country that large numbers of the inmates of sanatoria and convalescent homes are continually being transferred, in accordance with "economic plans", in some cases repeatedly, till eventually, after some weeks, a notification of their decease is received by relatives. The similarity of these measures and their accompanying circumstances in different regions leave no doubt that they are being undertaken as part of a massive scheme for the elimination of thousands of lives "not worth living". The view is held that in the interests of national defence these useless mouths should be put out of the way. It is also urged to be absolutely necessary for the improvement of the German breed to get rid as soon as possible of imbeciles and other incurable invalids, as well as abnormal and anti-social persons and those incapable of integration in the community. Over a hundred thousand individuals, it is estimated, would be affected by these measures. Professor Kranz, writing in the April number of the National Socialist paper *Volksdienst* ("Public Service"), actually puts the figure of those whose elimination is probably desirable at a million. At the present moment, therefore, it is likely that thousands of German citizens are being liquidated, or are facing imminent death, without the slightest legal justification. It is urgently necessary to put a stop to these proceedings with the least possible delay, for they are most seriously endangering the very foundations of German morality. The inviolability of human life is one of the corner-stones of any political system. If lethal measures are to be taken they must be supported by duly passed legislation. It is intolerable that invalids should be regularly liquidated in this way for the sake of mere expediency, without scrupulous examination or any judicial safeguard, against the will of their relatives and with no opportunity for legal representation. . . .

A further serious question arises. How far is the annihilation of the so-called "lives not worth living" to go? The comprehensive measures hitherto taken have proved that many people have been seized whose minds had a considerable degree of clarity and discrimination. In one case particularly well known to me six girls were to have been transferred who were about to be released from the Institution for employment as domestic servants in Labour Institutes. Are only the utterly incurable, congenital idiots, to be taken? The Instruction Leaflet, as I have already mentioned, refers to senile maladies. The latest decree of the same authorities orders the inclusion of children with serious hereditary diseases or deformities of any kind. They are to be collected and placed in special institutions. Such an arrangement is bound to arouse serious misgivings. Are tubercular patients, for instance, to be exempt? Apparently euthanasia has already started in the case of those in protective custody. Are other abnormal and anti-social persons now to be apprehended? Where is the line to be drawn? What sort of people are to be regarded as abnormal, anti-social or incurable?

Or incapable of integration in the community? What will happen to the soldiers who received incurable injuries while fighting for their country? They themselves are already asking such questions.'

In August 1941 the Bishop of Limburg wrote, *inter alia*:

[DOC. 615—PS.]*

'About 8 kilometres from Limburg in the little town of Hadamar, on a hill overlooking the town, there is an Institution which had formerly served various purposes and of late had been used as a nursing home. This Institution was renovated and furnished as a place in which, by consensus of opinion, the above-mentioned euthanasia has been systematically practised for months—approximately since February 1941. The fact is, of course, known beyond the administrative district of Wiesbaden because death certificates from the Hadamar-Moenchberg Registry are sent to the home communities. (Moenchberg is the name of this Institution because it was a Franciscan monastery prior to its secularization in 1803.)

Several times a week buses arrive in Hadamar with a considerable number of such victims. School children of the vicinity know this vehicle and say: "There comes the murder-box again." After the arrival of the vehicle the citizens of Hadamar watch the smoke rise out of the chimney and are tortured with the ever-present thought of the poor sufferers, especially when the nauseating odours carried by the wind offend their nostrils.

The effect of the principles at work here is that children call each other names and say, "You're crazy; you'll be sent to the baking oven in Hadamar." Those who do not want to marry, or find no opportunity, say "Marry, never! Bring children into the world so they can be put into the bottling machine!" You hear old folks say, "Don't send me to a State hospital! When the feeble-minded have been finished off, the next useless eaters whose turn will come are the old people."

Cardinal Faulhaber, Archbishop of München-Freising, addressed a long memorandum on the subject, dated the 6 November 1940, to Dr Gurtner, the then Minister of Justice. The closing paragraph is quoted below.

[DOC. 846.]

'It is intelligible that in wartime extraordinary measures are taken to ensure the safety of the country and the feeding of the population. We tell the nation that it must be ready in time of war to make great sacrifices, and even shed its blood, in a spirit of Christian generosity. We reverence the black-veiled women we meet in the streets who have made the sacrifice of beloved lives for the sake of the Fatherland. But the inalienable foundations of morality and the basic rights of the individual should never be abrogated, even in wartime.'

Pastor Schlaich, director of the combined sanatorium and nursing home at Stetten, gave his opinion as follows:

[DOC. 520.]*

'Since from the Institution under my direction altogether 150 of the patients entrusted to me are to be transferred to such an institution (seventy-five on the 10th and seventy-five on the 13th of September) I take the privilege of asking: Is it possible for such a measure to be carried out without a pertinent law having been promulgated? Is it not the duty of every citizen to resist under all circumstances an act not justified by law, even forbidden by law, even if such acts are carried out by State agencies?

On account of the complete secrecy and camouflage under which the measures are carried out, not only are the wildest rumours circulating among the people (for example, that people unable to work on account of age or injuries received during the World War have also been done away with or are to be done away with), but it seems as if the selection of the persons concerned is performed in a wholly arbitrary manner.

If the State really wants to carry out the extermination of these or at least of some mental patients, shouldn't a law be promulgated, which can be justified before the people—a law which would give everyone the assurance of careful examination as to whether he is due to die or entitled to live and which would also give the relatives a chance to be heard, in a similar way, as provided by the law for the Prevention of Hereditarily Affected Progeny?'

R

The number of such communications emanating from every social sphere, caused the Minister of Justice to consult the Minister of the Interior and Hitler himself. For a work published by Dr Gürtner, entitled *Future German Criminal Law*, contains the following passage, edited by Dr Graf Gleispach:

[DOC. 706.]

'There can be no question of freedom to destroy so-called "lives not worth living". The main category here is that of complete or nearly complete imbeciles. The National Socialist State seeks to prevent the occurrence of this sort of deterioration in the nation as a whole by taking comprehensive steps to ensure that examples of it grow steadily rarer. But the validity of the ethical standard implied in the prohibition of murder should not be weakened by allowing exceptions to it on grounds of mere expediency in the case of those afflicted by serious maladies or accidents. . . . On the other hand the view has come to be recognized as legitimate under existing legislation, though there is no special prescription to that effect, that genuine assistance to the dying or euthanasia, is not to be regarded as murder, i.e. when the physician refrains from artificially prolonging a tortured existence already on the point of extinction or when he changes the death agony to a smooth transition from life to death. The force of the prohibition of murder must not be diminished except in this one restricted sense. The law must always take care that the confidence of invalids in the medical profession is not shaken.'

The following attitude is taken up in the *Commentary on the Penal Code* published by Ohlshausen in 1944:

[DOC. 709.]

'The right to assist the dying (euthanasia), to inhibit the painful and possibly prolonged onset, rooted in a disease or wound, of certain dissolution, by administering a painless alternate death, even considering the legal impunity of such action, is not conceded under existing laws either to the physician or to any other person. Nor is it permissible even at the last stage, when death is imminent, nor again if the dying patient himself longs for death. Punishment is only mitigated in such a case by the provisions of Section 216. On the other hand a doctor incurs no penalty if in these circumstances he abstains from using special stimulants like camphor injections. For his duty to prolong life in all cases by every means in his power can then no longer be invoked. Other methods of destroying lives not worth living, for example the extinction of life in incurable imbeciles, could only be rendered legally guiltless by the alteration of existing laws.'

The reply received from national headquarters by the Minister of Justice is evident from his letter to Dr Lammers, Head of the Chancellery.

[DOC. 238.]

'. . . According to the information you gave me yesterday the Führer has declined to issue a decree. Consequently I feel it to be essential to suspend forthwith the secret extermination of the insane. One of the chief reasons for the rapid and wide-spread revelation of the present procedure was the attempt made to camouflage it. You will see from the enclosed papers what embarrassing results followed. There will be more and more of such inquiries. It will be extraordinarily difficult to answer them officially, as neither the fact of a decree by the Führer nor the content of any such document can be announced. It will be impossible for the Ministry of Justice to profess ignorance of the whole affair in the face of its own authorities.'

Himmler himself considered it time to intervene. In December 1940 he wrote to Brack, Bouhler's chief clerk:

[DOC. 018.]*

'I hear there is great excitement on the Alb because of the Institution Grafeneck.

The population recognizes the gray automobile of the SS and think they know what is going on at the constantly smoking crematory. What happens there is a secret and yet is no longer one. Thus the worst feeling has arisen there, and in my opinion there remains only one thing, to discontinue the use of the

Institution in this place and in any event disseminate information in a clever and sensible manner by showing motion pictures on the subject of inherited and mental diseases in just that locality.

May I ask for a report as to how the difficult problem was solved.'

In March 1941 the Secretary of State at the Ministry of Justice, Dr Schlegelberger, again consulted Lammers.

[DOC. 681—PS.]

'. . . I feel, however, that I must call your attention to the effect of these proceedings on a number of the fields of administration controlled by the Ministry, leading to troublesome confusion in their work. The departments affected are mainly those mentioned below. Difficulties have arisen for trustees in cases where judges have opposed the transfer of insane persons in the charge of guardians or trustees to other asylums. Often the courts were given no official information as to the whereabouts or the decease of insane wards, though the personal and financial affairs of any body of trustees, the communications between trustee and ward and the regular inquiries by relatives must enable the authorities to state the address and subsequent circumstances of any such ward. . . . Public Prosecutors have also been embarrassed when relatives or third parties have lodged charges of the murder of persons who have disappeared. One Prosecutor-General intends to cross-examine an official physician accused of having falsified the medical history of a patient who had "died". Details of problems which have arisen for criminal lawyers may be found in Enclosure 2. Serious doubts have affected the minds of authorities conducting trials under the legislation against malicious attacks on State and Party when defendants have alleged the killing of persons in good physical health. As the liquidation measures are kept secret, the most various rumours have been spreading among the population, have been encouraged by subversive elements and have reached immoderate dimensions. The secrecy involved and public ignorance of the extent of the measures are proving fertile soil for the spread of rumours that even perfectly sane inmates of penal establishments and actually persons

suffering from war injuries, as well as elderly German citizens
past work and the politically undesirable are being included in
the scheme. Trials in camera of persons accused of malicious
gossip in the dissemination of such talk would also appear to
involve special risks, as the investigation of individual features
of the case would bring the whole problem of the extermination
of lives not worth living into the open. In these circumstances,
too, unscrupulous agitators would escape the punishment they
deserve. Confidence in the medical profession, especially in the
Directors of sanatoria and convalescent homes, is being severely
shaken. People are saying that the deaths reported are due to
doctors' blunders and that insane patients are being used for
military experiments, such as the testing of poison gas and
other weapons of war. Other rumours reveal anxiety over the
food situation which it is felt must be precarious if remedies are
already being sought in the liquidation of some hundreds of
thousands of the mentally afflicted.'[1]

It may seem surprising that in addition to the numerous
written protests from theological and legal quarters no data
were forthcoming on a similar scale from the medical side in
those days. But the fact is accounted for by the methods of
those who carried out the programme. Its direction was not in
medical but in Party hands, those of a special department—
'T 4'—set up for this purpose by the Chancellery. 'T 4' was
associated with the office of the 'Controller of Sanatoria and
Nursing Homes' under Dr Linden, a direct subordinate of
Conti in the latter's capacity as Secretary of State for Civil
Health Services at the Ministry of the Interior. Conti was
described in Court by several witnesses as 'obsessed with power',
'ambitious' and 'a political expert'. He had, for instance,
drawn up a plan for the extermination of the Polish intelli-
gentsia by sterilization. [PROT. p. 4624.]

Both he and Linden have already been referred to in connection with the typhus experiments on human beings. Conti

1. Further 'Documents on the Murders of the Insane' and evidence of
opposition to them, divided under the headings of 'The Christian Objection', 'The Juristic Protest Against Lawlessness', 'Natural Horror' and
'The Withdrawal of a Doctor' appeared in the second and third issue of the
monthly magazine *Die Wandlung* for 1947 edited by Dolf Sternberger and
published by the Carl Winter University Press, Heidelberg.

had agreed to the subordination of the entire German medical profession to a Health Service scheme proposed by Robert Ley, the Government's organization specialist, to bring all Germans under a national insurance system. Conti's assent was given with a view to the establishment of a still non-existent Ministry of Health. As well as being Secretary of State he was head of the medical profession and had in this last capacity been provided by Hitler with a deputy in the shape of Professor Kurt Blome. But witnesses in Court agreed that Blome had opposed Conti and tried to keep the medical profession free from interference in its own affairs. When Blome objected that euthanasia was illegal, Conti retorted that the management of the profession and the profession as a whole had nothing to do with the euthanasia programme. Only a few doctors employed by the Ministry of the Interior had been informed of the plan, and, like those few appointed to carry it out, had been sworn to secrecy. They had mostly been chosen for their 'political reliability'. The physicians in charge of the sanatoria and nursing homes knew only of the 'transfers' and the profession as a whole merely heard 'rumours' of what was going on.

Of the doctors proved to have objected we need only mention here the psychiatrists Professors Ewald and Kleist and the specialist in tuberculosis Professor Kurt Klare. The opposition of most psychiatrists to this so-called 'further development of psychiatry' and their attempts to prevent the transfer of patients as soon as suspicion had been aroused by the attitude of the personnel of the 'Limited Company for Transport in the Public Interest', who were mostly SS men, are particularly evident from an official French report.[1]

A German translation was issued by the Schröder Verlag, Baden-Baden, entitled 'Were the murdered guilty?' The report was the result of six months' investigation. It summarizes the events in Württemberg and Baden.

The following paragraphs may be quoted:

'This monstrous plan was the very essence of hypocrisy and mendacity. Continuous efforts to camouflage it were made. The relatives of the patients and the doctors themselves were made fools of.

1. *"Rapport sur la destinée de l'Assistance Psychiatrique en Allemagne du Sud-Ouestpendant le Régime Nationalsocialiste."*

As soon as it was no longer possible to doubt the true character of the transfers, psychiatrists began, in the utmost excitement, to turn in all directions. The institution doctors applied for support wherever they believed they could get a hearing. But the universities remained silent, the local authorities told them, with threats, that it was their duty to keep the secret and the courts were found to be powerless. Only the Church and the Army made any direct attempts to intervene, in order to keep down the growing unrest in the provinces affected, where there was great alarm.

We are aware of the struggle of many universities against the new doctrine. Scientists of high moral standing were regularly "axed". No more was heard of them and thus their criticism was silenced.'

Professor Büchner of Freiburg spoke out to his students against the film on euthanasia entitled 'I accuse'. Professor Sauerbruch also protested against the plan, as recorded by Pastor Braune in the Home Mission Magazine for May/June 1947.

Certain psychiatrists, including Professor Kurt Schneider, declined positively to publish any further work on their subject.[1]

Hitler was sufficiently impressed by such unforeseen public

1. During the trials held at the Assize Courts of Düsseldorf and Freiburg, when certain doctors were accused of participation in the euthanasia proceedings, it was ascertained that many psychiatrists had opposed the idea. At the same time Judgments proved that the course of action in different provinces depended on the attitudes of the chief local medical officers.

At Freiburg the former head of the Health Department of the Baden Ministry of the Interior, Dr Sprauer, was sentenced to life imprisonment for having unreservedly supported the execution of the euthanasia programme, leaving the directors of the local institutions in complete ignorance and preventing the adoption of all appropriate counter-measures.

At Düsseldorf the former Secretary for Health of the Rhineland, Professor Walter Creutz, was discharged. It was stated in Judgment that his 'unmistakably proved opposition and consequent action led to equally unmistakable success'. He had saved 'at least 3,000' invalids from transfer as against 946 transferred. At the same trial Professors Pohlisch and Panse were also discharged, as their 'proved counter-measures had met with considerable success, to the benefit of patients'.

Appeals were lodged at the time against both Judgments, which also discharged two other doctors and sentenced two doctors and two nurses to imprisonment.

reaction to order Karl Brandt verbally, in August 1941 at his Headquarters, to 'put a stopper on' the euthanasia proceedings. Brandt passed on the news to Bouhler by telephone. No written evidence of these 'events' was ever found, nor does it seem ever to have existed.[1] But it was asserted by several witnesses that the gassing of the mentally afflicted in the institutions cited did in fact cease in the autumn of 1941.

Karl Brandt quoted a number of figures in Court showing the extent of the action taken in executing the plan. He said that the total of insane and weak-minded persons was 'about three million'. Of these 600,000 were under continuous medical treatment and 250,000 ward-patients: 70–80 per cent of the latter were schizophrenic. The figures relating to those who were subjected to euthanasia before the proceedings were suspended were given as follows.

[PROT. p. 2481.]

'I should like first to give the result of calculations in proportional form as 1,000 : 10 : 5 : 1, where 1,000 represents the number of healthy persons, 10 the figure of those under medical care, 5 those permanently confined in Institutions and 1 the patient who was given euthanasia. Thus this treatment was applied to one out of about 1,000 people in normal health, in other words some 60,000 in a population of sixty millions.'[2]

Brandt was told by Bouhler that between 4 and 6 per cent of the patients transferred to observation stations and euthanasia institutions were returned to their base. Responsibility within the programme was distributed, according to an extract from Brandt's evidence on his own behalf, as follows:

[PROT. p. 2436 ff.]

'Each doctor took personal responsibility for what he had to do within the framework of these measures, which culminated

1. The Judgment of the Düsseldorf assize court referred to above mentions that in September 1941 a memorandum by Professor Heyde was issued to the effect 'that the proceedings were to be discontinued for technical reasons'.

2. In the Judgment of the Düsseldorf Assize Court referred to the total of insane persons liquidated was not precisely given, but stated to be certainly over 100,000.

finally in euthanasia. The individual doctor took full responsibility for his judgments as assessor, as the surveyor also did in his. Doctors at both the observation and the euthanasia centres also assumed full responsibility for their actions. In no circumstances is it to be understood that any doctor serving under this scheme was ever obliged to perform euthanasia in a case where he himself had not decided that it was necessary. On the contrary, it was his duty, if he did not agree with any such decision, to decline altogether to perform the operation.

With these powers alone the doctor had to bear a heavy responsibility. But he was not only burdened with the responsibility for deciding on life or death. He also shared responsibility for the continued existence of his patient. This point should perhaps be borne in mind in order to form a correct estimate of the extent of responsibility laid upon individuals in this connection.

This responsibility was taken by all those concerned in the scheme. There may have been ten, fifteen or even twenty assessors who worked on instructions and explanations given them from time to time by the surveyor. . . .

Possibly the decisive factor, in my own view, was that the Head of the State had himself assigned the task to me. I could certainly not suppose that the execution of such a decree could have been dictated to me for any criminal purpose. Moreover, in the subsequent course of events it appeared to me, as it did to all the others concerned, that the matter was handled in every direction as if it were really a normal procedure, which was how in fact we regarded it.'

In reply to his Defence Counsel, Brandt gave his own views of euthanasia as follows:

[PROT. p. 2447 ff.]

'*Defence Counsel:* Do you not consider, when you take a comprehensive view of this whole business of euthanasia, that there was something cruel about it?

Brandt: Possibly. It certainly looks as if it might appear so. It may seem to have been inhuman in its actual operation. But it cannot be judged from that angle alone. It is absolutely necessary to realize what led to its execution and continued to influence it. The underlying motive was the desire to help individuals who could not help themselves and were thus prolonging their lives in torment. That consideration cannot be regarded as inhuman. Nor did I ever feel it to be in any degree unethical or immoral. I know that the external circumstances of the procedure, chiefly and repeatedly the feature of secrecy, led to certain regrettable incidents in spite of all the efforts of the centre concerned to prevent them. It has been stated in Court that two urns were on one occasion sent to a certain office. Another office was caused embarrassment by erroneous ascriptions of the cause of death. Such occurrences are regrettable, but do not affect the principle involved and cannot even in my opinion call it in question. A frank discussion of this problem of euthanasia and efforts at mutual understanding of it seriously based upon consideration of the facts would lead in my opinion to the working out of some system for adopting the procedure even for the future. The problem as such is no novelty. It has always existed and has been discussed for centuries. Professor Leibbrand, in the course of his evidence from where I now stand, referred to Hippocrates. He was thinking of the paragraph in which a doctor is forbidden to administer poison to an invalid even upon demand. But this prohibition, as formulated by Hippocrates, can assuredly no longer be regarded as valid in view of modern advances in diagnosis and prognosis and our present recognition of the limitations of therapy. I am convinced that if Hippocrates were alive today he would change the wording of his Oath. He was not in favour of the preservation of life under any circumstances. When he was asked for his help during the plague which raged at Athens in 430 B.C., he retorted quite simply that the plague-stricken should be left to lie where they were, since nothing could be done for them. He did not give this advice because he had any notion of infection, for at the same time he allowed the Athenians to build walls in the valleys so that contrary winds could not reach the city. He spoke as he did because he understood instinctively the nature of health and of any disease that has to take its course. To quote Hippocrates today is to proclaim that invalids and persons in great pain should never be given poison. But any modern doctor who makes so rhetorical a declaration without qualification is either a liar or a hypocrite. No physician today would deny narcotics to a patient in agony or refuse to alleviate the last moments of the dying. It may be objected that such a proceeding is not euthanasia. But it is nevertheless contrary to the meaning of the Oath of Hippocrates. It begins when a patient whose death is inevitable is no longer treated with stimulants and cordials. The next step is to administer a narcotic. Accordingly, whatever copies of the Oath of Hippocrates may be framed and hung up in the consulting-room of a pharmaceutical factory, no one adheres to it in practice. Furthermore, both the patient and his relatives expect him to be helped and surely such help has been given if the obituary subsequently states that the sick man has at last been released from his sufferings. Such reflections have nothing to do with the notion conveyed by Professor Leibbrand's phrase 'fiendish-ness by order'. For even today, possibly actually at this moment, the question of euthanasia is again being debated in foreign countries by gatherings of ecclesiastics both Evangelical and Methodist and the medical bodies attached to them. I know it is said that if a doctor is known to have practised euthanasia his patients may lose confidence in him. But the confidence of a patient, once acquired, is not like a capital sum handed over on which the doctor may obtain interest. On the contrary it is in my view his duty to acquire it afresh every time he meets his patient. An Institution should do the same. One can't say that an Institution has lost its reputation. An Institution does not exist in order to preserve reputation but to take care of and assist invalids. In talking of Institutions one has to realize what they are. These important establishments began to be erected about a hundred years ago. I remember the name of Forell of Zürich. But they are really nothing more than golden cages. One can say without exaggeration that life within their walls is as cruel and shameful as any to which human beings can be exposed.

During the last few months and weeks illustrations have been published in magazines which are of exactly the same character as those shown to us as exemplifying life in concentration camps. Not only is this the case. It is also stated to be so. The inmost feelings of the population are deeply hostile to these nursing homes. Their establishment always ran into difficulties and there is no modern State in which they are not under constant discussion. It is deplorable that such places should be necessary. For no State should be burdened with the expense involved when positive assistance can really be rendered to such people and they can be guaranteed accommodation fit for human beings.

It has often also been asserted by churchmen, in particular by Luther, that the life led by an idiot can certainly not have been part of the Divine plan. For it is felt to be unnatural. During the euthanasia scheme we put through in the years 1940 and 1941 we received a great number of letters expressing perfect understanding of and agreement with our work. That is again evidence in favour of the scheme. I should not like you to call attention to great quantities of written discussions of euthanasia. In many cases they copy one another and constantly evade the real problem. But one thing I do think necessary. If anyone wishes to form an opinion and pronounce judgment upon euthanasia, he should go to a lunatic asylum and if possible spend some days among the inmates. He can then be asked two questions, firstly whether he himself, as a human being, would care to live like that, and secondly whether he would be prepared to persuade a relative, possibly his own child or his parents, to prolong their existence under such conditions. The answer will have nothing to do with the idea of "fiendishness by order". It will be simply a clear expression of heartfelt gratitude by the speaker for his own health. As for the question of humanity, whether it is more humane to help such a being to end its life in peace or continue to keep watch and ward over it, surely the answer goes without saying. In this connection I was sent a study in which it was stated that a child with hereditary dementia, having an innate cerebral deficiency, was kept alive for three and a half years, during the whole of which time it never stopped screaming. I cannot see any special virtue, which can be described as humane, in this performance. It can certainly be affirmed that it was not a pretty one and that the end of a human life, whatever other feelings one may have about it, can be terrible. But not everything of a biological nature is agreeable. It can be disgusting, hideous and vile. One can apply such epithets to eating, right down the final act of digestion. Yet in the last analysis life itself arises from such action and is a necessary thing. Again, operational treatment in an unpleasant business, though it may be expedient. Nor, assuredly, is the bloody process of birth an attractive one, any more than any kind of death or the struggle against it that goes on for days. But everything depends on the view taken of these things. We can bear them and recognize them for what they really are if we simply regard them as in many respects a kind of transfiguration. I believe that if one adopts this standpoint one's reflections on euthanasia, which really go far beyond this limited earthly sphere, will include the consideration of poor, suffering humanity. They will then be associated with what existence in general implies and with imaginative thought, if I may once more refer to Hippocrates, in whose time people talked about the *Logos*, by which they meant regulative reason. I believe that future doctors will be able to lay down a sound scientific basis for the theory of euthanasia, that the theologian will help by incorporating it in his statements and finally that the jurist, as representing the authority of the State over the doctor will again enable him to render assistance to mankind, including even such unfortunate creatures. . . .

Q. When you consider this matter as a whole, do you feel that you yourself today are in any way to blame for the practice of euthanasia?

A. No. I do not feel myself to blame. I have a perfectly clear conscience about the part I played in the affair. I was actuated by purely humane sensibility. I never intended anything more than or believed I was doing anything but abbreviating the tortured existence of such unhappy creatures. I only regret that their relatives were caused unjustifiable pain as a result of external circumstances. But I am convinced that today they have overcome their distress and personally believe that the dead members of their families were given a happy release from their sufferings.'

Karl Brandt and Viktor Brack were found guilty on this and other counts of the indictment and sentenced to death. Judgment in Brandt's case included the following paragraphs:

[Judgment p. 49 ff.]*

'Shortly after the commencement of operations for the

disposal of "incurables", the programme was extended to Jews, and then to concentration camp inmates.[1] In this latter phase of the programme, prisoners deemed by the examining doctors to be unfit or useless for labour were ruthlessly weeded out and sent to the extermination stations in great numbers.

Karl Brandt maintains that he is not implicated in the extermination of Jews or of concentration camp inmates; that his official responsibility for euthanasia ceased at the close of the summer of 1941, at which time euthanasia procedures against 'incurables' were terminated by order of Hitler.

It is difficult to believe this assertion, but even if it be true, we cannot understand how this fact would aid the defendant. The evidence is conclusive that almost at the outset of the programme non-German nationals were selected for euthanasia and exterminated. Needless to say, these persons did not voluntarily consent to become the subjects of this procedure.

Karl Brandt admits that after he had disposed of the medical decisions required to be made by him with regard to the initial programme, which he maintains was valid, he did not follow the programme further but left the administrative details of execution to Bouhler. If this be true, his failure to follow up a programme for which he was charged with special responsibility constituted the gravest breach of duty. A discharge of that duty would have easily revealed what now is so manifestly evident from the record; that whatever may have been the original aim of the programme, its purposes were prostituted by men for whom Brandt was responsible, and great numbers of non-German nationals were exterminated under its authority.

We have no doubt but that Karl Brandt—as he himself testified—is a sincere believer in the administration of euthanasia to persons hopelessly ill, whose lives are burdensome to themselves and an expense to the State or to their families. The abstract proposition of whether or not euthanasia is justified in certain cases of the class referred to is no concern of this Tribunal. Whether or not a state may validly enact legislation which imposes euthanasia upon certain classes of its citizens is likewise a question which does not enter into the issues. Assuming that it may do so, the Family of Nations is not obligated to give recognition to such legislation when it manifestly gives

1. See pp. 275 and 285.

legality to plain murder and torture of defenceless and powerless human beings of other nations.

The evidence is conclusive that persons were included in the programme who were non-German nationals. The dereliction of the defendant Brandt contributed to their extermination. That is enough to require this Tribunal to find that he is criminally responsible in the programme.'

After the termination in the autumn of 1941 of the euthanasia programme as directed from headquarters some of the gas-chambers built for the purpose, for instance that at Hadamar, were dismantled and re-erected in eastern cities such as Lublin. There the overwhelming majority of victims were Polish Jews. On the other hand it was frequently stated in evidence supported by documents obtained from various institutions that even after the official proceedings had ended the mentally afflicted were liquidated at certain establishments at the orders of the Ministry of the Interior acting independently. In all the cases that came to light morphine or barbiturates were the means by which life was destroyed.

(ii) LIQUIDATION OF DEFORMED AND IDIOTIC CHILDREN

In contrast with the 'mercy killing' of adults, which had been abandoned at Hitler's orders, deformed and idiotic children continued to be liquidated until the end of the war.

The process was organized by the 'National Committee for the Scientific Study of Serious Hereditary Ailments' in Berlin.

By a decree of the Ministry of the Interior under reference IV b $\frac{3088/39}{1079\ \text{Mi}}$ and dated August 1939 municipal health officials, nurses, private doctors and hospital staff had to send Berlin answers to questionnaires about the children under their care. The assessors and surveyors of the Committee decided in certain cases upon euthanasia and drew up so-called 'authorizations' which were then dispatched to various 'Children's Sections of the Committee'. One of the latter, for example, was established at the Eichberg institution. According to its former Chief Physician [Prot. p. 1844] the children later delivered there were examined and after their disabilities had been checked were given 'assistance in dying'. From 1941 to 1944, according to the same witness, Dr Schmidt, some eighty children were disposed of at Eichberg by administration of 'morphine-hydrochloral or luminal'. Original lists of the victims, just as they were drawn up by the Committee already mentioned at the Ministry of the Interior, have survived. They include the serial number, name, date of birth, diagnosis, date of 'authorization' and date of death in each case. [DOC. 1146.]

In addition to Eichberg, institutions at Idstein, Kantenhof and Görden are named in the documents as centres for the extermination of deformed and mentally afflicted children.

The prosecution asked why any distinction was made between euthanasia for adults and that applied to children. Brandt replied:

[PROT. p. 2545.]

'Because in the case of the children it was desired, if only on account of the trouble they would cause their families and for similar reasons, to prevent their growing up. The object was to obtain possession of these abortions and destroy them as soon as possible after they had been brought into the world.'

In contrast with the procedure as regards adults the consent of parents was always, according to Brandt's evidence, sought before 'authorization' to liquidate was issued. But in no case is there any documentary evidence of such a thing. Brandt said he believed he had seen written consents. But he added that 'not all of them were delivered in writing. Some were given orally to the doctor or other competent authority concerned.' [PROT. p. 2559.]

This statement by Brandt, however, is contradicted by Doc. 890, a letter marked 'confidential', from the 'Committee' already mentioned to Dr Schmidt of the Eichberg Centre.[1]

1 Dr Schmidt was sentenced by the Frankfurt am Main Provincial Court at the Eichberg Trial. An extract from Judgment and a commentary by Professor Radbruch may be read in the *Süddeutsche Juristenzeitung*, 2/11, November 1947, published at Heidelberg by Lambert Schneider.

[DOC. 890.]

'With reference to a letter which has been addressed to Professor Brandt on the above subject I should be glad to receive a detailed medical report on the female patient named A. .... G. ..., who is alleged to be at present in your care. The Provincial President of Wiesbaden has already been taking an interest in this matter. It seems that the relatives of A. ... G. ... are pressing for her release if it can possibly be arranged. If medical responsibility can be taken for such release at the present juncture it is for consideration whether this demand should not in fact be met in order to safeguard the Institution's reputation.'

It appears from the statement in evidence of Dr Fritz Mennecke, a former Director of the Eichberg Provincial Sanatorium and Nursing Home, that the Committee referred to also continued on a reduced scale the original plan for the euthanasia of adults.

[PROT. p. 1903 f.]

'The programme was not resumed in its original form. But the activities of the National Committee were extended. The committee had originally dealt only with children up to 3 years old. This limit was later raised to 8, 12 and, I believe, actually to 16 or 17 years. This extension accordingly represented a substitution to some extent for the abandoned programme. I heard, moreover, in conversation with other participants in the scheme that no objection would be raised to any doctor in the institutions considering himself free to liquidate a patient by injection or overdosing if he were convinced that death would ensue in any case. In that event he could act entirely on his own responsibility. . . .'[1]

(iii) "DIRECT ELIMINATION" OF UNDESIRABLE
NATIONAL ELEMENTS AND UNDESIRABLE INVALIDS IN
EUTHANASIA CENTRES

At a later date the 'Children's Sections of the Committee' were also the scene of the deaths of children who were neither

1. The liquidation of deformed children by starvation was reported in the first section of this chapter.

S

hereditarily defective nor injured by external means, but had been condemned for racial reasons. This point is proved by the affidavit of a Head Sister serving at the Hadamar Institution.

[DOC. 1427.]

'In May 1943 certain hybrids (half-Jews), all of them children, were brought to Hadamar. I cannot say exactly how many there were, but to the best of my recollection they comprised some fifteen or twenty girls. They were almost all healthy. A few had skin eruptions. All these children were liquidated by injection. When I returned to Hadamar in October 1943 after twenty-four days' leave, I was told that they had been all disposed of.'

If there were no strictly medical excuse for 'assisting the dissolution' of mentally afflicted, deformed or idiotic children, further 'eliminating' operations were undertaken on undisguisedly political or ideological grounds, by designating the victims 'undesirable national elements' or persons rendered unable to work. The camouflaging of such homicidal intentions is revealed with special clarity by the proved fact that in the concentration camps prisoners were selected by the very same medical assessors who were at the same time deciding the fate of the inmates of sanatoria and nursing homes. The defendant Dr Waldemar Hoven, formerly camp doctor at Buchenwald, declared in an affidavit, *inter alia*:[1]

[DOC. 429.]*

'I became aware in 1941 that the so-called euthanasia

1. It appeared from the statements of witnesses in Court that Hoven attended both the SS and the political prisoners in the camp and was thus able to save several of the latter from execution. But a great many others, all of them said to have been reported as 'traitors to the cause of the prisoners' by the political prisoners at Buchenwald, were killed by Hoven with phenol injections. He admitted having treated sixty of them personally in this way. As early as September 1944 proceedings were taken against him by the SS for murder, in fact for a whole series of homicides. The investigating magistrate specially noted that the 'decision lay only between a capital sentence and life imprisonment.' The Trial, however, was deferred at that time. The Nuremberg Tribunal sentenced Hoven to death. (See the further reference on a later page of this section.)

programme for the extermination of the mentally and physically deficient was being carried out in Germany. At that time, the camp commandant Koch called all the important SS officials of the camp together and informed them that he had received a secret order from Himmler to the effect that all mentally and physically deficient inmates of the camp should be killed. The camp commandant stated that higher authorities from Berlin had ordered that all the Jewish inmates of the Buchenwald concentration camp be included in this extermination programme. In accordance with these orders 300 to 400 Jewish prisoners of different nationalities were sent to the euthanasia station at Bernburg for extermination. A few days later I received a list of the names of those Jews who were exterminated at Bernburg from the camp commandant and I was ordered to issue falsified death certificates. I obeyed this order. This particular action was executed under the code name "14 f 13".'

The defendant Viktor Brack denied that the euthanasia officials had any conscious connection with this '14 f 13' process. But an extract from his own statements under examination by his Defence Counsel showed clearly how the euthanasia programme came to be applied to the concentration camps.

[PROT. p. 7635 ff.]

'If I had ever been informed of the character of this process, camouflaged under the designation "14 f 13", I would not only never have consciously associated myself with any such proceeding, but would also have made it impossible for anyone else to support it in any way.

Q. What then, in fact, was the state of affairs?

A. The witness Hielscher stated in Court on the 16 April 1947 that the concentration camp prisoners, of whom I myself only met very few indeed after their release, looked like spectres. He described most of them as mental wrecks who had been ill for the greater part of their lives and whose minds, I might almost say, vitality, had broken down. It is possible that Himmler and also those who inspected the camps were aware of the condition of these people.

I am not in a position to judge the extent, if any, to which Hielscher's statement represents the truth when he asserts that

Himmler personally, through the system he controlled, broke the backbones, psychologically speaking, of these prisoners.

I should like in this connection to refer again to the discussion I had with Himmler in January 1941, when I was so deeply shocked by what he said about his plans for sterilization and about Jews in general. I had certain doubts at that time whether the idea I had hitherto formed of Himmler was the correct one. But later on I dropped these doubts to some extent, as I heard nothing more of his plans for dealing with Jews and thought he had given them up. Accordingly, I considered it a confirmation of my assumption that Himmler had recovered his humanity when Bouhler told me in the summer of 1941 that Himmler intended to order a thorough check-up, physically and mentally, of the severest cases of illness in the concentration camps. Himmler had requested Bouhler to obtain doctors of impartial views for him, as he himself did not altogether trust the professional knowledge of the camp doctors. Bouhler therefore instructed me at that time to get in touch with T 4 and inquire whether they would allow some experienced psychiatrists to be detailed for examination of prisoners in the concentration camps. I complied with these instructions myself. But I really cannot now say whether I passed them on to Nitsche, Heyde or Allers.'

'14 f 13' was an official symbol used by Himmler's Inspector of Concentration Camps, otherwise Group D of the SS Headquarters for Economic Administration in Berlin and Oranienburg. The symbol accordingly indicates links between a rather large number of documents. Two letters from the Inspector illustrate the activity of the 'Medical Committee'.

On the 10 December 1941 he gave the following instructions to several of his camp commandants:

[DOC. 1151—PS.]

'To the concentration camp commandants at Dachau, Sachsenhausen, Buchenwald, Mauthausen, Auschwitz, Flossenbürg, Gross-Rosen, Neuengamme and Niederhagen.

As the camp commandants at Dachau, Sachsenhausen, Buchenwald, Mauthausen and Auschwitz have already been informed in communications on this subject, medical commissioners will shortly visit the above-named camps for the purpose of examining prisoners. Visits to the camps at Flossenbürg, Gross-Rosen, Neuengamme and Niederhagen are expected to take place during the first half of January 1942. . . .

A specimen of the form to be completed at this stage is enclosed. Copies are to be photostated for completion. The form contains certain questions underlined in red. Only these need be answered, in accordance with the following instructions;

"The question referring to incurable bodily disease should not be answered merely by Yes or No but by a brief diagnosis. The question referring to war injuries is also to be answered specifically, as this information will substantially facilitate the work of examination by the medical committee. . . ."

All available papers and medical documents are to be held ready for inspection by the Committee on demand. . . .

On conclusion of the examinations a report is to be forwarded to the Inspector of Concentration Camps in which the number of prisoners subjected to the special "14 f 13" treatment must be stated. The exact date of the arrival of the Committee will be communicated in due course.

(*Signed per pro*) LIEBEHENSCHEL,
SS Obersturmbannführer.'

It appears from the second letter that Dr Mennecke, SS Obersturmbannführer and Director of the Provincial Sanatorium and Nursing Home at Eichberg and, already frequently mentioned, belonged to this 'Medical Committee'. The letter is dated 10 January 1942 and so incidentally proves that the destruction of 'lives not worth living' was proceeding independently of the original 'mercy killings' ordered by Hitler.

[PROT. p. 1739.]

'In pursuance of the above-mentioned arrangements SS Obersturmbannführer Dr Mennecke will undertake the examination of prisoners in the Gross-Rosen concentration camp as from the 16 or 17 January 1942. The necessary forms have already been transmitted to the camp. They are to be completed as instructed in the covering letter before Dr Mennecke's arrival if possible. . . .

(*Signed per pro*) LIEBEHENSCHEL.'

The apparent efficiency of the 'Medical Committee' was very frankly described by Dr Mennecke in his testimony under examination by Brandt's Defence Counsel. The following is an extract from the record of 17 January 1947:

[PROT. p. 1913 f.]

Q. Now you also stated, did you not, that questionnaires were completed for prisoners in the concentration camps as well?

A. Yes.

Q. You said, further, that political prisoners and Jews were also examined?

A. Yes.

Q. What determined the decisions in that process?

A. Will Counsel please note that this matter has already been discussed? Decisions with regard to the Jews were not taken on grounds of health but on the basis of the reasons for their arrest.

Q. You mean political and racial considerations?

A. Yes.

Q. Who instructed you to proceed on those lines?

A. This question, too, has already been answered by me. Different persons instructed me, at one time Professor Nitsche, at another Professor Heyde and at yet another Herr Brack.

Q. Did not such instructions constitute a complete break with what had been stated at the outset?

A. Yes. At any rate, it had nothing to do with the euthanasia of the insane.

Q. When did racial and political ideas first make their appearance in this affair? Was that already the case when you first visited a concentration camp?

A. No.

Q. Then when did it happen?

A. I think it may have started at Buchenwald or Dachau.

Q. What happened before that, then? How were you then supposed to proceed in the concentration camps?

A. I had to examine the prisoners brought before me to determine whether they were psychotic or psychopathological cases.

Q. So at first it was a matter of people of unsound mind?

A. It was a medical matter.

Q. Then later it became a political and racial matter?

A. Yes. But in addition to the political and racial aspects of the matter I had also, even at this later stage, to take purely medical decisions.

Q. So at that time you had two kinds of cases to deal with, those of persons of unsound mind, who were judged on medical grounds, and those who were to be judged on political and racial grounds?

A. It was not possible to make any distinction, learned Counsel. There was no question of any definite separation between the two.

Q. Do you mean that when you examined a large number of Jews you certified them all as being of unsound mind?

A. I have already expressed my view that they were neither at all sick nor of unsound mind either.

Q. All the same, you filled in the questionnaire?

A. Yes, for I had been ordered by Berlin to do so.

Q. Whose business was it to take action on these questionnaires?

A. I've no idea.

Q. Did you suppose that a decision would be taken by another doctor?

A. I couldn't say what conclusions any particular doctor might draw from the reports on Jews.'

Practical details were given by the same witness in a letter dated 25 November 1941 to his wife, while he was still 'medically' active in the camp at Buchenwald.

[DOC. 907.]*

'Afterwards we continued our examination until about 4 o'clock. I myself examined 105 patients, Mueller 78 patients, so that finally a total of 183 reports were ready as a first group. As a second group a total of 1,200 Jews followed, all of whom did not need to be "examined", but where it was sufficient to take the reasons for their arrest from the files (often very voluminous!) and to transfer them to the reports. Therefore, it is merely theoretical work which will certainly keep us busy until next Monday inclusive, perhaps even longer. We went on with this second group (Jews) today. I myself did seventeen, and Mueller fifteen. At five o'clock sharp "We threw away the trowel" and went for supper.

*   *   *

Exactly as the day I described above, the following days will pass—with exactly the same programme and the same work. After the Jews, another 300 Aryans follow as a third group who will again have to be "examined". Therefore, we are busy here until the end of next week.'

Dr Mennecke does not seem to have been the only euthanasia psychiatrist employed to pick out victims at a concentration camp. The same activities were later proved by the Prosecution to have been carried out by the Chief Surveyor Professor Heyde, described by Brack as a 'fine, sterling character'. The proof is contained in an affidavit by Dr Muthig, senior camp doctor at Dachau.

[DOC. 2799.]

'. . . In the autumn of 1941 Dr Lolling paid an official visit to my sick bay, during which he informed me that a committee of four doctors headed by Professor Heyde would shortly visit the camp at Dachau. He said that the committee's object was to select for euthanasia prisoners incapable of work and send them to the concentration camp at Mauthausen for gassing. The committee arrived soon after my conversation with Dr Lolling. The members comprised four psychiatrists under the direction of Professor Heyde, who accompanied them. Neither I myself nor any of the other camp doctors at Dachau had anything to do with the committee or its work. I saw, however, that the four psychiatrists occupied four separate tables in two huts and interviewed several hundred prisoners. The incapacity of the prisoners for work and their political activities were checked and they were registered accordingly. I know that the committee only stayed a few days in Dachau and during that brief period it was impossible for them to examine medically so many prisoners. The examination consisted merely of checking their papers in their presence. The men registered during these proceedings were of German and other nationalities or else Jews. I can state with absolute certainty that Professor Heyde directed the proceedings and was present at them. But I have forgotten the names of the other doctors.

Some weeks after the committee had left the camp at Dachau the first transport of several hundred prisoners who had been registered by the psychiatrists was dispatched, in December 1941, to Mauthausen concentration camp for gassing. A second convoy of several hundred prisoners, also registered by the committee, was sent in January 1942 to the same camp. I cannot swear that further convoys followed, as shortly after the second had left I was transferred from Dachau. The operation of selecting for euthanasia prisoners in Dachau concentration camp who were incapable of work was known as the 'Heyde Operation'.

An example of the fulfilment of the order of the 10 December 1941 sent to camp commandants was found in the internal correspondence files of the Gross-Rosen camp.

[DOC. 1151—PS.]

'The enclosed list forwarded by the Preventive Arrest Camp shows the prisoners now due for convoy:

70	selected from the Sick Bay
104	selected from the Blocks
119	Jews
293	Total as of 15 12 1941

The number demanded is exceeded by forty-three in order to leave a margin for the possible dispatch of prisoners in the convoy arranged for a later date.

Commandant,
Preventive Arrest Camp.'

Of these 293 prisoners in protective custody at the Gross-Rosen camp the head office in Berlin selected 214 for extermination.

The list of these 214 prisoners, which still exists, was passed on to the euthanasia centre at Bernburg. That establishment then communicated with the Gross-Rosen camp in order to arrange transport.

[PROT. p. 1740.]

'We consider the 24 March 1942 as the most suitable date for arrival, as we shall meanwhile be receiving consignments from other concentration camps and an interval will be required for organization of the work involved. If you are able to deliver the prisoners in buses, we suggest delivery in two convoys of 107 prisoners each, to arrive respectively on Tuesday the 24 March and Thursday the 26 March 1942.

Please let us know what you think of these proposals and inform us of your final decision, so that we can make further necessary arrangements accordingly.'

It seems from a further document that as the war went on prisoners were selected for extermination 'with an eye to the labour projects imposed on the concentration camps' and therefore more and more on account of their incapacity for work. Apparently this consideration even took precedence of the racial motive. As a sample of the degree of office organization at the administrative headquarters of the camps we may quote the entire heading of a circular from Oranienburg.

[DOC. 1007.]*

'SS Economic and Administrative Main Office,
Division Chief D Concentration Camps
D 1/1 File No.: 14 f 13/L/S—
Secret Journal No. 612/43.
                              Oranienburg, 27 April, 1943

Subject: Action 14 f 13 in Concentration Camps.
Re: Our Order—D/1/1 File No. 14 13/ot/S—Secret Diary No.
      32/43 of 15 January 1943.
Enclosures: None.

                                        (Stamp)
                                        Top Secret

                                        . . . . .th copy

To: the Camp Commanders of the Concentration Camps.
Dachua, Sachsenhausen, Buchenwald, Mauthausen, Neuen-
gamme, Auschwitz, Gross-Rosen, Natzweiler, Strutluf,
Ravensbrück, Riga, Herz-Lublin and Bergen-Belsen.
Copy to: Chief of Amt. D II, III in the building.

The Reich Leader SS and Chief of the German Police has
decreed that in future only insane prisoners can be selected for
the Action 14 f 13 by the medical commissions appointed for
this purpose.

All other prisoners unfit for work (persons suffering from
tuberculosis, bedridden invalids, etc.) are definitely to be excluded from this action. Bedridden prisoners are to be given
suitable work which can be performed in bed.

The order of the Reich Leader SS must be strictly observed
in the future.

Requests for gasoline for this purpose will therefore be discontinued.

(Signed) GLUECKS,
SS Brigadeführer and Generalmajor of the Waffen SS'

But even the prisoners taken to the euthanasia centres as a
result of the '14 f 13' process were not the only groups, in addition
to the original 'incurable invalids', to which the 'mercy killings'
were restricted. For the affidavit mentioned above of the Head
Sister at Hadamar contains, as well as the extract then quoted,
the following material, also substantiated by other testimony
given in Court: [PROT. p. 1791.]

[PROT. p. 1952.]

'From July 1944 until the final collapse 400 Russians and
Poles, men, women and children, all allegedly suffering from
tuberculosis, arrived at the Hadamar Sanatorium and Convalescent Home. They were always killed by injection immediately after arrival.'

The defendant Viktor Brack gave the following summary
account of euthanasia and its abuse:

[PROT. p. 7632 f.]

'It was natural for the Prosecution to designate euthanasia as the preliminary stage of a plan for mass-murder. In view of the witnesses and documents put at the disposal of Prosecuting Counsel I can well understand such an assumption by a disinterested representative of the United States. The secrecy that was maintained about Hitler's decree of the 1 September 1939 and the liquidation of political adversaries, prisoners of war and foreigners and, to crown all, the murders of millions of Jews might and indeed perhaps must have given Prosecuting Counsel the impression that the German Government, even before the war began, intended to turn the arrangements which had been made for euthanasia into an effective weapon against all the real or imagined enemies of Germany and to operate this instrument under cover of an ostensibly requisite euthanasia scheme.

But this assumption is certainly false if it implies that euthanasia was initially regarded as an instrument of some kind or even that anyone had conceived the idea of freeing the entire German people forthwith from the so-called "useless mouths" with a view to the later annihilation of both the internal and external enemies of Germany on the pretext of euthanasia.

We sincerely welcomed euthanasia on its introduction. For it was founded on the moral principle of compassion, on the very same humane considerations as those to which its adversaries themselves laid claim in their own views. I admit that shortcomings and mistakes occurred in the operation of the scheme. But this circumstance does not affect the character of the original idea as it was understood by Bouhler, Brandt or myself.'

Konrad Morgen, the former SS investigating magistrate, who was charged with the elucidation of crimes committed in the concentration camps during 1943 and 1944, stated in evidence:

[Doc. Karl Brandt 20.]

'I discovered in the course of my inquiries that the liquidation of physically enfeebled elderly persons and incurable invalids had been proceeding for a long time in the concentration camps. The process was known as euthanasia, or possibly "14 f 13". I found that in some cases obviously irresponsible action had been taken by doctors and that in others positively criminal, homicidal, intentions had been at work. I therefore reported the matter to Dr Grawitz and Professor Heyde. But I had no sooner begun to indicate my findings when Grawitz sprang up in a rage and said that he knew all about it but that not another word was to be wasted on the subject, since he had himself put a stop to the whole thing. Heyde expressed a similarly pained reaction. He had explicitly cited euthanasia, in his expert evidence at Hoven's trial,[1] as an idea responsible for obliterating in the mind of such a man the distinction between right and wrong. Both men accordingly felt, I imagine, that their subordinates were getting out of hand. It was an extraordinarily disagreeable experience for them to be reminded of it.

Eventually I identified the instructions issued by the office at Tiergartenstrasse 4. But in all my investigations I never came across the name of Professor Karl Brandt or any evidence of his participation or that of his Department in the matter. When my researches led me to Tiergartenstrasse 4, the Chancellery of the Führer, and I received other proofs of the responsibility of a very high authority acting under direct orders from the Führer, it was of course impossible for me to continue investigations carried out in the interests of a criminal prosecution.

(Signed) DR MORGEN'

Operations entirely separate from the liquidation in Germany itself of the mentally afflicted or otherwise incapacitated or labourers from the East suffering from infectious disease were carried out in the occupied regions to the East, where massmurders of Jews, Poles and Russians took place without any attempt to justify them on medical grounds. These 'eliminations' will not therefore be discussed. But as already remarked it should be noted that the euthanasia gas-chambers and staff were 'diverted' to such operations and used in them the experience acquired in gassing the mentally afflicted. The evidence of the SS magistrate Morgen [Doc. 2614], for example,

1. Hoven was at that time on trial for the murder by poison of a leading SS authority in the camp at Buchenwald.

agrees with another affidavit in describing the dreadful conditions, 'exceeding all imagination', which prevailed in the
extermination centre at Lublin. This camp was controlled by
the Criminal Law Commissioner Wirth of Stuttgart, who had
'performed his first experiments' at the euthanasia centre of
Brandenburg. Brack declared in Court that neither he nor
Bouhler had any idea, when the euthanasia personnel were
first handed over to the SS Brigadeführer Globocnik, of the
real intentions of that director of the entire process of the
extermination of Jews in the East. It was not until Globocnik
had obtained Bouhler's assent to a second supply of staff that,
according to Brack, Bouhler was let into the secret. He had
already, Brack continued, expressed 'the strongest disapproval'
of Hitler's and Himmler's plans in this respect. He suspected
Reinhardt Heydrich, in particular of initiating them and
believed they would be 'the beginning of the end'. Bouhler,
Brack said, therefore immediately opposed Globocnik's request
on the ground that:

[PROT. p. 7613.]

'there could be no question of employing people in the execution
of the euthanasia scheme who had previously been concerned
in work of so inconceivable a nature. For there could be no
doubt of the utterly brutalizing effects of such duties as
Globocnik had been carrying out. Globocnik, however, assured
Bouhler that any staff the latter put at the speaker's disposal
would not be set to such tasks but would merely act as over-
seers in the labour camps. On this assurance Bouhler consented
to supply the staff required.'[1]

But in a secret memorandum dated the 25 October 1941
[Doc. 365] by an 'official expert of the Department for Administration of the Occupied Regions of the East' it is stated:

[DOC. 365.]*

'Referring to my letter of the 18 October 1941, you are
informed that Oberdienstleiter Brack of the Chancellery of the
Führer has declared himself ready to collaborate in the manufacture of the necessary shelters as well as the gassing apparatus.

1. Brack's sentence is noted in the section on mass sterilization.

I draw attention to the fact that Sturmbannführer Eichmann, the Referent for Jewish questions in the RSHA, is in agreement with this process.'

An extract from Judgment of the International Military Tribunal [Doc. 2737] asserts:

[IMT—PROT. p. 16495 ff.]

'Adolf Eichmann, who had been entrusted by Hitler with the execution of this programme, estimated that in the course of the policy in question six million Jews were killed and that of this number four million perished in the extermination camps.'

While the surviving leaders of the euthanasia movement were being tried at Nuremberg, certain other officials concerned, such as the administrative and medical officers of various districts, the members of medical committees and the medical staff of the euthanasia and so-called intermediate stations appeared before German courts. A special problem of general significance therefore arose, in addition to the particular details completing the picture of events, at all these trials.

The question of the legal validity of Hitler's euthanasia decree was fully discussed in the Judgment of No. 4 Criminal Court at Frankfurt am Main, presided over by the County Court Judge Wirtzfeld, during proceedings which lasted from the 24 February 1947 to the 21 March against the medical, nursing and other staff of the euthanasia establishment at Hadamar.[1]

[4 a Js 3/46—4 KLs 74/7.]

'As to the legal basis referred to, it is clear that neither Hitler's decree nor any other law was ever published. Every step, on the contrary, was taken to keep these enactments strictly secret. It was forbidden under the severest penalties to mention them in public. Accordingly, the relevant papers remained in the hands of very few persons who were not allowed to part with them under any circumstances.

1. Parts of this Judgment are cited in the *Süddeutsche Juristenzeitung*, 2/11, November 1947 (Verlag Lambert Schneider, Heidelberg), with a commentary by Professor Gustav Radbruch.

In consequence of this secrecy the Prosecution has already denied these laws any formal validity. It has described them as null and void legislation and thus the action of the accused as objectively illegal. The Court is of opinion, however, that such secrecy was at least intelligible in view of the Government policy of the day and cannot therefore be regarded, of itself, as invalidating the laws passed. Both the announcement of the 1 September 1939 and the secrecy were orders by the then Head of the State, who had actually been invested with comprehensive administrative powers. In consideration of these constitutional conditions purely formal legal validity may perhaps be conceded to these so-called laws. The Court nevertheless denies them any validity in law and consequently any compulsory character, for the reasons stated below.

Every law has a material aspect, that of its content, as well as a formal one. It may be acknowledged that as a rule formal legal force is enough to lend the law validity and oblige all citizens to obey it. It is not therefore usually open to the jurists and moralists of a country to inquire into the validity of such a law. It is an urgent duty in the interests of the preservation of the uniformity and stability of law to recognize this circumstance explicitly. Such recognition of the positive character of law is essential. For otherwise legal instability, arbitrary action and eventually revolution would become permanent conditions and any communal life based upon law and order would be rendered impossible. It is, however, equally essential to insist that there are certain limits to the positive character of law which must not be transgressed. These boundaries exist because the State is never the sole source of all law and can never arbitrarily determine what is right or wrong. There is one law superior to all formal legislation, one ultimate standard for assessment of the latter. This is the law of nature, which sets irrevocable and final limits to the legal enactments of men. There are certain legal maxims so deeply rooted in nature that every legal and moral obligation must in the end be adjusted to conform with the law of nature that stands superior to it. Such legal maxims exert compulsory force because they are independent of the vicissitudes of time and human beliefs millennium after millennium, remaining constant and valid for every era. Accordingly, they necessarily compose an essential and permanent element of law as ultimately conceived by humanity in its regulations and opinions. The idea of a necessary equation between law and justice is basically acceptable, but only if the single limitation referred to is implied. If any legislation contravenes in any way the eternal standards of natural law, the content of such legislation will prevent its being equated with justice. It not only loses its obligatory force for the citizen but is actually invalid in law and must not be obeyed by him. For its content of injustice is then so considerable that it can never acquire the dignity of law, though the lawgiver may have endowed it with outwardly valid legal form.

One of these ultimate legal maxims, deeply and inextricably rooted in nature, affirms the sanctity of human life and the individual's right to it, forfeit to the State only after sentence passed in court or in time of war. But Adolf Hitler's so-called euthanasia laws grossly violated this particular assertion of natural right. They disregarded the law of the sanctity of human life and in so doing passed out of the sphere of law altogether. They offended every principle of justice, custom and morality and dissolved the foundations of society by ordering one part of it to die and another to live. They ceased therefore to remain adjusted to the eternal standards of natural law and could never acquire the dignity and efficacy of law owing to the crude injustice of their content.

Consequently, the decrees and laws passed on the subject of so-called euthanasia were legally null and void. They did not create law and thus never possessed the material force of legislation. It follows that the conduct of the accused was wrong and directed to contravention of the law. Their actions must therefore be described as objectively illegal.'

Elsewhere in the Judgment it is stated:

'Final recognition of right or wrong is not obtained by the consideration of external circumstances, such as laws or the assent of other persons, but only from the individual conscience.

If the defendant had been a man of high moral character or a strong upholder of the ethics of his profession he must have recognized these events as intolerable both from a medical standpoint and from that of common humanity.'

In a 'judicial assessment of the facts ascertained' the Court declared that the nursing, technical and administrative staff:

T

'all co-operated in one way or another in the execution of the so-called euthanasia programme and the killing of the mentally afflicted. The main question is not whether one of the accused collaborated to a greater extent than another but whether any of the accused can be said to have participated in any way in any measure connected with the liquidation of the patients. In the opinion of the Court such action contributed to the killing of each individual patient, because the steps taken were all systematic and prescribed parts of a whole proceeding which, by their combined working, necessarily and inevitably led to the previously planned deaths of many human beings. Failure to take any such steps would entail failure to bring about death by the methods adopted.

The first point, therefore, which is established in the case of all the accused is that they took purely external steps criminal in principle and accordingly to be regarded as evidence of penal offence.'

But in considering the question of statutory guilt the Court decided that the administrative staff accused had not intended to aid in the perpetration of a criminal act by others or known of it. It was possible accordingly that they were not aware of anything wrong or illegal in their actions.

'But the premeditation required to prove accessory guilt is in the opinion of this Court absent. The defendants belonging to the office staff are accordingly discharged for lack of evidence of possible premeditation.'

The same conclusion was reached regarding the three members of the technical staff accused. On the other hand those directly concerned, two doctors and nine male and female nurses, were found guilty of criminal action. Judgment stated:

'Affirmation of the statutory guilt of the accused is required if it is clear that they recognized the illegality of the so-called euthanasia laws and the proceedings involved in them to be so basic and serious as to render execution of them morally wrong and reprehensible in the defendants' own view, despite the support of their conduct by a law they themselves considered valid.

The profoundest feelings of the Court and the facts which came to light at the main trial have led . . . to the pronouncement of such affirmation.'

The important points which emerge from these extracts are

the criticism of Government action by the judiciary, its view of participation in proceedings in themselves criminal and its separate consideration of the question of the guilt involved in such participation. In this case the administrative staff's participation rendered the staff accessory in an objective sense to murder. Yet it incurred no criminal guilt in so doing. This point, however, merely serves to distinguish legal from moral guilt. For in all probability the circumstances were clear enough to most of the minor employees engaged to carry out certain duties. They wrote letters, for instance, to the relatives of the victims and knew that the causes of death therein specified were false. As compared with the legal guilt determined in the case of certain individuals, others appeared 'collectively' guilty in the sense that the individuals found legally guilty could only have been rendered so by the participation, the agreement, the voluntary or compulsory connivance, of many 'fellow-travellers'.

The former director, and also the resident physician, of the combined sanatorium and nursing home at Scheuern near Nassau were discharged by Criminal Court No. 3 of Coblenz, presided over by the County Court Judge Zündorf, after proceedings which lasted from the 29 September 1948 to the 4 October.

Scheuern was one of the so-called intermediate stations designed partly to camouflage later stages of the euthanasia programme and partly for the purpose of assembling and subjecting to cursory personal examination the patients on their way to the extermination centres. Judgment noted the following details of the medical proceedings.

[3 KLs 36/48.]

'The position of the directors and resident physicians of these intermediate stations was not altogether identical in various parts of the country. The regulations governing the extent of their tasks were in some cases obscure. Certain of these men were officially entrusted with the scheme and the duty of carrying it out, while others only had to attend the patients in a medical sense for the time being, the final decision to "eliminate", as the phrase went, being left to roving committees of doctors which subjected patients to cursory examination. In

these cases it was only open to the resident physician occasionally to prevent the inclusion of some invalid, for instance one
with a war decoration awarded on active service, in a convoy
already organized. But as a rule such a doctor would not be
allowed to exert any influence, on medical grounds, on the
patient's future fate. Such was the situation at Scheuern among
other centres. . . .'

It was proved that 1,323 patients passed through Scheuern
'mostly to Hadamar, but in some cases to Kalmenhof bei
Idstein, where killings also proceeded at a later date.'

Of these 1,000 had been delivered by the 'Limited Company
for the Transport of Patients in the Public Interest', perhaps
with the knowledge of the accused. In considering the question
whether the defendants 'participated in responsibility for the
unnatural deaths of these unfortunate beings and if so should
be punished, or whether any subsidiary causes might be held
to annul or at least mitigate their culpability' the Court discussed at length the problem of a 'conflict of duties'.

Judgment dealt point by point with the items of the indictment. Extracts are given below in view of the importance of
the general question raised.

[3 KLs 36/48.]

'The accused cannot be blamed for having accepted the so-
called intermediate patients. This step did not accelerate the
annihilation of the prospective victims, but on the contrary
postponed it and gained time. It was the social, professional
and not least the Christian duty of the defendants to take in
and care for these poor pitiable creatures, who often arrived
at Scheuern utterly debilitated, in disgraceful circumstances,
some of them besmeared with filth and even half starved. At
Scheuern they were not in the slightest degree ill-treated. At
any rate the evidence available gives no hint of any such thing,
nor do the characters of the accused or the spirit in which the
station was managed. . . . The facilitation of further transport
and the surrender to such convoys of the station's own patients
represent in an objective sense the promotion of lethal activities,
the abandonment of those in the care of the station and their
delivery to a fate which, after the 1 April 1941 . . . could no

longer be unknown and was in fact recognized. . . . If the defendants nevertheless dispatched convoys from their station, they unquestionably participated in the criminal conduct of the culprits and formed a link in the chain of cause and effect whereby those who perished met their fate. . . .

The accused were accessory by their conduct to the treacherous and cruel killing, for base motives, of about a thousand human beings. They had no intention personally of killing their patients. But they knew that what they did facilitated the action of the murderers. As proved by the statements of many witnesses whose names have already been mentioned, the accused suffered greatly from the consciousness of their share in this responsibility. It may be admitted in their favour that the details of the intermediate steps in the scheme were unknown to them. But they are sufficiently condemned by their indubitable recognition that the patients they dispatched were to die unnatural deaths. There is no need for the premeditation of an accessory to include such features of the crime as its base motives, trickery and cruelty. For the rest, the existence of such characteristics of the whole planning and execution of the scheme for liquidation of the mentally unsound needs no further emphasis. The lack of any legal basis for it, of any care in the selection of patients for elimination, of any consultation of their legal representatives together with the deception of the prospective victims and of the public regarding the purpose and aim of the measures planned and finally the incredible brutality of their infliction are all perfectly clear.

Yet at the same time the conduct of the defendants amounted to action accessory to a crime against humanity within the meaning of Regulation 10 of the Control Commission. . . .'

The following points were made in justification of the verdict:

'(1). The defendants' claim to have obeyed orders was considered. . . . But the fact that they did so can only mitigate, not set aside, the penalties incurred. For a criminal order can never bind the recipient to carry it out and release him from the verdict of his own conscience. . . .

(2). The state of emergency, in particular the so-called 'enforced emergency', was not considered on behalf of the defendants. The threats of the Third Reich authorities . . . of shooting or incarceration in a concentration camp, related only to the infringement of the enforced obligation of silence. Such menaces could not have prevented the accused from resigning their posts.'

These considerations, as well as the inapplicability of the so-called 'overriding emergency' and the record of oral evidence made it requisite to 'examine the problem of the so-called "conflict of duties", to which no solution has hitherto been found by German courts. In particular no proof has ever been adduced by the Defence in any previous trial relating to euthanasia that the accused, when faced with such a conflict, did everything humanly possible, by acts of sabotage, to avert a greater disaster. . . .'

In this connection it was noted in particular:

'The Supreme Court had already laid it down that the higher duty must be performed at the expense of the less important. But when two duties of equal standing are in opposition, should the effort to save individual lives, even a great many, of itself involve collaboration in the surrender of others to death? At the very least a tragic conflict of duties will then arise, when the accessory—for his case alone, not that of the perpetrator of the crime, is here being considered—will be obliged to shoulder a burden of guilt in order to avert a greater calamity. It must be emphasized in this connection that it was only the events taking place under a tyranny of the most recent past which have taught us the utterly unvarnished truth in all its pitiless, inescapable reality. Eugen Kogon refers in his epoch-making work, *The SS State* (Munich, 1946), to situations which arose in concentration camps when the senior members of the Red Party, i.e. the political prisoners, had to agree to organize death convoys in case authority in the camp should be acquired by the Green Party, that of the criminal offenders, when far worse consequences would certainly have followed. Similar cases are reported by Gilbert Dobrise in the periodical *Lancelot*, Vol. 2, 1946, pp. 60–62 and the Lorraine Catholic priest François Goldschmid in his book *Western Witnesses*. . . . The Court is therefore confronted for the first time with the question whether and under what conditions an act of sabotage can be held, not indeed to justify, but to excuse the statutory guilt of an accessory to lethal activities when he is involved in a conflict of duties. In conformity with the principles argued by von Weber in the two publications mentioned[1] the Court admits exculpation in the following circumstances:

(1). The accessory must have been faced with a true dilemma, i.e. human judgment could not have envisaged any possibility of saving the lives of at least some of those endangered except by the surrender of the rest.

(2). The accessory must not have become involved in such a situation, obliging him to interfere in other people's lives, voluntarily or from motives of self-interest. On the contrary, he must have been forced by circumstances to take a decision.

(3). The collaboration of the accessory in surrendering lives to the perpetrators of the crime must be limited to the smallest possible extent which the situation allows.

(4). The accessory must be proved to have acted in order to avert a greater evil. He must have reached his decision to act in that way only after the most careful and conscientious examination of all the circumstances. He must have intended by his act to save as many as possible of the endangered lives for which he was responsible.

(5). The accessory must have risked his own safety by doing

---

1. Professor Helmut von Weber stated in an article entitled *Legal Responsibility for Action under Orders* in the *Monatschrift für Deutsches Recht* for February 1948:

'It must be admitted that a greater degree of moral courage was often displayed in maintaining a firm attitude and conniving at the obstruction of orders and that proved behaviour of this kind by responsible men prevented a great deal of mischief under National Socialist rule. This point should not be neglected even by a strictly legalistic judgment. Nor can it be reasonably objected that all the harm done by National Socialism might have been prevented if all subordinates had refused to carry out orders. In this connection it is not the collective guilt of a certain class which is at issue but individual responsibility before the law. Judgment of it must be based on the fact that there could be no such thing as the refusal of a whole class, without exception, to carry out orders.'

The same author, in concluding his essay, entitled '*The Conflict of Duties in Criminal Law*' (Publication in honour of W. Kiesselbach, Gesetz und Recht Verlag, Hamburg, 1947) remarks, after observing that the person concerned would in every case be tragically conscience-stricken, that 'The resolution of such conflicts can only be achieved on purely spiritual lines, between one's conscience and one's God. Justification in law cannot help. For this reason no decision to which anyone may come in such a dilemma, after serious consultation with his conscience, should ever be made the subject of legal proceedings.'

all he could in the way of effective sabotage of the assistance he was called upon to render to the scheme. Mere recourse to the legal measures open to him would not be sabotage.

(6). The sabotage undertaken by the accessory must continue throughout the pressure brought to bear on him to such an extent that the number of lives so rescued bears at least a recognizable relation to the number of lives sacrificed.'

After exhaustive inquiry into the applicability of these conditions in the case of the two defendants the Court discharged them.

'In view of all these circumstances the Court holds it to be proved that the attitude of the two defendants was such as to justify their exemption from legal penalty in the present case.

But this Judgment arises from the consideration of a particular situation. It must not be taken, as was that of the earlier pronouncement of the Supreme Court on legal emergency, as indicative of generally applicable grounds of justification. For in this case the accused deliberately rendered themselves objectively and subjectively guilty, but with no other intention than that of averting a greater evil by their conduct as a whole. Whether they may now feel themselves in their hearts to be completely innocent is a matter for their own consciences. The Court therefore, in consciously developing the decision of the Supreme Court on the question of overriding emergency, concluded that assistance rendered under certain conditions to the perpetrator of a crime may be regarded as legally excused, though not justified, by acts of sabotage on the part of the accessory. This conclusion accordingly recognizes the idea of the conflict of duties'.[1]

By way of contrast with the Judgment in this special case No. 2 Criminal Court of Coblenz, under County Court Judge Grafe, sentenced two out of three doctors of the Andernach sanatorium and nursing home, tried from the 13 to the 29 July 1947, to eight and five years' penal servitude respectively, with deprivation of civil rights for five years, for mutually engaging in crimes against humanity coincident with mutual action accessory to murder in an unspecified number of cases.[2]

Judgment included the following passages:

1. Appeal was lodged against this Judgment.
2. This sentence was later quashed, as it was proved that the two doctors in question had in fact worked successfully to avert crimes.

[5 KLs 41/48.]

'The accused undertook this task voluntarily, as much so as
any other voluntary participant in the scheme, and not as
"compulsory volunteers" like so many who collaborated with
the National Socialist régime. . . . The witness Dr Schmidt for
instance'[1] 'remained quite unmolested after telling Brack himself, in Berlin, that he would not co-operate. Brack did no more
than insult him, though hardly for the reason that he had
declined to co-operate. It was mainly because Schmidt had not
notified his refusal at an earlier date, so that he had now been
needlessly initiated into the project. The only compulsion
imposed, and naturally enough in the sternest terms imaginable,
was the obligation not to breathe a word about the mass murder
which the euthanasia programme involved. . . . But the existence of secret opposition to the scheme has of itself no significance in the legal aspect of the matter. Its influence depends
upon whether it extended beyond those immediately concerned
and whether the fact of its existence caused the defendants to
decide either not to participate in the project or to work against
it. Essentially, however, they did all that Berlin expected of
them as responsible physicians in residence at the Andernach
intermediate station. They thus promoted the euthanasia
programme and in particular the murders at Hadamar. . . .
Nor can it be held in favour of the accused that the consciousness of breaking the law, which would have been a necessary
condition for the establishment of their guilt, was absent in
their case. . . . The National Socialist leaders, from the Führer
downwards, had themselves a bad conscience in this very respect. They knew that they were committing the most monstrous
crimes, for they never dared to allow their misdeeds to become
known to the people at large, though they were otherwise
cynically frank in what they told the country and in the demands
they made upon it. . . . The defendants had led innocent and
respected lives until the advent of the Third Reich and would
probably have continued to do so if that régime had not come to
power. But they made no resistance to what it required of them,
as men of firm moral principle and scrupulous conscience would
have resisted. They had been weakened by this fundamental

1. Dr Schmidt was employed at the Bonn sanatorium and nursing home.

defect and through this weakness they incurred guilt. In their case the guilt in which so many Germans were entangled by National Socialism turned to crime. That "inertia of the will", mentioned in Judgment of the Hadamar case, proved fatal to the accused in the present instance.'[1]

(iv) PLANS FOR "SPECIAL TREATMENT" FOR TUBERCULAR POLISH PATIENTS

Medical opinions and decisions were influential in connection with the question what was to be done with Poles suffering from open tuberculosis. The first documentary evidence of the plan to exterminate them appears in a letter dated the 1 May 1942 from Greiser, Federal Representative for the Wartheland District, to Himmler.

[DOC. 246.]*

'Reich Leader,
    The special treatment of about 100,000 Jews in the territory of my district, approved by you in agreement with the Chief of the Reich Security Main Office, SS Obergruppenführer Heydrich, can be completed within the next two to three months. I ask you for permission to rescue the district immediately after the measures taken against the Jews, from a menace which is increasing week by week, and to use the existing and efficient special commandos for that purpose.
    There are about 230,000 people of Polish nationality in my district, who were diagnosed to suffer from tuberculosis. The number of persons infected with open tuberculosis is estimated at about 35,000. This fact has led in an increasingly frightening measure to the infection of Germans who came to the Warthegau perfectly healthy. In particular, increasingly serious reports are received concerning the risk of infection of German children. A considerable number of well-known leading men, especially of the police, have been infected lately and are not available for the war effort because of the necessary medical treatment. The ever-increasing risks were also recognized and appreciated by the deputy of the Reich Leader for Public Health, Comrade

1. Appeal was lodged against this Judgment.

Professor Dr Blome, as well as by the leader of your X-ray battalion, SS Standartenführer Prof. Dr Holfelder.

Though in Germany proper it is not possible to take appropriate draconic steps against this public plague, I think I could take responsibility for my suggestion to have cases of open tuberculosis exterminated among the Polish race here in Warthegau. Of course only a Pole should be handed over to such an action who is not only suffering from open tuberculosis, but whose incurability is proved and certified by a public health officer.

Considering the urgency of this project I ask for your approval in principle as soon as possible. This would enable us to make the preparations with all necessary precautions now to get the action against the Poles suffering from open tuberculosis under way, while the action against the Jews is in its closing stages.

Heil Hitler!

(*Signature*) GREISER'

The then Chief of the Security Police, Heydrich, wrote on the 9 June 1942 that for his part he would not hesitate to agree that:

[DOC. 245.]

'refugees and Stateless persons of Polish nationality resident in the Wartheland District and suffering from open tuberculosis should be included, if their disease is medically certified incurable, in the "special treatment" proposed by District Leader Greiser.'

Himmler assented to this view for the first time in a letter of the 27 June 1942 to Greiser. [DOC. 244.]

But the 'special treatment' proposed rendered it necessary for the entire population to be X-rayed first. This project was undertaken by the SS Röntgen-Sturmbann under Professor Holfelder. Meanwhile, the deputy chief of the National Socialist Centre for Public Health, Professor Blome, expressed certain doubts to Greiser. His letter reveals the complete subordination of medical opinion to national policy and propaganda in order

to meet the demands of the Government. The letter is therefore
given in full below.

[DOC. 250.]*

'Dr med, Kurt Blome,
    Deputy Head,
    NSDAP Main Office for Public Health.
                                    18 November 1942
                            Berlin SW 68, Lindenstrasse 42
To the Reichsstatthalter and Gauleiter, Party Member Greiser,
    Poznan.
Reference: Tuberculosis action in the Warthegau.

Dear Party Member Greiser.
    Today I return to our various conversations concerning the
fight against tuberculosis in your district, and I will give you—
as agreed on the 9th of this month in Munich—a detailed picture of the situation as it appears to me.
    Conditions for quickly getting hold of all consumptives in
your district exist. The total population of your district
amounts to about 4·5 million people, of which about 835,000
are Germans. According to previous observations, the number
of consumptives in the Warthegau is far greater than the
average number in the old Reich. It was calculated that in
1939 there were among the Poles about 35,000 persons suffering
from open tuberculosis, and besides this number about 120,000
other consumptives in need of treatment. In this connection it
must be mentioned that, in spite of the evacuation of part of
the Poles farther to the East, the number of sick persons is at
least as great as in 1939. As, in consequence of the war, living
and food conditions have deteriorated steadily, one must expect
an even higher number.
    With the settlement of Germans in all parts of the district
an enormous danger has arisen for them. Several cases of
infection of children and adults occur daily.
    What goes for the Warthegau must to a certain degree also
hold true for the other annexed territories, such as Danzig-
West Prussia and the administrative districts of Zichenau and
Katowice. There are cases of Germans settled in the Warthegau

who refuse to have their families follow because of the danger of infection. If such behaviour is imitated, and if our compatriots see that necessary measures for combating tuberculosis among the Poles are not carried out, it is to be expected that the necessary further immigration will come to a halt. In such a way the settlement programme for the East might reach an undesired state.

Therefore, something basic must be done soon. One must decide the most efficient way in which this can be done. There are three ways to be taken into consideration:

1. Special treatment of the seriously ill persons.
2. Most rigorous isolation of the seriously ill persons.
3. Creation of a reservation for all TB patients.

For the planning, attention must be paid to different points of view of a practical, political, and psychological nature. Considering it most soberly, the simplest way would be the following: Aided by the X-ray battalion we could reach the entire population, German and Polish, of the district during the first half of 1943. As to the Germans, the treatment and isolation are to be prepared and carried out according to the regulations of tuberculosis relief. The approximately 35,000 Poles who are incurable and infectious will be "specially treated". All other Polish consumptives will be subjected to an appropriate cure in order to save them for work and to avoid their causing contagion.

According to your request I made arrangements with the offices in question, in order to start and carry out this radical procedure within half a year. You told me that the competent office agreed with you as to this "special treatment" and promised support. Before we definitely start the programme, I think it would be correct if you would make sure once more that the Führer will really agree to such a solution.

I could imagine that the Führer, having some time ago stopped the programme in the insane asylums, might at this moment consider a "special treatment" of the incurably sick as unsuitable and irresponsible from a political point of view. As regards the euthanasia programme it was a question of people of German nationality afflicted with hereditary diseases. Now it is a question of infected sick people of a subjugated nation.

There can be no doubt that the intended programme is the most simple and most radical solution. If absolute secrecy could be guaranteed, all scruples—regardless of what nature—could be overcome. But I consider maintaining secrecy impossible. Experience has taught me that this assumption is true. Should these sick persons, having been brought, as planned, to the old Reich supposedly to be treated or healed, actually never return, the relatives of these sick persons in spite of the greatest secrecy would some day notice "that something was not quite right". One must take into consideration that there are many Polish workers in the old Reich who will inquire as to the whereabouts of their relatives; that there are a certain number of Germans related to or allied by marriage with Poles who could in this way learn of the transport of the sick. Very soon more definite news of this programme would leak out which would be taken up by enemy propaganda. The euthanasia programme taught in which manner this was done and which methods were used. Politically, the new programme would be even more exploited, as it concerns persons of a subjugated nation. The Church will not remain silent either. Nor will people stop at discussing this programme. Certain interested circles will spread the rumour among the people that similar methods are also to be used in the future for German consumptives—even, that one can count on more or less all incurably ill being done away with in the future. In connection with this I recall the recurring recent foreign broadcasts in connection with the appointment of Professor Brandt as commissioner general, spreading the news that he was ordered to attend as little as possible to the healing of the seriously sick, but all the more to healing the less sick. And there are more than enough people who listen to illegal broadcasts.

Furthermore, it is to be taken into consideration that the planned proceeding will provide excellent propaganda material for our enemies, not only as regards the Italian physicians and scientists, but also as regards all the Italian people in consequence of their strong Catholic ties. It is also beyond all doubt that the enemy will mobilize all the physicians of the world. And this will be all the more easy as the general age-old conception of medical duty practice is "to keep alive the poor and guiltless patient as long as possible and to allay his suffering".

Therefore, I think it necessary to explain all these points of view to the Führer before undertaking the programme as, in my opinion, he is the only one able to view the entire complex and to come to a decision.

Should the Führer decline the radical solution, preparations for another way must be made. An exclusive settlement of all Polish consumptives, both incurable and curable, would be one possibility of assuring an isolation of the infected. One could settle with them their immediate relatives, if they so desire, so that nursing and livelihood would be assured. As regards labour commitment, besides agriculture and forestry certain branches of industry could be developed in such territories. I cannot judge whether you can conceive such a possibility within your district. I also could imagine the creation of a common area for the settlement of the consumptives not only of your district but also of the districts of Danzig-West Prussia, of the administrative district of Zichenau and of the province of Upper Silesia. In order to avoid unnecessary overtaxing of public means of transport the transfer could be accomplished by walking. This would be a solution that world propaganda could hardly use against us, and one, on the other hand, that would not arouse any of those stupid rumours in our own country.

Another solution to be taken into consideration would be a strict isolation of all the infectious and incurable consumptives, without exception, in nursing establishments. This solution would lead to the comparatively rapid death of the sick. With the necessary addition of Polish doctors and nursing personnel, the character of a pure death camp would be somewhat mitigated.

The following Polish accommodation possibilities are at present available in your district:

Nursing Home "Waldrose"	400 beds
Nursing Home "Grosse Wiese"	300 beds
Smaller establishments	200 beds
Leslau as of 1 January 1943	1,000 beds
Total	1,900 beds

Should the radical solution, i.e. proposal No. 1, be out of the question, the necessary conditions for proposals 2 and 3 must be created.

We must keep in mind that war conditions deprive us of the possibility of arranging for a fairly adequate treatment of the curable consumptives. To do so would require procuring at least 10,000 more beds. This figure, under the condition that the programme is to be carried out within half a year, could not be met.

After a proper examination of all these considerations and circumstances, the creation of a reservation, such as the reservations for lepers, seems to be the most practicable solution. Such a reservation should be able to be created in the shortest time by means of the necessary settlement. Within the reservation one could easily set up conditions for the strict isolation of the strongly contagious.

Even the case of the German consumptives represents an extremely difficult problem for the district. But this cannot be overcome, unless the problem of the Polish consumptives is solved at the same time.

Heil Hitler!

Yours,

(*Signed*) Dr Blome'

Even Himmler could not close his mind to these arguments. Accordingly, in a second letter to Greiser dated the 3 December 1942, he suggested that 'a suitable district be found for the reception of incurable cases of tuberculosis.' [DOC. 251.]

Blome stated in Court that he was obliged to deal with Greiser, as the latter's approval was necessary for all X-ray procedure on the scale of mass radiography. The work itself was arranged and carried out by Blome himself and others. He explained that he had written the letter just quoted after consulting Professor Holfelder and the Chief Medical Officer of the Wartheland District, Dr Gundermann, since he could only expect results from the kind of communication which would please those then in power. He added:

[PROT. p. 4616.]*

'I would have preferred merely to have pointed out the criminal aspects of this proposal in my letter, but I knew the mentality of these men, and it was quite clear to me that the expression of any such point of view could only have had a negative result. . . . I had, however, realized, and it was also the opinion of Professor Holfelder, that I would have to make it appear as if I agreed to the plan if I wanted to have any success with my counter-proposals. I was convinced that the mention of all the political aspects which might involve danger would be the only effective weapon.'

An affidavit by Dr Gundermann, put in by the defence, declared, *inter alia*:

[DOC. Kurt Blome 1.]*

'I concluded, mainly from the development in the fight against tuberculosis in the Wartheland, that the letter from Dr Blome to Gauleiter Greiser had been successful. The regulation about tuberculosis relief having become effective for the whole Reich territory on the 1 April 1943, a similar regulation for protection against tuberculosis could be decreed in the Wartheland in favour of the Polish population. A central office for the fight against tuberculosis was established under the management of a specialist. This office gave the same treatment to German and Polish cases.'

There was no documentary evidence of the transfer of Poles suffering from tuberculosis.

Professor Kurt Blome was discharged by the Court.

(v) EXPERIMENTAL PREPARATIONS FOR MASS STERILIZATION

The origin of the sterilization experiments can also be precisely traced. As the war went on the intention of the Party to destroy the defeated peoples of the East became less and less disguised. In the course of time several methods were independently devised for rendering whole populations barren. Experiments were carried out with sterilization by (*a*) drugs, (*b*) X-rays and (*c*) intra-uterine irritants.

U

(*a*) The idea of sterilization by drugs can be traced back to a letter of October 1941 from the defendant Dr Adolf Pokorny to Himmler.

[DOC. 035.]*

'Led by the idea that the enemy must not only be conquered but destroyed, I feel obliged to present to you, as the Reich Commissioner for the Consolidation of German Folkdom, the following:

Dr Madaus has published the result of his research on medicinal sterilization (both articles are enclosed).[1] Reading these articles, the immense importance of this drug in the present fight of our people occurred to me. If, on the basis of this research, it were possible to produce a drug which, after a relatively short time, effects an imperceptible sterilization on human beings, then we would have a new powerful weapon at our disposal. The thought alone that the three million Bolsheviks at present German prisoners could be sterilized so that they could be used as labourers but be prevented from reproduction, opens the most far-reaching perspectives.

Madaus found that the sap of the caladium seguinum, when taken by mouth or given as injection to male and also to female animals, after a certain time, produces permanent sterility. The illustrations accompanying the scientific article are convincing.

If my ideas meet your approval, the following course should be taken:

1. Dr Madaus must not publish any more such articles. (the enemy listens!).
2. Multiplying the plant (easily cultivated in greenhouses!).
3. Immediate research on human beings (criminals!) in order to determine the dose and length of the treatment.
4. Immediate research on the constitutional formula of the effective chemical substance in order to

1. The reference is to a contribution entitled *Experiments with Animals in Relation to Sterilization by Drugs* in Vol. 109, I, of the *Zeitschrift für die gesamte experimentelle Medizin*. The periodical *Umschau* (38, 1941) dealt with the same subject in an article entitled *Wonder-working Plants in the Light of Experimental Research*.

5. Produce it synthetically if possible.'

The following is a summary of the arguments of the defendant and the attitude of the Court.

[Judgment p. 240 f.]*

'The defendant has attempted to explain his motives for sending the letter by asserting that for some time prior to its transmittal he had known of Himmler's intentions to sterilize all Jews and inhabitants of the eastern territories, and had hoped to find some means of preventing the execution of this dreadful programme. He knew, because of his special experience as a specialist in skin and venereal diseases, that sterilization of human beings could not be effected by the administration of caladium seguinum. He thought, however, that if the articles written by Madaus could be brought to the attention of Himmler, the latter might turn his attention to the unobtrusive method for sterilization which had been suggested by the articles and thus be diverted, at least temporarily, from continuing his programme of castration and sterilization by well-known, tried and tested methods. Therefore the letter was written—so explained the defendant—not for the purpose of furthering, but of sabotaging the programme.

We are not impressed with the defence which has been tendered by the defendant and have great difficulty in believing that he was motivated by the high purposes which he asserted impelled him to write the letter. Rather are we inclined to the view that the letter was written by Pokorny for very different and more personal reasons.

Be that however as it may, every defendant is presumed to be innocent until he has been proved guilty. In the case of Pokorny the prosecution has failed to sustain the burden. As monstrous and base as the suggestions in the letter are, there is not the slightest evidence that any steps were ever taken to put them into execution by human experimentation. We find, therefore, that the defendant must be acquitted—not because of the defence tendered, but in spite of it.'

The discovery of the sterilizing effect of caladium seguinum also seems to have appealed to another official as affording a favourable method of ensuring mass sterilization. On the 24

308 THE DEATH DOCTORS

August the deputy District Leader of the Lower Danube wrote to Himmler as follows:

[DOC. 039.]*

'Since the prevention of reproduction by the congenitally unfit and racially inferior belongs to the duties of our National Socialist racial and demographic policy, the present Director of the District Office for Racial Policy, Gauhauptstellenleiter Dr Fehringer, has examined the question of sterilization and found that the methods so far available, castration and sterilization, are not sufficient in themselves to meet expectations. Consequently, the obvious question occurred to him whether impotence and sterility could not be produced in both men and women by the administration of medicine or injections. So he came to the studies of the Biological Institute of Dr Madaus, in Dresden-Radebeul, on animal experiments for medical sterilization, which became accessible to him through the Madaus Annual Report, seventh year, 1940, and are of the greatest interest for our demographic policy. Madaus and Koch found that caladium seguinum used in homoeopathic doses, that is, administered in infinitesimal quantities, favourably affects impotence, sterility, and frigidity (sexual indifference), so that clinical and medical research should not proceed without regard to this fact. It was established by an extensive series of experiments on rats, rabbits, and dogs that, as the result of the administration or injection of caladium extract, male animals became impotent and females barren, and the differences in effect of the various methods of applying the drug could be seen. From the animal experiments, it seems that a permanent sterility is liable to result in male animals and a more temporary one in females.

It is clear that these observations could be of tremendous importance if alterations of potency or fecundity could also be successfully brought about in human beings by the administration of a caladium extract. Research on human beings themselves would, of course, be necessary for this.

The director of my race policy office points out that the necessary research and human experiments could be undertaken by an appropriately selected medical staff, basing their work on the Madaus animal experiments in co-operation with the pharmacological institute of the Faculty of Medicine of Vienna, on the persons of the inmates of the gipsy camp of Lackenbach in the Lower Danube region.

It is quite clear that such research must be handled as a nationally important secret matter of the most dangerous character, because enemy propaganda could work tremendous harm all over the world by the knowledge of such research, should it come by such knowledge.

Since these considerations are only a theory, the fundamental accuracy of which has already been established by animal experiments and the possibility of the application of which to human beings is highly probable, a mere indication only can be given of the prospects of the possibility of the sterilization of practically unlimited numbers of people in the shortest time and in the simplest way conceivable.'

But Himmler had already followed up the first suggestion. He had at once instructed Obergruppenführer Pohl, head of the SS Economic and Administrative Head Office, and the SS Surgeon-General and Gruppenführer Grawitz to get in touch with Dr Madaus on his behalf and

[DOC. 036.]*

'to inform him, on my behalf, that he should not publish anything else on these questions of medicinal sterilization, and offer him possibilities of doing research, in co-operation with the Reich Physician SS, on criminals who would have to be sterilized in any case.'

But in practice it turned out that the cultivation of the plant in question, native to South America, presented difficulties. A hothouse was established for the purpose. Himmler insisted that:

[DOC. 044.]

'sterilization experiments should in any case be carried out in the concentration camps with the aid of such constituents of this plant as may become available.'

Dr Koch of the Madaus Laboratory testified in court that

caladium seguinum had never been supplied to the SS and that the experiments his Institute had been ordered to carry out on drosophila melanogaster, mice and rats had been deliberately prolonged until the middle of 1944, by which date no further interest in the matter on either side was apparent. All the experiments had proved fruitless. They had been arranged and performed in such a way that:

[PROT. p. 10291.]

'they have no scientific value today. The reason is that we suspected the SS or Pohl of possibly cherishing certain intentions with which we could not agree. We accordingly set about the experiments in this manner from the start, planning and conducting them in similar fashion.'

(b) X-ray sterilization. The defendant Viktor Brack, formerly administrative head of Bouhler's office, the Chancellery, referred in an affidavit to certain reasons for and particulars of these experiments.

[DOC. 426.]

'By 1941 it was an open secret in high-ranking Party circles that those in power intended to exterminate the entire Jewish population in Germany and the occupied regions. I myself and my colleagues, especially Dr Hevelmann and Herr Blankenburg, considered this project of the Party Leaders to be unworthy of Germany and of humanity as a whole. We therefore determined to find some other solution of the Jewish problem, less drastic than the complete extermination of an entire race. We conceived the idea of deporting the Jews to some distant country. I can remember that Dr Hevelmann suggested Madagascar in this connection. We drew up a plan for the purpose in my office and submitted it to Bouhler. Apparently it could not be accepted[1] and consequently we came to the conclusion that sterilization might be the answer to the problem. The plan would be one of considerable complexity, so we decided to use X-rays. I presented this proposal to Bouhler in

1. This plan was submitted to and rejected by Hitler.

1941. But it was declined. Bouhler told me that such a programme would not be feasible, as Hitler was against it. I then did some more work on the project and finally submitted a revised version to Himmler. . . .'

Brack's 'Report on Experiments with Röntgen Castration' was included among the documents before the Court. It had been forwarded by Brack to Himmler in March, with a covering note, and read as follows:

[DOC. 203.]*

'The experiments in this field are concluded. The following result can be considered as established and adequately based on scientific research:

If any persons are to be sterilized permanently, this result can only be attained by applying X-rays in a dosage high enough to produce castration with all its consequences, since high X-ray dosages destroy the internal secretion of the ovary, or of the testicles, respectively. Lower dosages would only temporarily paralyse the procreative capacity. The consequences in question are for example the disappearance of menstruation, climacteric phenomena, changes in capillary growth, modification of metabolism, etc. In any case, attention must be drawn to these disadvantages.

The actual dosage can be given in various ways, and the irradiation can take place quite imperceptibly. The necessary local dosage for men is 500–600 r., for women 300–350 r. In general, an irradiation period of two minutes for men, three minutes for women, with the highest voltage, a thin filter and at a short distance, ought to be sufficient. There is, however, a disadvantage that has to be put up with: as it is impossible unnoticeably to cover the rest of the body with lead, the other tissues of the body will be injured and radiologic malaise will ensue. If the X-ray intensity is too high, those parts of the skin which the rays have reached will exhibit symptoms of burns— varying in severity in individual cases—in the course of the following days or weeks.

One practical way of proceeding would be, for instance, to let the persons to be treated approach a counter, where they could be asked to answer some questions or to fill in forms,

which would take them two or three minutes. The official
sitting behind the counter could operate the installation in such
a way as to turn a switch which would activate the two valves
simultaneously (since the irradiation has to operate from both
sides).

With a two-valve installation about 150–200 persons could
then be sterilized per day, and therefore, with twenty such
installations as many as 3,000–4,000 persons per day. In my
estimation a larger daily number could not in any case be sent
away for this purpose. As to the expenses of such a two-valve
system, I can only give a rough estimate of approximately
20,000–30,000 RM. Additionally, however, there would be
the cost of the construction of a new building, because adequately extensive protective installations would have to be
provided for the officials on duty.

In summary, it may be said that, having regard to the
present state of radiological technique and research, mass
sterilization by means of X-rays can be carried out without
difficulty. However, it seems to be impossible to do this in such
a way that the persons concerned do not sooner or later realize
with certainty that they have been sterilized or castrated by
X-rays.

(*Signed*) BRACK'

In connection with the diversion of Brack's staff to speed up
Brigadier Globocnik's anti-Jewish measures the former reminded
Himmler a year later, on the 23 June 1942, of his sterilization
proposals, on the following grounds:

[DOC. 205.]*

'Among ten millions of Jews in Europe there are, I figure, at
least two to three millions of men and women who are fit
enough to work. Considering the extraordinary difficulties the
labour problem presents us with, I hold the view that those two
to three millions should be specially selected and preserved.
This can, however, only be done if at the same time they are
rendered incapable to propagate. About a year ago I reported
to you that agents of mine had completed the experiments

necessary for this purpose. I would like to recall these facts once more. Sterilization, as normally performed on persons with hereditary diseases, is here out of the question, because it takes too long and is too expensive. Castration by X-ray, however, is not only relatively cheap, but can also be performed on many thousands in the shortest time. I think, that at this time it is already irrelevant whether the people in question become aware of having been castrated after some weeks or months once they feel the effects.

Should you, Reich Führer, decide to choose this way in the interest of the preservation of labour, then Reichsleiter Bouhler would be prepared to place all physicians and other personnel needed for this work at your disposal. Likewise he requested me to inform you that then I would have to order the apparatus so urgently needed with the greatest speed.'

At Himmler's request Blankenburg, Brack's deputy in the Chancellery, communicated with Pohl, head of the Central Concentration Camp Control Office. But the collaboration of Brack's doctors with the SS in the camps was only substantiated by the following letter of 1944:

[DOC. 208.]*

'Dear Reich Leader:

By order of Reich Leader Bouhler I submit to you as an enclosure a work of Dr Horst Schumann on the influence of X-rays on human genital glands.

Previously you have asked Senior Colonel Brack to perform this work, and you supported it by providing the adequate material in the concentration camp Auschwitz. I point especially to the second part of this work, which shows that by those means a castration of males is almost impossible or requires an effort which does not pay. As I have convinced myself, operative castration requires not more than six to seven minutes, and therefore can be performed more reliably and quicker than castration by X-rays.

Soon I shall be able to submit a continuation of this work to you.'

In 1939–40 Dr Schumann had been in charge of an euthanasia

institution and had also acted as assessor in the organization of the programme. His activities and the experimental castrations by X-ray in 1943 were described by a former Jewish prisoner in an affidavit and also from the witness stand.[1] [DOC. 819.]

'I had been working for a month on road-making when one evening the Block clerk suddenly called out: "All Jews between 20 and 24 who are fit for work are to report." But I did not report. Of those who did twenty were ordered to report to a doctor two days later. They returned the same day and were obliged immediately to start work. No one knew what was to be done with them. A week later another twenty Jews of the same age-group were selected. But this time they were chosen alphabetically. I was one of the very first. We were sent to a women's labour camp at Birkenau. There we were met by a tall doctor in a grey Air Force uniform. We had to undress and put our sexual organs under a machine for fifteen minutes. The apparatus made these parts and the adjoining regions of the body quite hot. Afterwards the parts turned black. We were obliged to go to work again immediately afterwards. A few days later the sexual organs of most of my comrades were suppurating and the men could hardly walk. But they had to go on working till they fell down. Those who fell were taken to the gas-chamber.

In my own case there was only a certain amount of moisture, no suppuration. Two weeks later, about October 1943, seven men of our group were taken to Auschwitz I. They had to walk the whole way. It was very difficult for them, because their sexual parts were painful. At Auschwitz I we were placed in the hospital building, Block 20, where we were operated on. We were given an injection in the back which anaesthetized the lower half of our bodies but left the upper half quite normal. Both testicles were removed. There was no previous examination of the seminal fluid. I was able to watch the process in the mirror of a surgical lamp. No one was asked to consent to

1. Dr Schumann's experiments at Auschwitz were also reported in the testimony of one Dr Vuysje, of which extracts are given in the 'Summary of Information No. 55' of the United Nations War Crimes Commission, London.

the operation. We were only told, "You're next." Then we were immediately put on the operating table without another word. The director of the sterilization and castration experiments at Auschwitz was a certain Dr Schumann. . . .'

'Please forgive me for crying, I can't help it. I was three weeks in the hospital at Auschwitz. Then 60 per cent of those in our Block were taken away for gassing. I got frightened and left the hospital to go to work, though I was only half fit. I went to work in the prisoners' tailoring department. There I had to work very hard and was often beaten. . . .' [PROT. 588.]

An affidavit by Gustawa Winkowska, a female Polish prisoner at Ravensbrück, confirms that X-ray sterilization was also attempted at that camp, in connection with the Auschwitz experiments.

[DOC. 865.]

'A doctor came from Auschwitz for a few days, perhaps a week. He spent the whole of each day, so long as he remained in the camp, sterilizing the gipsy children with X-rays. He did not use anaesthetics. The children used to come out crying after being sterilized and ask their mothers what had been done to them. . . .'

Dr Robert Levy, head surgeon of a hospital block at Birkenau, a camp subsidiary to that at Auschwitz, had been a prisoner since 1943. He also described X-ray sterilizations that were followed by operative castration.

[PROT. p. 602.]

'At Birkenau I saw people who had been sterilized. I found out in September that when people arrived about 100 of the younger persons were selected. They were Poles who had been living near Auschwitz. They came shortly before we did and the well built, robust youngsters in the best of health were picked out. At the time we didn't know what they were wanted for. From December or possibly January onwards some of them were brought to me for medical treatment. They complained of circulation trouble in the abdominal region. By asking them questions I discovered that in September 1943 they had undergone X-ray treatment and been operated on a month later. Either one or both testicles had been removed. The men showed symptoms of ulceration which I identified from their typical aspect as radio-dermatitis. The suppurations did not tend to heal, mainly because we had so few medical remedies available. Nevertheless, we managed to give some of the patients the treatment required, though most of them eventually disappeared in the periodical extermination measures. . . .

. . . I surmised that the testicles had been removed for microscopic examination of the results of X-ray treatment. I assume that the subjects were exposed to radiations of varying strength, with a view to determining the best concentration for the purpose in hand. . . .'

The defendant Viktor Brack made full use of his right to give evidence on his own behalf. To cut a long story short, he alleged that his meticulously laid plans were 'desperate measures' to stop the 'mass murder' of Jews. He said he had known Himmler a long time and could not believe him responsible for these destructive designs, which he always regarded as emanating from Bormann and, in particular, Heydrich. Brack described his first report to Himmler on 'Röntgen Sterilization' [Doc. 203] as one of these 'wild and desperate' measures, as he had been convinced in consultation with an expert that the plan was impracticable and could only be the subject of diversionary and delaying tactics. [PROT. p. 7582 ff.]

He added that as soon as Himmler told him that Hitler had 'ordered the annihilation of the Jews' and that 'in the interests of camouflage they would have to work as fast as possible' he had reported for active service. He said he wanted to 'get away from the office of a Führer whose radicalism was increasingly getting on my nerves'. He declared that his second letter [Doc. 205] had been written while he was on leave for Heydrich's funeral ceremonies (6 September 1942), as after Heydrich's death he thought he saw further opportunities of 'putting a stop to the mass murders even at the eleventh hour'.

But it is today certain, despite the evidence of many affidavits testifying to Brack's good intentions and admirable qualities, that his planning of and participation in the euthanasia and sterilization proceedings led to innumerable killings and mutilations. The Court sentenced him to death.

(c) Sterilization by intra-uterine irritants. This method, whereby irritant fluid is introduced into the womb, was developed solely by Professor Clanberg of Königshütte in Upper Silesia.[1]

In a letter of the 7 June 1943 Clauberg reported to Himmler on the level of development and effectiveness so far attained by his method.

[DOC. 212.]*

'The method I contrived to achieve the sterilization of the female organism without operation is as good as perfected. It can be performed by a single injection made through the entrance of the uterus in the course of the customary gynaecological examination known to every physician. If I say the method is "as good as perfected", this means:

1. Still to be worked out are only minor improvements of the method.

2. Already today it could be put to practical use in the course of our regular eugenic sterilization and could thus replace the operation.

As to the question which you, Reich Leader, asked me almost one year ago, i.e. how much time would probably be required to sterilize 1,000 women by using this method. Today I can answer you with regard to the future as follows:

If my researches continue to have the same results as up to now—and there is no reason to doubt that—then the moment is not far off when I can say:

1. The 'Summary of Information No. 5' of the United Nations War Crimes Commission in London contains a statement by Dr Vuysje regarding the Auschwitz experiments which suggests the derivation of the method. According to this evidence Clauberg had originally been experimenting on women, in collaboration with a chemist, in order to find a substitute for iodine, of which there was a shortage in Germany. Some 400 women were subjected to these experiments, not at the time intended to sterilize, though in many cases they had that effect.

"One adequately trained physician in one adequately equipped place, with perhaps ten assistants (the number of assistants in conformity with the speed desired) will most likely be able to deal with several hundred, if not even 1,000 per day."'

Himmler's inquiry, referred to in this letter, concerning the rate at which sterilization by Clauberg's method could be expected, is confirmed by another document. Rudolf Brandt wrote on the 10 July 1942 to Clauberg in an officially secret communication from the 'Personal Staff of the Reichsführer SS':

[DOC. 213.]*

'1. To Professor Clauberg,
     Koenigshuette.

Dear Professor!

Today the Reich Leader SS charged me with transmitting to you his wish that you go to Ravensbrück after you have had another talk with SS Obergruppenführer Pohl and the camp physician of the women's concentration camp, Ravensbrück, in order to perform the sterilization of Jewesses according to your method.

Before you start your job, the Reich Leader SS would be interested to learn from you how long it would take to sterilize a thousand Jewesses. The Jewesses themselves should not know anything about it. As the Reich Leader SS understands it, you could give the appropriate injections during a general examination.

Thorough experiments should be conducted to investigate the effect of the sterilization largely in a way that you find out after a certain time, which you would have to fix, perhaps by X-rays, what kind of changes have taken place. In some cases a practical experiment might be arranged by locking up a Jewess and a Jew together for a certain period and then seeing what results are achieved.

I ask you to let me know your opinion about my letter for the information of the Reich Leader SS.
                    Heil Hitler!

                              (*Signed*) BRANDT,
                         SS Obersturmbannführer ([1])

2. To SS Obergruppenführer Pohl, Berlin, for information.

SS Obersturmbannführer Koegel has also received a carbon copy from me for the appraisal of the camp doctor. Further carbons have been received by the Reich Physician SS and the Reich Security Head Office.

(*Signed*) BRANDT,
SS Obersturmbannführer

3. To SS Gruppenführer Grawitz, Reich Physician SS.

(*Signed*) BRANDT,
SS Obersturmbannführer

4. To SS Obersturmbannführer Koegel, Economic and Administrative Head Office, for information and appraisal of camp doctor.

(*Signed*) BRANDT,
SS Obersturmbannführer

5. To Reich Security Head Office, Berlin (SS Sturmbannführer Guenther IV B 4 Jewish Affairs Department for information.

(*Signed*) BRANDT,
SS Obersturmbannführer'

Dr Zdenka Nedvedova-Nejedla, a prisoner employed on medical work at Ravensbrück concentration camp, gave an account, as eyewitness, of this sterilization process by the injection of fluid into the uterus.

[DOC. 875.]

'I saw gipsy women prisoners going into the X-ray room and coming out again. They were sterilized there in accordance with a system which I know was tried out at "Osviecim" (Auschwitz). The method is based on the injection into the uterus of a liquid causing inflammation. It was most probably silver nitrate combined with a contrasting fluid, designed to

1. All these signatures are those of Rudolf Brandt, Himmler's personal consultant.

facilitate subsequent X-ray checking of the operation. All the women sterilized were exposed to X-ray treatment immediately afterwards. I examined the photographs with Dr Mlada Taufrova and am therefore in a position to state that in most of these cases the Fallopian tube was blocked and in several even the abdominal cavity. In only about the last ten cases were anaesthetics administered on the insistence of the SS Sister Gerda. I attended the children the whole night after their operations. They were all bleeding from the sexual organs and were in such pain that I was obliged to give them sedatives surreptitiously. In the morning, before roll-call, I took the children back to their Blocks with the assistance of the girls working in the sick bay. . . .'

The fact that Clauberg had been authorized by Himmler to perform his experiments at that camp is proved by a letter of July 1942 from the Führer's headquarters. It too came from Himmler's personal adjutant.

[DOC. 216.]*

'On the 7 July 1942 a discussion took place between the Reich Leader SS, SS Brigadeführer Professor Dr Gebhardt, SS Brigadeführer Gluecks and SS Brigadeführer Clauberg, Koenigshütte. The topic of the discussion was the sterilization of Jewesses. The Reich Leader SS promised SS Brigadeführer Professor Clauberg that Auschwitz will be at his disposal for his experiments on human beings and animals. By means of some fundamental experiments, a method should be found which would lead to sterilization of persons without their knowledge. The Reich Leader SS wanted to get another report as soon as the result of these experiments was known, so that the sterilization of Jewesses could then be carried out in actuality.

It should also be examined, preferably in co-operation with Professor Dr Holfelder, an X-ray specialist in Germany, in what way sterilization of men could be achieved by X-ray treatment.

The Reich Leader SS called the special attention of all gentlemen present to the fact that the matter involved was most secret and should be discussed only with the officers in charge and that the persons present at the experiments or discussions had to pledge secrecy.'

The scale as a whole of the sterilization undertaken by X-ray treatment and Clauberg's method cannot be ascertained from the documentary material available.[1] It is certain, however, that the military position after 1943 no longer permitted *genocidium*—race extermination—by these methods.[2]

1. The editors were not given access to any papers dealing with proceedings taken in Poland against Professor Clauberg or with the trial of the Auschwitz SS staff.

2. The word *genocidium* was coined by the American scholar Raphael Lembkin and means, according to the international definition arrived at by the Legal Committee of the United Nations Assembly, 'the persecution of national, ethnic, racial, religious and political groups for the purpose of wholly or partly exterminating them as such'. In the draft agenda of the United Nations Plenary Committee for Human Rights a distinction is made between 'physical, biological and cultural genocidium'. The Legal Committee's definition was submitted to the Assembly. Its ratification carries the recognition of genocidium as an offence against international law.

x

CHAPTER ELEVEN

GENERAL EVIDENCE FOR EXPERIMENTS ON HUMAN BEINGS AND MEDICAL CONDUCT

In the course of court proceedings the accused took full advantage of the opportunity offered them to contest the Prosecution's case and record their general attitude to experiments on human beings and the question of medical ethics.[1]

The defence supported this testimony by many extracts from the works of medical writers of several nations. The prosecution objected to the introduction of comparative material of this kind. The objection gave rise to a number of disputes in Court, when the views of each side were argued at length. The first evidence which led to such a difference of opinion concerned experiments in connection with malaria carried out on 800 inmates of a prison in the State of Illinois, who had voluntarily submitted to the tests.[2] A report of the affair was published in the periodical *Life*. The Prosecution sought to prevent recognition of this evidence on two grounds.

In the first place it was argued that the Prosecution would be obliged to undertake meticulous checking of the experiments in question, in order, for example, to ascertain whether participation of the subjects was in fact voluntary, whether they had been made fully aware of the risks involved and whether it had been absolutely necessary to use human beings as subjects in these particular experiments, etc.

Secondly, the following reasoning was advanced.

[PROT. p. 2784 f.]

'*Mr McHaney:* Nevertheless, I don't see how the matter can be considered relevant and of any value as evidence. Even if it is assumed that experiments were carried out abroad and in certain cases against the will of the subjects, that would not

1. In this connection the previously cited statements should also be noted.
2. For details of this voluntary submission see p. 346.

322

justify, in my opinion, any of the crimes now under investigation.' [PROT. p. 2784.]

'Crimes may be committed in the United States and elsewhere just as they may be in Germany. And the fact that proof exists of the commission of such a crime in the United States in any given case is not, in my view, a point in favour of the Defence in the present proceedings.' [PROT. p. 2786.]

The Defence for its part was concerned to clarify the idea of 'crime'. In order to do so it was alleged that one would have to be 'clear about what is generally regarded as humane behaviour, so as to be able to make comparisons'. Defence Counsel declared this view in emphatic terms.

[PROT. p. 2789 f.]

'The Prosecution has invoked the criminal law of all countries as providing the basis for judgment of conduct and has summoned an expert to spend a whole day giving his views on the ethical aspect of the matter. The object was to provide a platform for the Prosecution. I must be allowed to indicate the argument against such tactics. There is no need to go into the question whether all the experiments described in articles and books were accurately reported. In my view the main point is that no voice was raised throughout the world against such proceedings. For example, Document 1, the article in *Life*, did not result in any American criticism of the action referred to. Nor is this a unique case. Such instances have been occurring in all countries for many years. In File 3 of the Karl Brandt papers I collected from printed sources a number of cases which will amaze anyone who reads them. Yet it is even more amazing that they aroused no indignation whatever in the world. When, therefore, in similar circumstances Prosecuting Counsel rises to invoke the laws of humanity, it is obviously of importance to be able to prove that they have never yet been understood in this sense.' [PROT. p. 2789.]

Another Counsel for the Defence added the following considerations:

[PROT. p. 2791.]

'Justice does not exist merely in a vacuum. In order to form a just judgment it is necessary to examine the actual conditions prevailing in the particular field under consideration. Accordingly, the Defence does not adduce evidence of this kind simply to prove that such crimes were committed in foreign countries such as the United States, France and elsewhere, but to add weight to the abstract content of a penal code. It is a fact that many such codes refer to criteria for the judgment of situations and that these criteria presuppose certain standards of value. Judgment, in particular, of the question whether medical experiment can be considered a crime is subject to these criteria. In such a case it has to be inquired whether medical experiment can be regarded as culpable, in other words reprehensible, conduct. In this inquiry it cannot be a matter of indifference how doctors in other countries have behaved in similar situations. It is therefore of decisive importance for the Defence to establish whether foreign physicians who share universally current medical and ethical beliefs have also felt it desirable to perform such experiments in the interests of a higher aim or in consideration of some special state of emergency. The evidence adduced by the Defence is therefore admissible to the extent that it enables the Court to adjust abstract penal regulations to real life and thus bring out their full implications Just as the actual behaviour of nations cannot be ignored in the framing of international law, so also the behaviour of doctors abroad cannot be wholly left out of account in deciding whether a certain medical experiment does or does not constitute a crime.'

The point at issue was therefore the necessity for or the needlessness of experiments on human beings. It also had to be decided whether it remained a doctor's duty to carry out such experiments when the subject would be exposed to grave or the gravest risks and was not a voluntary participant but coerced by the State.

At a later stage in the Trial, when similar evidence was submitted, the Prosecution declared:

[PROT. p. 5532 f.]

'The physicians and scientists in the dock have not been

charged simply with performing experiments on human beings. We for the Prosecution take the view that such experiments are necessary and recognized means of medical research. But we nevertheless charge the accused with criminal behaviour. Their crimes were mostly in connection with their use of subjects who were not volunteers, as well as with negligence and ignorance in the conduct of their experiments and with related action which we claim to have been illegal. There is, moreover, a good deal of difference between the abstracts and data submitted by these physicians—' the reference is to abstracts from printed sources—'and the matters here under consideration. The documents they submitted differ from those relating to their own cases which we have examined in this Court. . . . The former experiments are not connected in any way with those of which we accuse the defendants.'

The Tribunal allowed the Defence to introduce accounts of experiments on human beings which had appeared in medical literature in order, as was later stated in Judgment,

[Judgment p. 4.]*

'. . . to allow each defendant to present his defence completely, . . . and to offer in the case all evidence deemed to have probative value.'

The number of such documents put in by the Defence and accepted by the Court was large, occupying several thick files, notably those of Karl Brandt, Gerhard Rose, Joachim Mrugowsky and Becker-Freyseng. Professor Hans Luxemburger and Dr Erich H. Hahlbach compiled an exhaustive treatise entitled '*Experiments on Human Beings in World Literature*' [Doc. Becker-Freyseng 60] in which medical experiments were formally classified. The authors distinguished the following types of experiments on human beings:

[DOC. Becker-Freyseng 60.]

'1. Clinical experiment on:
(*a*) persons suffering from diseases of natural origin,
(*b*) persons artificially infected with disease for the purpose of either (i) ascertaining the cause of the disease (clinical

experiments of an aetiological nature), or (ii) ascertaining the correct treatment (clinical experiments of a therapeutic nature).

2. Physiological experiment with a view to:
(a) examining a normal vital process as such (research on fundamentals),
(b) ascertaining the limit of normal resistance to strain (often necessary for decisions upon practical aims and proposed action).'

Subjects were divided into the following categories:
'1. Healthy persons, viz. (a) soldiers, (b) certain elements of the population such as immigrants, (c) children, (d) nurses and sanitation employees, (e) convicts.

2. Invalids, with a view to clinical experiment on:
(a) persons suffering from diseases of natural origin (in order to study the causes or treatment of the disease),
(b) sick persons artificially infected with a disease other than that already existing in order to study the artificially induced malady,
(c) invalids to be subjected to physiological experiment (investigation of normal vital process) if their disease bore no relation to the problem calling for experiment.'
In each class the authors referred to examples and printed sources noted in an Appendix, which listed fifty-four.
They dealt with the problem of voluntary participation as follows:
'A peculiarly difficult question is that of the voluntary consent of the subject. It does not arise in the cases of children and the mentally afflicted. In the case of soldiers, especially in war, it should probably be considered to a great extent as part of their normal duty. It is equally questionable whether poor persons who offer their services for agreed financial compensation can be regarded as volunteers. In clinical experiment the matter of the invalid's consent is rarely discussed. In the case of prisoners consent is sometimes specially insisted on, while on other occasions the point is not raised at all.
Out of fifty-three printed sources quoted seventeen state that the subjects consented. In thirty-six the matter was not men-

tioned in any way and in several of these cases it appeared that the subjects might not have presented themselves willingly. The following report is not intended to convey any personal views on the question or to lay down any ethical principles in connection with it but merely to record the situation so far as it can be ascertained from existing international literature and to attempt to account for it. We had to assume that in all cases some mention was made of voluntary participation. The fact that in nearly 70 per cent of the examples the matter was not referred to allows two main conclusions to be drawn (i) that consent was so self-evident that there was no need to give it special emphasis and that consequently enough volunteers had been found without difficulty, (ii) that it is nevertheless conceivable that an experiment should have been undertaken, camouflaged as therapy or some other ordinary measure, without troubling to obtain the consent of the subject beforehand.'

Reference to examples follows.

The authors continue:

'Special attention is required by the terms of this report to experiments on prisoners. The fact that of the fifty-three quotations nine are concerned with such experiments, without counting those mentioned in the historical introduction, is alone remarkable. In view of the importance of these nine cases they are briefly indicated below.

1. Eight hundred convicts from three American prisons were artificially infected with malaria after having voluntarily presented themselves without expectation of reward.[1]

2. Eleven prisoners under sentence of death were subjected to toxicological experiments. No mention of consent was made in the report of this case.

3. A large number of prisoners sentenced to death were infected with typhus in Turkey. No mention of consent in the report.

4. Pellagra was induced by Goldberger in twelve American convicts after they had been promised remission of punishment.

5. The first experiments with reduced cultures of plague bacilli were made by Strong at Manila on several criminals sentenced to death. No mention of consent.[2]

1. See p. 339 for the question of consent.
2. See statement of the defendant Rose on p. 140.

6. In Hawaii a criminal named Keanu under sentence of death was infected with leprosy. The consent of the culprit was obtained and the death sentence remitted. Keanu fell ill and died of leprosy.

7. Twenty-five American prisoners were injected with streptococci after voluntarily presenting themselves.

8. The Manila Worcester Institute tested a series of new medical remedies on convicts in the Bilibid prison, who were rewarded.

9. Experiments with hashish were performed on seventy-seven American prisoners on the responsibility of a committee appointed by the Mayor of New York.

The question arises why these nine experiments were carried out on prisoners. Were the tests so dangerous that no one else volunteered?

They included some in which the highest risks were run, viz. with plague, leprosy and typhus, and others which entailed a certain amount of risk, as with malaria and streptococci, and others again which were practically harmless, being curative remedies. Goldberger's experiments with pellagra may be regarded as controllable tests which involved little danger, though this was not known prior to the experiment, which was undertaken primarily to ascertain the nature of the disease. It failed to achieve its purpose, though the subjects suffered severely from pellagra. The tests of medical remedies must have been on the whole without risk. In the case of the hashish experiments it must be emphasized that they involved the risk of addiction. To familiarize people with a narcotic cannot be regarded as a harmless proceeding, especially as experience shows that seventy-seven convicts must include a not inconsiderable percentage of unbalanced persons and psychopaths with a high liability to addiction. On the other hand, the hashish tests may have been performed on certain prisoners for the very reason that the risk of addiction could in practice be excluded in the case of those condemned to penal servitude for many years or for life. Such persons would, of course, be designated as positively ideal subjects for the experiment.

Our investigation shows, therefore, that the risk of an experiment is not always the only reason why prisoners were used as subjects. They were preferred, rather, because (a) it was known that they would be available over a definite period for this one purpose, from which they would not be diverted by any other business or duty, (*b*) almost any given number of them lived under absolutely standardized conditions, always open to supervision, as regards, for example, their accommodation, diet, hours of sleep, employment, and clothing (*c*) owing to the great range of selection possible, subjects of closely similar ages, physical characteristics and mentalities could be chosen, thus permitting a certain uniformity of psychological treatment during the experiment.

It is probable that most of the scientists who decided to experiment on prisoners were more influenced by the above-mentioned considerations than by any thought of the risks which might be run. The number of measures, for instance, which would have had to be taken if it had been resolved to apply the malaria experiment to ordinary American citizens instead of 800 prisoners is almost beyond computation. It would have been impracticable to take all the steps requisite for the uniformity and control, and accordingly for the success, of an experiment on this vast scale. But under prison conditions such organization presented no obstacle.

Nor should it be forgotten that the participation of prisoners in many of these experiments was rewarded by mitigation of punishment or in some other way. This circumstance must also have influenced a physician in deciding to choose prisoners for experiment. For example, remission of sentence was granted to subjects who made a good recovery in the case of Goldberger's pellagra experiments on twelve prisoners in the State of Mississippi. Again, the criminal infected by Arning with leprosy in Hawaii was reprieved from execution, while the inmates of the Bilibid prison at Manila, on whom the Worcester Institute tested certain medical remedies, received compensation which took the form of mitigation of punishment when any considerable risk was involved.

But in all cases prisoners submitting to experiment could count on better treatment and the recognition of their endeavours to acquire a good reputation in this way.'

From a subsequent passage it appears that experiments on prisoners reported in both scientific and lay publications were 'recognized as permissible and even meritorious not only by the learned world but also by the public at large'.

In a chapter on the conditions to be observed in these cases the authors list the most important as the character of the scientist in charge, the necessity of the experiment, and thorough prior experiments on animals and medical men themselves, together with calculations of risk and of the requisite number of subjects. The actual result of the experiment should not be regarded as decisive for its permissibility.

'The formulation of the problem is the only decisive factor in judgment of the necessity . . . even a negative result may be of great value.'

Some of the reports put in dated back to the eighteenth century and beyond. As a rule they did not refer to the voluntary participation, or otherwise, of the subject. But a few hint clearly enough, sometimes only at the end, that participation was involuntary. The majority of the experiments were concerned with infection and in these the proceedings make a very deep impression on the reader. The following may be quoted:

[DOC. Karl Brandt 3, p. 109.]

'J. Ssusikoff, an assistant medical officer, aged 20, in perfect health, submitted in February 1852 to inoculation with a smear taken from a syphilitic . . . I placed a Spanish fly on his left thigh and after removing the epidermis by this expedient transferred the smear material to the exposed spot with the scoop, covering the place with *charpies* [threads of worn-out rag] soaked in the same material. . . . In the fifth week roseola eruptions appeared on the chest and abdomen and syphilis then began to develop rapidly. I kept the patient in that state for a whole week in order to show him to as great a number of doctors as possible and give them the opportunity to convince themselves of the actual circumstances. I then resorted to mercury treatment and healed the patient in three months.' (Professor Ch. von Hübbenet, '*Observations and Experiments Concerning Syphilis*', Journal of Military Medicine, Th. 77, 186, pp. 423–427.)

Professor W. A. Manassein states: 'In reading this one cannot decide which is the more astonishing, the cold-blooded way in which the experimenter allowed syphilis to develop till a clear picture of it could be obtained and 'shown to the greatest possible number of doctors' or the peculiar logic, characteristic of a principal, by which he considered himself entitled to inflict a serious, sometimes fatal disease upon a subordinate without even troubling to demand his consent. I should very much like to know whether Professor Hübbenet would have inoculated his own son with syphilis, even if the latter consented.' ('*Lectures on General Therapy*', Th. I, St Petersburg, 1879, p. 66.)

A further collection of documents is concerned with theories of eugenics and the pioneers of the idea of euthanasia. Thus an extract from *The Passing of the Great Race* by Madison Grant (New York, 1923, 4th ed.) reads:

[DOC. Karl Brandt 3, p. 118 ff.]

'... A drastic weeding out of the feeble-minded or incapable members of society, in other words its refuse, would solve the whole problem within a century and enable us to get rid of the undesirable elements which at present fill our prisons, hospitals and lunatic asylums. Individuals could be supported, trained and protected by the State in their lifetime, but also sterilized in order to ensure that they would have no posterity. Otherwise future generations would be as burdened as our own with the curse of an ever-growing number of the victims of a misguided and extravagant sentimentality.'

In *Erbgesundheitsrecht* ('The Right to Inherited Health') by E. Ristow (Stuttgart, 1935, Verlag Kohlhammer) it is stated that:

'... The United States may claim the credit of having been the first of nations to exert conscious influence, by the practice of sterilization, upon the spread of inherited disease in the world's posterity. In the State of Michigan a scheme, which did not, however, become law, was introduced in 1897. It was the State of Indiana which first passed a law on the subject, dated the 9 March 1907. Many other States followed its example. ...'

'Thomalla strikingly refutes the objections of the Roman Catholic Church. "As against this view it may be in the first place pointed out that until late in the nineteenth century the choirboys of the Sistine Chapel were not only sterilized but actually castrated, in order to preserve the quality of their clear childish sopranos. The grave consequences of this operation, wrecking the entire lives of the boys, may be imagined." '

Extensive extracts are quoted from *Release Through the Destruction of Life Not Worth Living*, by Binding and Hoche, in which such phrases as 'empty human husks', and 'ballast lives' laid the intellectual foundation of euthanasia.

The following answer is given by the authors to the question: What sort of people should be subjected to euthanasia by order of the State?

'. . . I will now put a preliminary question. Are there people with so little sense of legal obligation that their continued existence has become permanently worthless both to themselves and to society? . . .

The question only needs to be asked in order to produce an uneasy feeling in the minds of those accustomed to assess the worth of an individual life to itself and to others. The painful realization of our prodigality with the most valuable, energetic and creative careers and personalities is then coupled with reflection upon the amount of hard work, patience and capital expenditure we devote, often quite fruitlessly, to the sole purpose of keeping lives not worth living in being until nature, often cruelly late in the day, deprives them of their last chance to endure. . . .[1]

There can be no doubt whatever that some people exist whose deaths would constitute a release to themselves as well as to society and in particular would free the State of a burden from which it derives not the slightest benefit, except the mere consciousness of setting an example of boundless altruism.

But if this is the case and there are in fact lives in the preservation of which no further reasonable interest can ever be taken, legislators are faced with the fateful question whether they are professionally obliged to take active steps for the prolongation of such lives at odds with society or on the contrary to permit their obliteration if certain conditions are fulfilled. . . .

So far as I can see, such persons should be divided into two main groups, with an intermediate group between them. The first group would consist of those suffering from incurable disease or injury, fully conscious of their situation and urgently

1. This sentence suggests the conclusion that one can at least be 'prodigal' with 'lives not worth living'.

desirous of release from it, as they have signified in some way
or another. . . .

I can find absolutely no reason in law, sociology, morality
or religion why those who request permission to kill incurables
who urgently demand death should not be granted such permission. In fact, I consider it to be the duty of the legitimately
compassionate to act in this way. . . .

The second group would consist of incurable imbeciles,
whether born so or having declined, like paralytics in the last
stage of their affliction, into such a condition.

They have no will either to live or to die. There is accordingly
on their part no discernible consent to annihilation, but on the
other hand this step will not be opposed by any will to live
which has to be broken down. Their lives are utterly pointless.
But they do not feel this circumstance to be unbearable. They
constitute a terribly heavy burden upon their relatives and
upon society. Their deaths would not leave the smallest gap
to be filled, except perhaps in the feelings of a mother or
devoted nurse. As they need a great deal of attention their
existence gives rise to a profession wholly concerned with the
prolongation, for years and decades, of lives not worth living.

It cannot be denied that such a situation represents an
appalling paradox in the sense of a misuse of vital energy for
deplorable ends.

Again I can find no grounds whatever in legal, social, ethical
or religious considerations for not granting permission to kill
such people, who represent so dreadful a contrast to normal
humanity and arouse horror in almost anyone who encounters
them. But such permission should not of course be granted to
all and sundry. It is probable that in a more scrupulous age—
for all heroic quality has disappeared from our own—these
unfortunate creatures would be released by the State itself
from the lives they live. . . .'

The economic side of the problem is also discussed.

'. . . If we take the average individual life as lasting fifty
years, it is easy to calculate what vast funds must be withdrawn
from the national income to provide food, clothing and heating
for an unproductive purpose. . . .'

. . . A nursing staff numbering several thousands is committed to this entirely fruitless task and prevented from taking

up useful work. It is painful to think that whole generations of such attendants grow old in the company of these empty husks of human beings, quite a number of them reaching ages of seventy and over. . . .

It will long remain extremely difficult to attempt to bring this situation to the notice of legislators. The proposal, moreover, to permit the obliteration of entirely worthless and mentally dead human beings and thus relieve the nation of this immense burden will at first and perhaps for many years to come meet with strenuous, predominantly emotional opposition, deriving its strength from very different sources, such as disinclination to novelty and unfamiliarity, religious scruples, sentimentality and so on.

. . . The type of compromise reached between these conflicting tendencies has hitherto been a guide to the level of humane feeling achieved at different periods and in different regions of the earth. Our present outlook in this matter is the culmination of a long and tedious process of development over millennia, in part substantially influenced by the growth of Christianity.

If we take a loftier view of the moral duty of a State, it seems tolerably certain that there has been some exaggeration in the effort to preserve under any circumstances lives not worth living. . . .

A survey of the numbers of lives which represent mere ballast proves, after brief reflection, that the majority must be retained. We shall never cease, even in the hard times which we can see ahead, to tend cripples and the infirm, so long as their minds survive. We shall never cease to do all in our power to relieve the physically and mentally afflicted, so long as any prospect remains of the improvement of their condition. But one day perhaps we shall be mature enough to see that the elimination from the world of those already dead to it is neither criminal, immoral nor brutally insensitive but a legitimate and beneficial proceeding.'

Nor do Binding and Hoche shirk the point that the legalization of euthanasia must be preceded by a change in the notion hitherto accepted of what constitutes humane conduct. The change would be more than questionable, as history has since proved.

'Nevertheless, in the face of this new situation, only a very slow process of adaptation to and acceptance of it can be expected. Realization of the insignificance of the individual in comparison with the interests of the whole community, recognition of the imperative obligation to concentrate every resource available and decline every unnecessary task, consciousness of a supreme responsibility for contribution to a difficult and most troublesome undertaking, will all have to exist among people in general to a far higher degree than they do today before the views here advanced can be fully appreciated. For most of us are only capable of very strong feeling on the rarest occasions and even then never for long. . . .

We must possess some small share at least of so heroic a temper before we can hope to attempt the practical initiation of such action as has here been considered in theory. . . .'

In *Racial Improvement and Christianity*, by the theologian Wolfgang Stroothenke (Leipzig, 1940, L. Klotz Verlag), it is pointed out that even Luther was in favour of the slaughter of imbecile children.

'In his day they were called changelings or monsters. It was believed that they had been substituted by the devil for abducted normal children or had even been directly procreated by the devil. Luther had adopted this attitude in consequence of an occurrence at Dessau. He had seen there a 12-year-old changeling which had the outward aspect of a normal child. But its activities were limited to the intake and excretion of victuals. Its reactions of laughter or tears were quite unrelated to its environment. Luther said that if it rested with him he would drown the child. For such creatures were merely lumps of flesh, without a genuine human soul. A few churchmen even today are in favour of euthanasia. . . . (See Meltzer, *Problem of the Abridgement of Lives Not Worth Living*.)'

The American Nobel prize-winner, Alexis Carrel, wrote in *Man the Unknown* (no year of publication given) *inter alia*:

'There still remains the problem of the countless inferior human types and born criminals. They represent a monstrous burden upon the normal part of the population. We have already referred to the vast sums at present spent upon the maintenance of prisons and lunatic asylums in order to protect the public from antisocial and insane persons. Why do we keep all these useless and dangerous creatures alive? For the abnormal, we must never forget, prevent the normal from developing their full potentialities. Why does society not deal more economically with criminals and the insane? It is absurd to attempt a precise distinction between "responsible" and "irresponsible" persons, punishing the former when they are guilty of crime and sparing the latter, as considered morally "irresponsible", when they are equally guilty. We are not, of course, entitled to sit in judgment upon our fellow creatures. But meanwhile the community must be protected against disturbing and dangerous elements. How is it to be done? Certainly not by building progressively bigger and more comfortable prisons, any more than true health can be promoted by bigger and more expertly directed hospitals. In Germany the Government has taken energetic measures against the multiplication of inferior types, the insane and the criminal. The ideal solution would be to eliminate all such individuals as soon as they are proved dangerous. Criminality and insanity can only be prevented by a thorough understanding of human nature, by the practice of eugenics, by improvement of social and educational systems and finally by the absolute exclusion of all sentimental considerations. . . . In the case of less important crimes the perpetrator could be given a salutary lesson with the cat or some rather more scientific means of correction. If it were followed by a brief spell in hospital the whole thing would probably be satisfactorily settled in this way. But in the case of murderers, robbers armed with automatics and tommy-guns, abductors of children, those who swindle the poor out of their savings and deliberately mislead people in important matters, a final settlement should be conducted on more humane and scientific lines, in certain small establishments for painless killing by gases suitable for the purpose. The same procedure would be appropriate in the case of insane persons found guilty of crime. The time has come for modern society to take decisive and drastic steps towards the ultimate goal of helping the normal individual to obtain his rights. Philosophic theory and sentimental prejudice are not entitled to a hearing in so urgent a matter. For the final aim of civilization is to bring the human personality to its highest stage of development. . . .'

All this material collected by the Defence no doubt illustrated for the Court the historical background of a small fraction of experimental research in medicine and medical thought. The picture is naturally made to appear one-sided. Yet the fact that even high authorities often held such theories, represented as an item in favour of the accused, must be queried. History has shown that the 'heroism' of which Hoche deplored the lack could not reinforce humane feeling but became an anachronism indicative of barbarous scorn for others. The 'ethical' view taken of the guilty, even Carrel's at this point, was not in advance of its time but behind it. The fact was eventually proved by the only too readily granted permission to take 'vengeance' on the weak. The intellectual impotence which the scientists could never have confessed was transferred in a physical guise to those victims. It was the kind of impotence which arises when the challenge of a period cannot be met as such and attempts are made by negative and destructive acts to amend what can no longer be either guided to a positive end or endured. The attitude and manoeuvres of the accused were illegal enough and scientifically on a low level. But they were also, on a wider view, antiquated. It was in this highly topical and instructive sense that they were interpreted by Viktor von Weizsäcker when he wrote:

'The indicted actions arose from an antiquated type of medical practice, not of its nature subject to moral inhibitions. It could not therefore either protect its practitioners from such dealings or warn them against the potential immorality involved.

For there can really be no doubt that the moral indifference to the sufferings of those selected for euthanasia and experiments was favoured by a medical ideology which put human beings on the level of a molecule, a frog or a guinea-pig. Today everyone is aware of the fact, with the exception, it may be feared, of certain doctors and pathologists who cannot recognize the truth owing to their special preoccupations.'[1]

The extension of documentary evidence to international medical literature only serves to throw into relief the question how far such historical examples, however shocking, may have appeared to afford legal justification for the behaviour of those

1. *Euthanasia and Experiments with Human Beings*, Psyche 1/1 (1947) p. 101 f., Verlag Lambert Schneider, Heidelberg.

who ordered and executed, at Himmler's directions or in collaboration with him, the above-mentioned procedures in the concentration camps and the carrying out of the euthanasia and other programmes of 'national politics'. Nothing can be less logical than to excuse one's own misdeeds by reference to other offences against humanity, no matter when and where they took place or by whom they were supervised. It was certainly a regrettable error on the part of certain Defence Counsel, though understandable in their position, to suggest, by a parade of such events in the past, which aroused no misgiving at the time, that it would be a mistake to regard as criminal the experiments on human beings then under discussion in Court. The various 'grounds of exemption' advanced on behalf of certain defendants also at most confuse instead of clearing up the issue. Since when has it been considered decent and lawful to employ inhuman methods simply because they have been declared 'necessary' by certain theorists in the interests of an aim itself in practice inhumane? Those who took this line of defence could, of course, hardly have been prepared to invoke all the evidence which proved in the majority of cases of experiments on human beings that conditions were all that could have been desired and that every consideration was shown for the subjects.

The feelings or fears to which talk of experiments on human beings gave rise under National Socialist rule are clear from the following brief order issued in those days:

[DOC. 1309.]

'At the desire of Field-Marshal Keitel the Army is not to take any responsible part in the experiments, as these may include experiments on human beings.'

Yet even as precedents the analogies drawn by the Defence from international literature differed essentially from the acts on trial at Nuremberg. The extent of the latter, the degree of their disdain for their victims and the arbitrary way in which their subjects were selected were all unique of their kind. For these reasons they were described in Judgment as follows:

[Judgment p. 21.]*

'Judged by any standard of proof the record clearly shows the commission of war crimes and crimes against humanity substantially as alleged in Counts 2 and 3 of the indictment. Beginning with the outbreak of the Second World War criminal medical experiments on non-German nationals, both prisoners of war and civilians, including Jews and "asocial" persons, were carried out on a large scale in Germany and the occupied countries. These experiments were not the isolated and casual acts of individual doctors and scientists working solely on their own responsibility, but were the product of co-ordinated policy-making and planning at high governmental, military, and Nazi Party levels, conducted as an integral part of the total war effort. They were ordered, sanctioned, permitted, or approved by persons in positions of authority who under all principles of law were under the duty to know about these things and to take steps to terminate or prevent them.'

Almost all the defendants and experts called were questioned in Court about the general principles of medical ethics and their personal views on the subject. Thus the evidence offered went beyond its main object of formal proof of responsibility in the individual and penetrated far into the roots of the problem.

The following extract from the Prosecution's cross-exami-nation of Karl Brandt gives an excellent idea of the way in which a citizen's personal responsibility could be surrendered to a national idol, the individual representing it being credited with a mystically based private capacity for leadership. The quotation also shows how under American law the accused gives evidence on his own behalf and the judges intervene with queries designed to throw light upon motive and situation.

[PROT. p. 2577 ff.]

'*Prosecuting Counsel:* Herr Brandt, do you consider experi-ments on a human being to be criminal, when they take place against his will?

Karl Brandt: That depends upon what sort of experiments they are. The question of consent is an important consideration, in my view, in arriving at a general judgment of the experi-ments. And if the word "criminal" is to be employed in such judgment, it is rendered more difficult by the consideration of that question.

Q. Why should you make any distinction between the various experiments? What does the kind of experiment matter, if the subjects have not consented to its performance?

A. The word "experiment" may be used when a new medical remedy is applied. In such a case one may be convinced that it will help, though one may not be absolutely sure that it will. Since a proceeding of this kind may also be regarded as experimental, I should like to draw a distinction in the formulation of the problem under discussion. Furthermore, the consent or otherwise of a prisoner introduces a significant psychological consideration as it also does in the case of insane persons. Accordingly, before giving the answer "criminal", as a matter of course, to such a question, one has to be clear what sort of an experiment is involved. The features which aggravate the judgment of experiments in general as criminal are three, lack of consent on the part of the subject, above all the needlessness of an experiment and thirdly the risk it involves.

Q. In other words, you consider that there may be situations in which an experiment is permissible, even from the legal and ethical standpoints, though the subject does not volunteer. Is that correct?

A. Yes, both these circumstances may be present.

Q. You are a physician and I suppose that you may be fairly familiar with cases of improper treatment and prescription in Germany. Let us assume that in pre-war Germany you tested a new drug on one of your patients without telling him about it or in any way obtaining his consent and that injury to him resulted. Would you not then be called to account for improper behaviour?

A. Yes, I would certainly be exposed to such a charge.

Q. In that case I don't quite understand in what circumstances you consider it would be permissible to treat a patient without his consent.

A. That was the point of my previous distinction, because in this case the question of risk would also arise. . . .

Q. Would the experiments charged in the indictment be regarded by you as criminal if the subjects did not consent? Answer the question, please.

Defence Counsel: Mr President, that is a purely legal question which in my opinion cannot be put to the accused.

The President: I should like to ask Prosecuting Counsel if he means to ask the witness whether the experiments he has in mind—I don't know what these may be—would be illegal or contestable if they had been carried out by a doctor or civilian having no sort of connection with military service.

Prosecuting Counsel: I beg to inform the Tribunal that such was my intention. I was trying to account for the moral value the witness sets upon such experiments.

Judge Sebring: Well, Mr McHaney, did you wish by your question to obtain the witness's opinion as to whether any of these experiments were illegal or criminal, or did you start from the premise that the assumption of the Prosecution in this case was correct, i.e. that the experiments were in fact illegal or criminal owing to the way, actually, in which they were carried out?

Prosecuting Counsel: Yes, I think so. The latter was the case.

Judge Sebring: I think perhaps it is not quite so certain.

Prosecuting Counsel: I am trying to ascertain the importance which the witness attaches to the consent of the subject in relation to the experiments charged in the indictment.

Judge Sebring: It seems to me that there are certain kinds of so-called medical experiments not of themselves likely to produce painful or shocking results. On the other hand, I can see that some experiments may assume a criminal character if they degenerate. So I should like to suggest that we shall arrive at our destination sooner if a difference is admitted in examining the witness.

Prosecuting Counsel: I believe, if the Tribunal pleases, that I would prefer to question him in relation to each experiment charged in the indictment rather than in general.

Q. You have heard the evidence given concerning the freezing experiments carried out at the Dachau concentration camp. I should like to ask you to assume in this case that the evidence submitted by the Prosecution represents the facts accurately and you will remember that there was a very great deal of spoken testimony that the subjects did not consent to the experiments. Will you give the Tribunal your views on the criminality of the experiments in question?

Judge Sebring: Mr McHaney, are you now dealing with the experiment as such or with the way in which it was conducted?

Mr McHaney: With the way in which the experiment was conducted.

Judge Sebring: With the way in which it was assumed from the evidence of the Prosecution that it was conducted?

Mr McHaney: Yes, certainly.

Q. Let us assume that the experiments were conducted in such a way as the Prosecution intended to prove that they were conducted. Would that have been in your view a criminal proceeding?

A. I cannot answer the question if it is put in that form. For it asks me to define criminality from a legal standpoint. I can only comment on the matter so far as the chilling experiments or their necessity are concerned if the general conditions which led to the performance of experiments in this field are made clear. I can thus only indicate my position on the ethical issue. It was influenced predominantly by the formulation of the problem which arose and the orders given in connection with it, which first brought up the general question of such experimental work. The most influential factor in deciding whether or not to carry out experiments is the importance or otherwise of such work. When this factor was considered in relation to the chilling tests proposed, their importance under war conditions was agreed, since in addition to the interests of the medical profession and of humanity at large those of the State were involved. It was therefore deduced that such experiments must be carried out. Then a point came up relating to their performance, whether only volunteers should be used or not. With regard to the related consideration of risk I would say, weighing my words with the utmost care, that a harmless experiment is possibly permissible if carried out by a doctor who takes account of the general principles of his profession and of common humanity. If risk is present, the doctor must be relieved of the responsibility for incurring it. This can only be done by some form of directive issued to him by a superior administrative authority or through a guarantee by the State. In that process, under war conditions, different interpretations of the national interest are possible. But I can express no opinion regarding such attitudes so far as the chilling experiment is concerned nor can I decide whether such experiments were criminal from a legal standpoint or not.

Q. Do you consider that the chilling experiments were dangerous?

A. Yes. Since fatalities occurred in consequence of them, they were indubitably dangerous experiments.

Judge Sebring: Mr McHaney, I would like to ask the witness a question. Herr Brandt, we are assuming for the sake of clarity that it would have been of the very greatest importance for the Army to ascertain definitely how long a human being could be exposed to cold before succumbing to its effects. You understand me? Well then, secondly, we are assuming that human subjects for such experiments were selected without their consent. Thirdly, we are assuming that these subjects were experimented on against their will in the tests concerned and perished as a direct or indirect consequence of them. Will you now please give the Court your opinion of such an experiment, either from a legal or from an ethical standpoint?

A. I had better begin by repeating the question, so that I may be properly understood. It is being suggested that supreme military importance, coercion of the subjects and possible fatalities would be involved in the organization of the experiment. In such a case I would say that in view of the existent military situation the person or the Government establishment which determined the importance of the experiment for war purposes must also relieve the doctor of any responsibility for a fatal outcome of the proceedings.

Judge Sebring: Well, in your view would it completely absolve the doctor of responsibility or share it with him?

A. In my opinion it would absolve him. For the doctor would be at that juncture a mere instrument, like an officer on active service, for instance, who on the receipt of an order puts a detachment of three or five of his men in a position where they must inevitably perish. The situation, when considered in relation to our circumstances in Germany during the war, is in principle the same. I do not believe that a doctor as such, in view of his professional code of conduct or moral sensibilities, would be capable of performing or would in fact perform such an experiment without the guarantee extended to him by an authoritarian State, a guarantee in formal legal terms, and furthermore the State's order to him to act in his professional capacity. That is obviously a more theoretical consideration when applied to the present case, where a particular matter is envisaged in a way which I cannot appreciate in connection with the chilling experiment. I do not know the form in which this order and guarantee were given. I would in principle distinguish between the organization of an experiment required mainly for medical reasons but where the State intervenes in certain circumstances to encourage medical action and the opposite case of State claims exploiting professional practice.

Judge Sebring: The Court has another question of some interest to put. Would, in your opinion, an order authorizing or instructing a subordinate Medical Service officer or group to carry out a certain medical experiment—let us assume for the moment that it involved these chilling tests—supposing it were also a general order directing a certain Institute to perform chilling experiments, without specifying any particular programme or details—would you then consider that such an order entitled the officer so instructed to select unwilling subjects and perform experiments on them which he knew for certain, or should know, would probably end with their deaths?

A. The question is a very difficult one to answer, since the reply would depend upon the intelligibility of the instructions given. Perhaps I had better quote an instance of such an order.

If Himmler directed Dr X to carry out a certain experiment, it might very well turn out that Dr X did not wish to obey. But in that case Dr X would not have himself been in a position to appreciate the importance of the experiment. He would be in the same position as a lieutenant who, on the receipt of a certain military order—and in Dr X's case the order would be a military one—cannot see why he and his detachment of eight men must at all costs hold a bridgehead and may perish in the attempt. Yet he and his eight men, to whom he duly communicates the order, will be ready to die at the post as ordered. In the same way Dr X, who has received this order from Himmler, may in certain circumstances have to carry out an experiment without being able to appreciate the principles and basic reasons which impelled a central department to take such a decision. Dr X would undoubtedly have been called to due account if he had failed to perform the experiment. In this case personal feelings of special obligation to a professional code of conduct—since we must bear in mind the authoritarian character of the Government—may well have had to yield to the demands of a "totalitarian" war. I can only repeat that such expressions of opinion on my part are mainly theoretical, stressing at the same time the difficulty of taking such decisions.

Accordingly, the result of an important experiment may render it unimportant. From that moment, in my opinion, it becomes criminal. For this reason it is also essential that if experiments on human beings are made at all their results should be given international publicity, so that those performed in Russia in one year may not be repeated in France or England the next. . . .

Judge Sebring: Herr Brandt, as to this question of the necessity of experiments, is it in your opinion a matter for the State to determine the urgent necessity of an experiment and that consequently those who serve the State are bound to carry out its decision in this respect? I believe you will be able to answer yes or no.

A. This Trial proves that it must be the task of the State, without fail, to settle this question once for all throughout the world for future generations.

Judge Sebring: Dr Brandt, I gathered from your statement a short while ago that a doctor, on entering the Army, must suppress his professional and ethical views in order not to find himself in opposition to a military order from higher Service quarters. Is that correct?

A. I did not mean to put it in that way. A doctor should not, of course, change his fundamental professional views the moment he enters the Army Medical Service. Such instructions may equally well be issued to a doctor who has no military obligations. My statement was intended to refer to the entire situation in Germany during the period of authoritarian leadership. The system made inroads upon the individual's personality and his consciousness of it. As soon as individual personality was lost in the idea of the collective entity, any claims upon the former were dropped in the interests of the latter. Consequently the claims of the community as a united body were set above those of the individual and he was fully exploited in its interest. . . . At bottom, the individual did not count any longer. This proved to be the case more and more definitely as the war went on. The situation became known eventually as "total war". . . .'

The other defendants expressed similar views of the problem of experiment on human beings and on general questions of medical conduct, speaking in each case from their particular official standpoint. The Oath of Hippocrates and various interpretations of it were also frequently discussed. Most of the speeches of Defence Counsel added their own observations on the relations between medicine and law.

The Prosecution's expert, Professor Andrew Conway Ivy of Chicago, stated, *inter alia*, that he had been chairman of a committee

[PROT. p. 9274.]

'appointed by the Governor of the State of Illinois to investigate the question of the ethical conditions under which convicts in the State prisons might be used as subjects for medical experiment. The question had arisen because remission of punishment had been mentioned as a reward for prisoners who had served as subjects for the malaria tests. . . .'

These 800 prisoners reported for experiment after a lengthy notice had been posted up describing in detail the nature of the tests required and the risks involved. No personal pressure was brought to bear on any of the prisoners. After reporting they were requested to sign the following document which Professor Ivy laid before the Court.:

[DOC. 3969.]

'I . . . . . ., No. . . . . . ., aged . . . . . ., hereby declare that I have read and clearly understood the above notice, as testified by my signature hereon, and I hereby apply to the University of Chicago, which is at present engaged on malaria research at the orders of the Government, for participation in the investigations of the life-cycle of the malaria parasite. I hereby accept all risks connected with these experiments and on behalf of my heirs and my personal and legal representatives I hereby absolve from such liability the University of Chicago——' a list of names follows— 'and all the technicians and assistants taking part in the above-mentioned investigations. I similarly absolve the Government of the State of Illinois in the United States of

America, the Director of the Department of Public Security of the State of Illinois, the Warden of the State Penitentiary at Joliet-Stateville and all employees of the above Institutions and Departments from all responsibility, as well as from all claims and proceedings or Equity pleas, for any injury or malady, fatal or otherwise, which may ensue from these experiments.

I hereby certify that this offer is made voluntarily and without compulsion. I have been instructed that if my offer is accepted I shall be entitled to remuneration amounting to .... dollars ($ ....), payable as provided in the above Notice.

Witnessed.........   Signed................

                      Dated................

Address...............................'

After this document had been read in Court the following exchange took place between Defence Counsel and Professor Ivy.

[PROT. p. 9319.]

'*Defence Counsel:* Professor, from the standpoint of medical ethics, do you believe that in America or any other civilized country the recognition of such a code can be reconciled with the carrying out of experiments involving a certain risk on prisoners who have previously been made to sign such a declaration, renouncing all future claims, even those by their heirs? In your opinion is such a proceeding compatible with medical ethics?

Professor Ivy: Yes. It can be regarded as in accord with the basic principles of medical ethics.'

Karl Brandt's Defence Counsel laid the following document before the Court as a very recent specimen of Government procedure and formalities prior to the performance of an experiment on human beings in Germany:

[DOC. KB 93.]

'Civil Governor, North Rhine Province   Düsseldorf,
M 632—III—C III/3   29 June 1946

To Federal Governors,
    Aachen, Düsseldorf, Cologne.

Subject: Medical Research Committee.
Text and Translation enclosed of a letter from the Military
    Government dated the 22 June 1946, NR/PH/2457.
I understand that the National Research Department will
be undertaking tests of kidney function. Will you therefore
please instruct the hospitals concerned to supply the necessary
reports?

(*Signed*) (per pro.)

COPY.
(Translation).
Headquarters, Military Government, North Rhine Region.
                    NR/PH/2547, 22 June 1946

Subject: Medical Research Committee.

To Civil Governor, North Rhine Province.
    1. Professor McCance and the members of his Medical
Research Department desire to be informed whether and if so
when children were born in Maternity Homes or the women's
wards of hospitals with meningocele or other abnormalities
rendering survival improbable or impossible for more than a
short time.
    2. Professor McCance and his Department desire to make
some experiments on such children which experience indicates
will be quite painless. But the Department does not feel justified
in performing such experiments on normal healthy children.
The births of suitable children should be at once notified by
telephone to Professor McCance, Wuppertal 36665.
                    (*Signed*)
                            for Brigadier.
                Deputy Regional Commissioner, North Rhine
                                            Region'

    The reply of the Cologne Government Department con-
cerned to an inquiry by the editors astonished them by its
unchanged attitude of bland indifference to the content of an

order for transmission. The Department answered that the order 'had simply been passed on to the hospitals. No comments were added nor were the hospitals informed of the nature of the proposed experiments, which obviously could not be carried out unless the parents consented.'[1]

Elsewhere Professor Ivy referred to similar prescriptions by the State of Illinois passed in December 1946 for the regulation of experiments on human beings. He also called attention in this connection to a circular dated the 28 February 1931 by the German Minister of the Interior.[2]

The German regulations of 1931 were never repealed and are therefore cited below:

[Circular.]

'Federal Government.

Ministry of Interior Circular of Instructions for Medical Treatment on New Lines and the Undertaking of Scientific Experiment on Human Beings.

28 February 1931

1. After a long correspondence with the British Military Government Department concerned and some help from the Düsselforf Ministry the editors eventually learned that the experiments had consisted of the 'taking of small quantities of blood and urine' from infants affected by incurable meningocele. A memorandum addressed by Dr R. A. McCance to the Legal Division of the Military Government explained that 'certain solutions' were used in the experiments and that it was also 'thought possible that the condition of the infants might be improved by solutions of salts and might then even permit operation'. These expectations, however, were not fulfilled. 'A certain minimum risk was involved in all the experiments and it was therefore considered more appropriate to perform them on infants who were certain to die in a few days, whatever was done for them.' Similar experiments were performed in England and the United States.

As to the question of 'consent' the same memorandum stated:

'In England the consent of the mother to such an experiment on her child was obligatory. In Germany the experiments were carried out with the consent and collaboration of the doctors responsible for the children. The mothers would have been consulted if that had been the custom in Germany. But it obviously was not.' There is, however, no difference between the customs of the two countries in this respect. (See the circular dated the 28 February 1931 by the Minister of the Interior quoted in the passage immediately following.)

2. *Reichsgesundheitsblatt*, 1931, p. 179. *Volkswohlfahrt*, the official journal of the Minister for Social Welfare, 1931, p. 607.

SUMMARY

The Department of Public Health considers it of special importance to ensure that all doctors should be made acquainted with the following Instructions and has therefore unanimously decided that all physicians employed in private or public institutions for the treatment or care of invalids pledge themselves, by signature on entry, to respect the Instructions in question.

Final Draft of Instructions for Medical Treatment on New Lines and the Undertaking of Scientific Experiment on Human Beings.

1. Medical science cannot, unless it is to be brought to a standstill, dispense with the application in suitable cases of new remedies and procedures not yet fully tested. Nor can it do entirely without scientific experiment on human beings in itself, for otherwise advances in diagnosis, cure and measures to obviate disease would be impeded or even rendered impracticable.

Physicians must always remain conscious, in the exercise of the rights here extended to them, of their special duty and their high responsibility in respect of the lives and health of all patients treated by them on new lines or subjected to experiment.

2. Treatment on new lines in the sense of these Instructions comprises operations on and methods of treatment of human beings which are in the interests of health, that is to say, are undertaken in any individual case in order to diagnose, cure or avert malady or suffering or to remove a physical defect, although the effects and consequences of such procedures cannot be forecast in their entirety so far as present experience goes.

3. Scientific experiment in the sense of these Instructions comprises operations on and methods of treatment of human beings undertaken in the interests of research without contributing to cure of the individual patient concerned and the effects and consequences of which cannot be forecast in their entirety so far as present experience goes.

4. All treatment on new lines must remain in accord with the principles of medical ethics and the precepts of medical art and science, both in its motivation and in its execution.

The greatest care should always be taken to consider beforehand whether any injury which may result is likely to bear a reasonable relation to the scientific advantage anticipated.

Treatment on new lines should only be undertaken if it has been tested, so far as practicable, by prior experiment on animals.

5. Treatment on new lines should only be undertaken after the patient or his legal representative has declared himself, after previous explanation of the procedure and its purpose, in unequivocal agreement with it.

In the absence of such consent, treatment on new lines should only be introduced if it is a matter of imperative necessity to save life or avert serious injury to health and the situation precludes the obtaining of prior consent.

6. The question of applying treatment on new lines must be examined with very special care if the patient is a child or a person under 18 years of age.

7. Medical ethics condemns without qualification the exploitation of social distress in the interests of undertaking treatment on new lines.

8. The greatest caution is recommended in cases of treatment on new lines with living microorganisms, especially live pathogenic agents. Such treatment is only to be regarded as permissible if it can be assumed that the procedure will be relatively harmless and the situation precludes the expectation of equal advantage by other methods.

9. In clinical hospitals, out-patients' departments and all other institutions for the treatment and care of invalids treatment on new lines should only be undertaken by the head physician himself, unless he expressly orders another doctor to undertake it and assumes full personal responsibility for the experiment.

10. A record is to be made of every treatment on new lines, clearly explaining the object of the measure, its motivation and the way in which it was carried out. In particular, a statement must be available to the effect that the patient, or if necessary his legal representative, has previously been instructed as to the procedure and consented to it.

11. Publication of the results of any treatment on new lines must take a form which pays due attention to the requisite

consideration for the patient and the principles of humane conduct.

12. Instructions 4 to 11 inclusive apply also to scientific experiment. (See Instruction 3.)

Scientific experiment is further to be subject to the following regulations:

(*a*) The undertaking of an experiment in the absence of consent is impermissible in any circumstances.

(*b*) Experiments which can equally well be made on animals are not to be carried out on human beings. Experiments on human beings are only to be undertaken if all the illustrative and supporting evidence is available which can be obtained by the biological methods at the disposal of medical science, consisting of laboratory research and experiment on animals. In these conditions all inadequately motivated and unsystematic experiment on human beings will be automatically ruled out.

(*c*) Experiments on children or persons under 18 years are inadmissible if they expose such patients to the slightest risk.

(*d*) Experiments on the dying are not in accord with the principles of medical ethics and are therefore forbidden.

13. Although the medical profession and in particular the responsible heads of hospitals are expected to prove by their observance of these Instructions that they are guided by a high sense of duty towards the patients entrusted to their care, there is no intention of depriving them of the satisfaction of feeling responsibility for attempting to provide relief, improvement or cure of or protection against malady by new methods when they are professionally convinced that those hitherto in use are likely to fail.

14. Every opportunity should also be taken in formal lectures to call attention to the special duties of a physician who embarks upon new lines of treatment or undertakes a scientific experiment and also in preparing the results of such procedures for publication.'

Judgment of the Tribunal summarized as follows all the precautions formulated at various times. The main points made appear suitable as a basis for future international agreement.

[Judgment p. 21 ff.]*

'The great weight of the evidence before us is to the effect that certain types of medical experiments on human beings, when kept within reasonable well-defined bounds, conform to the ethics of the medical profession generally. The protagonists of the practice of human experimentation justify their views on the basis that such experiments yield results for the good of society that are unprocurable by other methods or means of study. All agree, however, that certain basic principles must be observed in order to satisfy moral, ethical and legal concepts:

1. The voluntary consent of the human subject is absolutely essential.

This means that the person involved should have legal capacity to give consent: should be so situated as to be able to exercise free power of choice, without the intervention of any element of force, fraud, deceit, duress, over-reaching, or other ulterior form of constraint or coercion; and should have sufficient knowledge and comprehension of the elements of the subject matter involved as to enable him to make an understanding and enlightened decision. This latter element requires that before the acceptance of an affirmative decision by the experimental subject there should be made known to him the nature, duration, and purpose of the experiment; the method and means by which it is to be conducted; all inconveniences and hazards reasonably to be expected; and the effects upon his health or person which may possibly come from his participation in the experiment.

The duty and responsibility for ascertaining the quality of the consent rests upon each individual who initiates, directs or engages in the experiment. It is a personal duty and responsibility which may not be delegated to another with impunity.

2. The experiment should be such as to yield fruitful results for the good of society, unprocurable by other methods or means of study, and not random and unnecessary in nature.

3. The experiment should be so designed and based on the results of animal experimentation and a knowledge of the natural history of the disease or other problem under study that the anticipated results will justify the performance of the experiment.

z

4. The experiment should be so conducted as to avoid all unnecessary physical and mental suffering and injury.

5. No experiment should be conducted where there is an *a priori* reason to believe that death or disabling injury will occur; except, perhaps, in those experiments where the experimental physicians also serve as subjects.

6. The degree of risk to be taken should never exceed that determined by the humanitarian importance of the problem to be solved by the experiment.

7. Proper preparations should be made and adequate facilities provided to protect the experimental subject against even remote possibilities of injury, disability, or death.

8. The experiment should be conducted only by scientifically qualified persons. The highest degree of skill and care should be required through all stages of the experiment of those who conduct or engage in the experiment.

9. During the course of the experiment the human subject should be at liberty to bring the experiment to an end if he has reached the physical or mental state where continuation of the experiment seems to him to be impossible.

10. During the course of the experiment the scientist in charge must be prepared to terminate the experiment at any stage, if he has probable cause to believe, in the exercise of the good faith, superior skill and careful judgment required of him that a continuation of the experiment is likely to result in injury, disability, or death to the experimental subject.'[1]

1. Consequent declarations by the Tribunal are given in its handling of the evidence submitted. (See next section, 'Evidence applicable to War Crimes and Crimes Against Humanity.' p. 361).

CHAPTER TWELVE

COURSE OF THE TRIAL AND LEGAL
BASES OF JUDGMENT

THE Tribunal was composed of the following Judges:

Chairman: Judge Walter B. Beals, LL.D., Chief Justice of the Supreme Court of the State of Washington.

Judge Harold L. Sebring, LL.D., Judge of the Supreme Court of the State of Florida.

Judge Johnson Tal Crawford, LL.D., Judge of the District Court of Oklahoma at Ada.

Deputy Judge Victor C. Swearingen, LL.D., Chief of the Office for War Crimes at the Pentagon.

The Introduction to Judgment summarized the development of proceedings and the legal bases of Judgment.

[Judgment p. 1 ff.][1]*

'Military Tribunal I was constituted on the 24 October 1946 by General Order 68 issued by the American Military Governor for Germany. This Tribunal was the first of several Military Tribunals created in the American Occupied Zone by Order 7 of the Military Government to deal with offences recognized as criminal by Regulation 10 of the Control Commission for Germany.

The Order setting up the Military Tribunal and appointing the undersigned as members of it provided for Military Tribunal No. 1 to meet at Nuremberg, Germany, and hear such cases as might be submitted by the Chief Counsel for War Crimes or his duly nominated deputy.

On the 25 October 1946 the Chief Counsel for War Crimes lodged an Indictment against the above-mentioned defendants in the office of the General Secretary of the Military Tribunals in the Hall of Justice at Nuremberg. A German translation of

1. The omissions indicated by dots are those of the original.

the Indictment was delivered to each of the defendants on the 5 November 1946. On the 21 November 1946 each of the defendants appeared before Military Tribunal I and pleaded Not Guilty to every count in the Indictment charged against him.

On the 9 December 1946 the Prosecution began the presentation of evidence in support of the charges laid in the Indictment. After the Prosecution had concluded its case the Defence began (on the 20 January 1947) the presentation of its evidence. The presentation of all the evidence in this case terminated on the 3 July 1947. During the week beginning the 14 July 1947 the Tribunal heard speeches for the Prosecution and for the Defence. Personal statements by the defendants were heard on the 19 July 1947, on which day the case finally closed.

The Trial was conducted in two languages, English and German. It lasted 139 days of session of the Tribunal including six days devoted to the closing speeches and the personal statements of the defendants. During the 133 days of the Trial occupied with the presentation of evidence thirty-two witnesses uttered spoken testimony for the Prosecution and fifty-three witnesses, including the twenty-three defendants, spoke for the Defence. In addition, the Prosecution presented altogether 570 sworn depositions, reports and documents as evidence. The Defence submitted altogether 901 documents. In other words, 1,471 items of evidence in all were admitted.

German translations of all the items of evidence delivered by the Prosecution in the course of its case were made available to the defendants before being admitted as evidence.

At the opening of the Trial and throughout the proceedings each defendant was represented by Counsel of his own choice. Whenever possible applications by Defence Counsel for the personal appearance of those who had provided the Prosecution with sworn statements were granted and such persons were brought to Nuremberg for examination or cross-examination by the Defence. During the Trial the Defence was allowed great latitude in the presentation of evidence, to such an extent that at times items of very slight evidential value were admitted.

The Tribunal adopted all these measures in order to permit each defendant to present his defence without restriction, in accordance with the meaning and intent of Order 7 of the

Military Government, which assures the right of a defendant to be represented by Counsel, to subject witnesses for the Prosecution to cross-examination and to present all the evidence to which evidential value can in any sense be attributed.

All the evidence has now been presented. The closing speeches have terminated and the Tribunal has heard the personal statements of each defendant. All that still remains to be done in this case is to pronounce Judgment and Sentence.

Competence of the Tribunal

The competence and powers of this Tribunal were specifically established by Regulation 10 of the Control Commission for Germany.[1] The fundamental stipulations of the Regulation concerning ourselves provide as follows:

ARTICLE II

1. The following actions are regarded as criminal. . . . . .

(b) *War Crimes.* Acts of violence or offences against the person, against life or property, committed in violation of the laws or usages of war, inclusive of the following, which do not, however, exhaust the above-mentioned category: murder, ill-treatment of the civil population of the occupied territories, their deportation to forced labour or for other purposes or the employment of slave labour in the occupied region itself, murder or ill-treatment of prisoners of war and persons on the high seas, the killing of hostages, the looting of public or private property, deliberate destruction in urban or rural districts or any devastation unjustified by military necessity.

(c) *Crimes Against Humanity.* Acts of violence or offences

---

1. In the Judgment of Criminal Court No. 3 of the Coblenz Petty Session (County Court Judge Zündorf) the following opinion was expressed by German authority regarding this law. 'Nor is the applicability of this enactment affected by the fact that the offences now to be judged took place several years before it was passed. Apart from the retrospective force conferred upon the law in question, the generally accepted juristic principle of *nulla poena sine lege* is not an indisputable legal privilege or outcome of natural law among all civilized nations. Exceptions to it are actually required, beyond all doubt, in the interests of law and order in the higher sense whenever, as in Germany under Hitler, an unscrupulous Government contemptuously rides roughshod over every principle of such law and order. . . .'

inclusive of the following, which do not, however, exhaust the above-mentioned category: murder, extermination, enslavement, forcible deportation, deprivation of liberty, torture, rape or other inhuman acts against the civil population, persecution on political, racial or religious grounds, irrespective of their infringement of the laws of the country in which such acts are perpetrated.

(d) *Membership of certain types of criminal associations or organizations the criminal character of which has been determined by the International Military Tribunal.*

2. Any person, irrespective of nationality or of the capacity in which he acted, will be considered guilty of crime in the senses defined . . . . . by this Article if he

(a) himself commits the act, or

(b) has collaborated as an accomplice in any such crime or ordered or provoked it, or

(c) participated therein by consent, or

(d) planned or executed any act in connection therewith, or

(e) belonged to any organization or association connected with its execution. . . . . .

4. (a) The fact that any person may have occupied an official post, whether that of the head of a State or that of any responsible Government employee, does not relieve him of responsibility for any such crime or constitute any ground for mitigation of sentence.

(b) The fact that any person may have acted at the orders of his Government or official superior does not relieve him of responsibility for a crime but may be considered as ground for mitigation of sentence.

The Indictment in the present case was drawn in accordance with these stipulations.

Counts of the Indictment

The Indictment comprises four Counts.

1. *Common Plan or Conspiracy.* The first Count accuses the defendants of having conspired and agreed, in accordance with a common plan, contrary to law, intentionally and consciously, to commit war crimes and crimes against humanity as defined by Regulation 10 of the Control Commission.

During the Trial the defendants disputed the first Count on

the ground that the fundamental statute gave the Tribunal no legal right to penalize the crime of conspiracy as a separate and substantial offence. This objection was formally debated between Prosecution and Defence Counsel. It was then allowed by the Tribunal at one sitting. In order to render the present Judgment continuous the decision reached on that occasion is incorporated herein. The following decree was then issued in consequence of the objection lodged:

"This Tribunal decides that neither the International Military Tribunal nor Regulation 10 of the Control Commission defined a conspiracy to commit a war crime or a crime against humanity as a substantial crime in itself. This Tribunal is accordingly not competent to arraign any defendant on a charge of conspiracy as a substantial crime in itself.

In addition to the actual charge of conspiracy, Count 1 also accuses the defendants of unlawful participation in the planning and execution of war crimes and crimes against humanity, which participation in fact covers the commission of such crimes. We cannot therefore actually cancel the whole of Count 1. But in so far as it charges the alleged crime of conspiracy as a substantial crime in itself, apart from any war crime or crime against humanity, the Tribunal will disregard the charge.

This decision is not to be interpreted as restricting the effective operation of Article 2 of Paragraph 2 of Control Commission Regulation 10 or as depriving the Prosecution or the Defence of the right to present any facts or circumstances as evidence which may have occurred before or after September 1939 if such facts or circumstances might serve to prove or to refute a charge brought against any defendant of having committed war crimes or crimes against humanity as defined by Regulation 10 of the Control Commission."

Counts 2 and 3. War Crimes and Crimes Against Humanity

The second and third Counts of the Indictment raise the charges of war crimes and crimes against humanity respectively. The Counts are identical in content except for the fact that Count 2 asserts that the acts constituting the basis of the charge were perpetrated on 'civilians and members of the armed forces of nations then at war with Germany . . . . . in the exercise of the latter's authority as a belligerent Power', while in Count 3 it is asserted that the crimes in question were committed 'against German civilians and the citizens of other countries'. Both Counts will be treated and considered as one, the above-mentioned distinction being borne in mind.

Counts 2 and 3 declare, in essence, that from September 1939 until April 1945 all the defendants 'were principal parties and collaborators in, instigators and promoters of, certain acts, consented to and were connected with certain plans and undertakings, concerned with medical experiments . . . . . without the consent of the subjects of such experiment, whereby the defendants in the course of these experiments committed murders, acts of brutality, cruelty, torture, atrocity and other inhuman actions.'

Counts 2 and 3 close with the affirmation that the crimes and abominations described 'represent transgressions of international agreements . . . . . the laws and usage of war, the general principles of penal legislation as codified by all civilized nations and the criminal laws of those countries in which the crimes in question were committed, as well as infringing Regulation 10 of Article 11 of the Control Commission.'

Count 4. Membership of Criminal Organizations.

The fourth Count of the Indictment charges the defendants Karl Brandt, Genzken, Gebhardt, Rudolf Brandt, Mrugowsky, Poppendick, Sievers, Brack, Hoven and Fischer with membership of an organization declared criminal by the International Military Tribunal, in that each of the defendants named belonged after the 1 September 1939 to the Security Detachments commonly known as SS, of the National Socialist German Labour Party and thereby transgressed Paragraph 1 (*d*) of Article 11 of Regulation 10 of the Control Commission.

"The Tribunal does not include the so-called Cavalry SS. . . . . . The Tribunal declares criminal in the sense of the Statute that group of persons officially enrolled, as enumerated in the preceding paragraph, in the SS organization or aware of the circumstances that they were being used for the promotion of actions declared criminal by Article 6 of the Statute, or who were involved as members of the organization in the commission of such crimes, but exclusive of those persons who were summoned to membership by the State in such a way that they had no other choice and who did not commit any such crimes. The present Judgment arises from the participation of the organization in war crimes and crimes against humanity in connection with the war. The group declared criminal cannot therefore comprise such persons as ceased, prior to 1 September 1939, to belong to any organization enumerated in the preceding paragraph."[1]

Evidence Applicable to War Crimes or Crimes Against Humanity

The evidence submitted, as assessed by any conceivable criterion, proves clearly that war crimes and crimes against humanity, as envisaged by Counts 2 and 3, were committed. From the outbreak of the Second World War onwards criminal medical experiments were carried out on persons not possessing German citizenship, on prisoners of war and civilians, including Jews and so-called anti-social elements, and moreover on a great scale, both inside Germany and in the occupied regions. The experiments were not isolated cases nor the casual work of a few doctors and scientists acting exclusively on their own responsibility. They were on the contrary the result of the uniform preparation of a certain policy and the formulation of plans on a high Government, military and National Socialist level and they were conducted as an essential part of the total war effort. They were ordered, approved, permitted or sanctioned by persons occupying positions of authority, whose duty it was, on every basic legal principle, to detect such occurrences and take measures to stop or prevent them.'

The statements quoted at the end of the last section on 'permissible medical experiments' are then repeated.

'Of the ten principles enunciated above we are naturally concerned, in passing Judgment, with those of a purely legal character or at any rate so closely related to the aims of law as to be of assistance to us in the establishment of penal guilt and the appropriate sentence. To enlarge on this point would be to go beyond the limits of our competence. But there is in fact no need to do so. It is clear from the evidence that in the medical experiments before us these ten principles were much more often disregarded than observed. Many of the inmates of

1. This passage is quoted from the Judgment of the International Military Tribunal.

concentration camps who died as the result of these atrocities were citizens of foreign countries. They were non-Germans, including Jews and so-called anti-social elements, both prisoners of war and civilians, who had been arrested and forced to submit to these tortures and barbarities without even the semblance of a trial. In every case reported subjects were used who did not volunteer. In some cases it was not even asserted by the defendants that the subjects had volunteered. In no case had any subject the opportunity to withdraw from an experiment at discretion. Many of the experiments were conducted by untrained persons. Such tests were initiated arbitrarily, in the absence of adequate scientific justification and under repulsive conditions. All the experiments were accompanied by unnecessary suffering and injury. Very little provision, or none at all, was made for the protection or preservation of the subjects from potential injury, lasting bodily damage or death. In every single case the subjects had to endure considerable pain or agony and in most cases they sustained permanent physical injury, mutilation or death, either as a direct consequence of the experiments or due to the lack of proper after-treatment.

It is quite obvious that all these experiments, with their cruelties, torments, crippling injuries and fatal results were conducted without the slightest regard for international agreements, the laws and usage of war and the general principles derived from the penal codes of all civilized countries as reflected in criminal law and Regulation 10 of the Control Commission. Experiments on human beings under such conditions clearly contravene "the principles of international law arising from the customary behaviour of civilized peoples, common humanity and the dictates of the public conscience".

Whether any of the defendants here charged may be guilty of these atrocities is, of course, a different question.

In Anglo-Saxon law every defendant charged with a penal offence is considered innocent, during his trial, until the prosecution submits a valid and credible proof of his guilt which eliminates all reasonable doubt. This assumption is made of the defendant at every stage of his trial until such proof is submitted. A 'reasonable doubt' is, as the name indicates, one which any reasonable person would entertain. In other words the phrase describes a case in which an impartial, fair-minded and

COURSE OF TRIAL AND LEGAL BASES OF JUDGMENT 363

scrupulously reflective person entrusted with responsibility for
the decision is obliged, after thorough-going comparison of and
full attention to all the items of evidence, to confess that he is
not permanently convinced, with the force of moral certainty,
of the truth of the indictment.

If any one of the defendants is to be found Guilty on Counts
2 or 3 of the Indictment, it must be because the evidence submitted showed beyond any reasonable doubt that the defendant,
irrespective of his nationality or position, was active as a principal party, collaborator, instigator or promoter in, consented
to or had some connection with plans and undertakings
concerned with at least a part of the medical experiments and
other atrocities envisaged by these Counts. Otherwise he
cannot be convicted.'[1]

1. The defendants Handloser and Genzken, not named in this report,
as well as the accused Karl Brandt and Schröder, were found Guilty,
among other reasons, because the Court decided that they had failed to
exercise their necessary duties of supervision. In Handloser's case the
Court's decision was formulated as follows:

[Judgment p. 70.]*
'The law of war imposes on a military officer in a position of command
an affirmative duty to take such steps as are within his power and appropriate to the circumstances to control those under his command for the
prevention of acts which are violations of the law of war. The reason for
the rule is plain and understandable. As is pointed out in a decision rendered by the Supreme Court of the United States, entitled Application of
Yamashita, 66 Supreme Court [Reporter] pp. 340–347, 1946–

"It is evidence that the conduct of military operations by troops whose
excesses are unrestrained by the orders or efforts of their commander
would almost certainly result in violations which it is the purpose of the
law of war to prevent. Its purpose to protect civilian populations and
prisoners of war from brutality would largely be defeated if the commander of an invading army could with impunity neglect to take reasonable measures for their protection. Hence the law of war presupposes that
its violation is to be avoided through the control of the operations of war
by commanders who are to some extent responsible for their subordinates."

What has been said in this decision applies peculiarly to the case of
Handloser.'

Handloser's Defence Counsel, in his 'Plea for Ratification of Judgment
to be Withheld', dealt fully with the applicability of this decision to Handloser's case.

Plea
'The decision of the Supreme Court does not apply to Handloser's case.

THE DEATH DOCTORS

For the facts are not similar nor is the legal concept underlying the Court's decision relevant.

1. In the case of Yamashita the accused was the military commander-in-chief of an army operating on foreign soil in its occupation.

2. The published regulations for protection of the civil population according to international law and the Hague Convention and for the protection of prisoners of war according to the Geneva Agreement of 1929 must be observed and guaranteed in the orders issued by the military commander-in-chief.

3. Experience shows that transgression of these regulations by the fighting troops must be expected. Such cases can therefore be anticipated and it is consequently the duty of the commander-in-chief to consider how he may best prevent them.

In Handloser's case these circumstances did not exist.

1. The perpetration of war crimes or crimes against humanity by medical officers of the German Army either in the field or on garrison duty in the occupied regions was neither asserted by the Prosecution during the Trial nor mentioned in Judgment.

2. The facts with which Judgment in Handloser's case was concerned, i.e. the freezing, sulphonamide and typhus experiments, took place in the native territory of the accused, viz. in concentration camps.

3. It was neither asserted during the Trial nor stated in Judgment that Handloser had any official dealings with the concentration camps, their management and direction or with the selection of prisoners to undergo the experiments.

4. After many years' experience, both as generally understood and personally encountered, of medical service in the Army, including the years of the First World War, reinforced by the proved circumstance that no case ever came to light of inadmissible experiments on human beings in any Institute within the purview of the Inspector of the Army Medical Service, Handloser had no conceivable reason for issuing any protective order in this field.

(Handloser was not a military commander. As a Public Health Inspector he was only competent to give instructions.)

The decision of the Supreme Court in the Yamashita case cannot be regarded as a precedent for that of Handloser, either directly or by way of legal analogy.'

It is significant that the ruling of the Supreme Court which was made to apply to Handloser's case was not mentioned in any way in the Judgment of Military Tribunal V at Nuremberg, dealing with the senior military commanders of the South-East Area.

CHAPTER THIRTEEN

JUDGMENT OF AMERICAN MILITARY TRIBUNAL I ON 20 AUGUST 1947 AT NUREMBURG [1]

In the matter of war crimes, crimes against humanity and membership of an organization adjudged criminal by the International Military Tribunal the following were found Guilty and sentenced:

To death by hanging:

Viktor Brack, Administrative Head of the Chancellery and SS Oberführer.

Karl Brandt, Professor and Doctor of Medicine, Commissioner of State for Public Health, Personal Physician to Hitler, Lieutenant-General of the Waffen SS.

Rudolf Brandt, Doctor of Laws, Personal Consultant to the Reichsführer SS, Director of the Ministerial Department in the Ministry of the Interior, SS Standartenführer.

Karl Gebhardt, Professor and Doctor of Medicine, Head Physician of the Hohenlychen Sanatorium, Senior Clinical Consultant to the Reichsarzt SS, Personal Physician to Himmler, President of the German Red Cross.

Waldemar Hoven, Doctor of Medicine, Camp Doctor at Buchenwald Concentration Camp, SS Hauptsturmführer.

Joachim Mrugowsky, Professor and Doctor of Medicine,

1. After Judgment had been pronounced the Defence filed applications for 'Verification of Judgment' and appeals for clemency with the American Military Governor in Germany and with the Supreme Court of the United States. In these petitions Counsel called attention, *inter alia*, to the Geneva Conventions and stated that the Closing Briefs submitted by the Defence after all the evidence had been heard had not been in the possession of the Court when Judgment was pronounced, so that 'a sufficient hearing of the arguments of the Defence, as provided by law, had not been granted'. The Closing Briefs, however, contained no new evidence. They merely summarized and assessed the documents before the Court in the case of each individual defendant.

The United States Supreme Court declined revision of Judgment by five votes to three.

Director of the Waffen SS Institute of Hygiene, Senior Hygienist, SS Oberführer.

Wolfram Sievers, General Secretary of the 'Ancestral Heritage' Society (SS Community for Research and Instruction), Director of the Institute for Practical Research on Military Science, SS Standartenführer.

To life imprisonment:

Fritz Fischer, Doctor of Medicine, Assistant Physician at Hohenlychen, Waffen SS Sturmbannführer.

Karl Genzken, Doctor of Medicine, Director of the Waffen SS Public Health Service, Lieutenant-General of the Waffen SS.

The following were found Guilty of war crimes and crimes against humanity, and sentenced:

To life imprisonment:

Siegfried Handloser, Professor and Doctor of Medicine, Director of the Army Public Health Service and Inspector of the Health of the Army, Surgeon-General in Chief.

Gerhard Rose, Professor and Doctor of Medicine, Director of the Tropical Medicine Department of the Robert Koch Institute, Consulting Hygienist and Tropical Medicine Adviser to the Director of the Luftwaffe Health Service, State Surgeon-General.

Oskar Schröder, Professor and Doctor of Medicine, Director of the Luftwaffe Health Service and since 1 January 1944 Inspector thereof, Surgeon-General in Chief.

To twenty years' imprisonment:

Hermann Becker-Freyseng, Doctor of Medicine, Consultant for Aviation Medicine in the Department of the Inspector of the Luftwaffe Health Service, Staff Surgeon.

Hertha Oberheuser, Doctor of Medicine, Camp Doctor at Ravensbrück Concentration Camp, Assistant Physician at Hohenlychen.

To fifteen years' imprisonment:

Wilhelm Beiglböck, Professor and Doctor of Medicine, Senior Physician of University Clinic 1 for Medicine in Vienna under Professor Eppinger, Staff Surgeon.

To ten years' imprisonment:

Helmut Poppendick, Doctor of Medicine, Senior Physician at the SS Headquarters for Racial and Settlement Administration, Director of the Private Office of the Staff of the SS State Physician, SS Oberführer.

The following were found Not Guilty of the charges raised against them in the Indictment:

Kurt Blome, Professor and Doctor of Medicine, Deputy Director of the State Health Services, Deputy Director of the State Chamber of Medicine.

Adolf Pokorny, Doctor of Medicine, Specialist in Skin and Venereal Diseases.

Hans Wolfgang Romberg, Doctor of Medicine, Departmental Chief at the German Aviation Research Institute.

Paul Rostock, Professor and Doctor of Medicine, Director of the University Clinic for Surgery at Berlin, Army Consultant Medical Officer, Director of the Centre for Medical Science and Research, Surgeon-General of the Reserve.

Siegfried Ruff, Doctor of Medicine, Director of the Pilots' Medical Institute at the German Research Centre for Aviation, Berlin.

Konrad Schäfer, Doctor of Medicine, Assistant in the Chemotherapy Laboratory of the Schering Company, Junior Surgeon on the Staff of the Research Institute for Aviation Medicine, Berlin.

Georg August Weltz, Professor and Doctor of Medicine, Director of the Institute for Aviation Medicine, Munich, Chief Field Service Medical Officer.